Dictionary of Veterinary Epidemiology

Dictionary of
VETERINARY
EPIDEMIOLOGY

Editors
Bernard Toma
Jean-Pierre Vaillancourt
Barbara Dufour
Marc Eloit
François Moutou
William Marsh
Jean-Jacques Bénet
Moez Sanaa
Pascal Michel

Associate editors
Philip H. Kass
Michel Bigras-Poulin

Translators
Pascal Michel
Jean-Pierre Vaillancourt

IOWA STATE UNIVERSITY PRESS / AMES

© Éditions du Point Vétérinaire, 9, rue Alexandre, 94702 Maisons-Alfort, Cedex, France
Dépot légal: 1ʳᵉ édition, août 1991

This edition of Toma, Bénet, Dufour, Eloit, Moutou, and Sanaa: *Glossaire d'épidémiologie animale* is published by arrangement with Éditions du Point Vétérinaire, 9 rue Alexandre, B.P.233, F, 94702 Maisons-Alfort Cedex, France. Web site: http://www.pointveterinaire.com. Publication realized with the assistance of O.I.E. (Office International des Épizooties)

© 1999 English language edition, Iowa State University Press

Iowa State University Press
2121 South State Avenue, Ames, Iowa 50014

Orders: 1-800-862-6657
Office: 1-515-292-0140
Fax: 1-515-292-3348
Web site: www.isupress.edu

First English language edition, 1999

International Standard Book Number: 0-8138-2639-X

Library of Congress Cataloging-in-Publication Data
Glossaire d'épidémiologie animale.   English
    Dictionary of veterinary epidemiology / editors, Bernard Toma, Jean-Pierre Vaillancourt . . .
    [et al.] ; translators, Pascal Michel, Jean-Pierre Vaillancourt. — 1st English language ed.
        p.   cm.
    Includes bibliographical references.
    ISBN 0-8138-2639-X (alk. paper)
    1. Veterinary epidemiology Dictionaries.   I. Toma, B. (Bernard)
II. Iowa State University Press.
SF780.9.G5813   1999
636.089′44—dc21   99-24920

The last digit is the print number: 9 8 7 6 5 4 3 2 1

Editors

Bernard Toma, DVM, PhD, received his DVM from the National Veterinary School of Alfort, France, and his PhD from the Pierre and Marie Curie University in Paris. Dr. Toma founded the European Association of Veterinary Schools as well as the Association for the Epidemiological Study of Animal Diseases. He is a professor of contagious diseases and is president of the International Society of Veterinary Epidemiology and Economics.

Jean-Pierre Vaillancourt, DVM, MSc, PhD, received his DVM and MSc from the University of Montreal and his PhD from the University of Minnesota. Dr. Vaillancourt is presently an associate professor of poultry health management in the College of Veterinary Medicine, North Carolina State University, and teaches health management and production medicine (population medicine for food animals).

Barbara Dufour, DVM, PhD, received her DVM from the National Veterinary School of Alfort and her PhD from the University of Paris-Val-de-Marne. She is the coordinator of epidemiological research at the National Veterinary and Food Research Center (CNEVA), Alfort, France.

Marc Eloit, DVM, PhD, received his DVM from the National Veterinary School of Alfort and his PhD from the University of Paris VI. He is professor of infectious diseases at the National Veterinary School of Alfort, France.

François Moutou, DVM, received his DVM from the National Veterinary School of Alfort. He is head of the epidemiology unit at the National Veterinary and Food Research Center (CNEVA), Alfort, France, with special interest in contagious diseases of domestic and wild animals.

William Marsh, MS, PhD, received his advanced degrees in agricultural economics and veterinary medicine from the University of Minnesota. He is presently president of Farm Wise Systems, Inc., Little Canada, Minnesota.

Jean-Jacques Bénet, DVM, received his DVM from the National Veterinary School of Lyon, France. He is professor of contagious diseases and vice president of the Association for the Epidemiological Study of Animal Diseases.

Moez Sanaa, DVM, PhD, received his DVM from the Tunis Veterinary School and his PhD from the University of Paris XI. He is an associate professor of biostatistics and epidemiology and is the head of the epidemiology and risk analysis unit at the National Veterinary School of Alfort, France.

Pascal Michel, DVM, MPVM, PhD, received his DVM from the University of Montreal, his MPVM in epidemiology and preventive medicine from the School of Veterinary Medicine, University of California, Davis, and his PhD in population medicine from the Ontario Veterinary College. Dr. Michel is presently an epidemiologist with the Health Protection Branch, Guelph Laboratory, Health Canada.

Associate editors

Philip H. Kass, MS, MPVM, DVM, PhD, received his advanced degrees in statistics, veterinary medicine, and epidemiology from the University of California, Davis. He is presently an associate professor of analytical epidemiology in the School of Veterinary Medicine, University of California, Davis.

Michel Bigras-Poulin, DVM, MSc, PhD, received his advanced degrees in veterinary medicine from the University of Montreal and in epidemiology from the University of Guelph, Ontario, Canada. He is presently professor of veterinary epidemiology as a member of the veterinary medicine faculty, University of Montreal.

Translators

Pascal Michel, Health Protection Branch, Guelph Laboratory, Health Canada.

Jean-Pierre Vaillancourt, College of Veterinary Medicine, North Carolina State University.

Contents

Contributors

The individuals listed below contributed either to the French glossary or to the English dictionary. Their contribution varied from reviewing some definitions to writing a few of them. Because they have not reviewed the entire work, their inclusion in this list should not be interpreted as their endorsement of all the definitions.

Glenn Almond, College of Veterinary Medicine, North Carolina State University
Geneviève André-Fontaine, École nationale vétérinaire de Nantes, France
Peter Bahnson, College of Veterinary Medicine, University of Minnesota
H. John Barnes, College of Veterinary Medicine, North Carolina State University
Donald Barnum, Ontario Veterinary College, University of Guelph
John Barta, Ontario Veterinary College, University of Guelph
Nicholas Barton, translator, Paris, France
Jean-Robert Bisaillon, Agriculture and Agri-food Canada
Jacques Cabaret, Institut national de recherche agronomique, Tours, France
Bruno Chomel, School of Veterinary Medicine, University of California, Davis
Richard Clifton-Hadley, Central Veterinary Laboratory, Surrey, United Kingdom
Maria T. Correa, College of Veterinary Medicine, North Carolina State University
Peter Cowen, College of Veterinary Medicine, North Carolina State University
Peter Davies, College of Veterinary Medicine, North Carolina State University
John Deen, College of Veterinary Medicine, North Carolina State University
Cate Dewey, Ontario Veterinary College, University of Guelph
Ian Dohoo, College of Veterinary Medicine, University of Prince Edward Island
Victoria Edge, Ontario Veterinary College, University of Guelph
Maryellen Elcock, School of Veterinary Medicine, University of California, Davis
Peter Farin, College of Veterinary Medicine, North Carolina State University
Robert Friendship, Ontario Veterinary College, University of Guelph
Carlton Gyles, Ontario Veterinary College, University of Guelph
Caroline Hewson, Ontario Veterinary College, University of Guelph
Martin Hugh-Jones, School of Veterinary Medicine, Louisiana State University
Bruce Hunter, Ontario Veterinary College, University of Guelph
Bruno Jactel, Conseil d'État, Paris, France
Richard Julian, Ontario Veterinary College, University of Guelph
Azad Kaushik, Ontario Veterinary College, University of Guelph
Luc Lengelé, Ministry of Agriculture, Brussels, Belgium

Jay Levine, College of Veterinary Medicine, North Carolina State University
David Ley, College of Veterinary Medicine, North Carolina State University
S. Wayne Martin, Ontario Veterinary College, University of Guelph
Guy Martineau, Faculté de Médecine Vétérinaire, Université de Montréal
Louis Massé, École nationale de la santé publique, Rennes, France
Monte McCaw, College of Veterinary Medicine, North Carolina State University
Scott McEwen, Ontario Veterinary College, University of Guelph
Alan Meek, Ontario Veterinary College, University of Guelph
Paula Menzies, Ontario Veterinary College, University of Guelph
Henri Hubert Mollaret, Institut Pasteur, Paris, France
François Monicat, Centre de Coopération Internationale en Recherche
    Agronomique pour le Développement, Département d'Élevage et de
    Médecine Vétérinaire, Montpellier, France
Roberta Morales, Virginia-Maryland Regional College of Veterinary Medicine
Laurent Msellati, The World Bank, Washington, D.C.
Rita Nespeca, Ontario Veterinary College, University of Guelph
Peter Physick-Sheard, Ontario Veterinary College, University of Guelph
Frank Pollari, Ontario Veterinary College, University of Guelph
Ashley Robinson, College of Veterinary Medicine, University of Minnesota
Sabine Separi, Université Paris I, France
Alexandra Shaw, AP Consultants, United Kingdom
Mohamed Shoukri, Ontario Veterinary College, University of Guelph
Barrett Slenning, College of Veterinary Medicine, North Carolina State
    University
Elizabeth Spangler, College of Veterinary Medicine, University of Prince Edward
    Island
Bret Territo, School of Veterinary Medicine, Louisiana State University
Dennis Wages, College of Veterinary Medicine, North Carolina State University
David Waltner-Toews, Ontario Veterinary College, University of Guelph
John Wilesmith, Central Veterinary Laboratory, Surrey, United Kingdom
Dave Wilson, College of Veterinary Medicine, North Carolina State University
Jeff Wilson, Ontario Veterinary College, University of Guelph

Foreword

S. Wayne Martin
Former Chair and presently Professor, Department of Population Medicine,
Ontario Veterinary College,
University of Guelph,
Guelph, Ontario, Canada

In 1992, Bernard Toma sent me a copy of a French glossary of veterinary epidemiology, which he had coauthored. I made this glossary available to Dr. Jean-Pierre Vaillancourt, who was, at the time, a faculty member in the Department of Population Medicine. As Chair, I was pleased to see that it led to a cooperative project between Dr. Vaillancourt and Dr. Toma's group. The project was ambitious: namely, to produce a dictionary of veterinary epidemiology, incorporating the translations of the French glossary, written for a large spectrum of the members of the animal health professions, and jointly presenting the French and the North American perspectives on definitions of terms. It was ambitious because of the time commitment required to discuss and agree on the terms to be included, and because of the numerous issues that were bound to arise in view of language, cultural, and even professional differences when defining the meaning of specific terms.

This completed effort indicates that the challenge was worth pursuing. A growing number of animal health workers are attempting to formally link epidemiologic principles and methods with their daily activities. Further, the global market economy offers new opportunities to animal-based industries. Indeed, the rapid development of new markets for animal products has fueled the already high-paced evolution of animal production. Concurrently, major outbreaks of diseases, such as influenza, classical swine fever, and BSE, have emerged or reemerged. Communication on all of these issues will be enhanced by the availability of a currently agreed set of terms that will help all of us to understand the situations and our individual and collective perspectives on them. For this reason, the scope of this book was extended, beyond epidemiologic terms, into the basic nomenclature of economics and biostatistics, two important disciplines associated with epidemiology and animal health.

The publication of this dictionary offers a quick reference for people with an interest in animal health issues. Its international perspective is noticeable in many of the words and expressions being defined and in the numerous comments and examples offered in support of the definitions. Certainly, there is, currently, no consensus within the veterinary epidemiology community on the meaning of several expressions in this book. The publication of this dictionary will not end the debates over these terms; however, it will at least provide a focus for discussions and guidance for people with an interest in population-based problem solving.

I offer my personal congratulations to the authors and the contributors to this dictionary for a job well done.

Jean Blancou
World Organization for Animal Health
Director General of the O.I.E. (Office International des Epizooties)
Paris, France

The history of veterinary medicine has frequently been marked by misunderstandings arising from the translation or the interpretation of documents dealing with animal diseases. In May 1921, during the International Conference that led to the creation of the Office International des Epizooties, the French representative, Doctor Vallée, said to his Italian counterpart, Doctor Bisanti:

"... We basically agree, but we do not speak the same language. There is quarantine and there is quarantine..."

Defining the principal terms used in veterinary epidemiology and translating them into the main Western languages used for scientific communication throughout the world could therefore be considered a major step forward in solving such problems.

However, such an important undertaking, selecting the terms to be defined, providing the best possible definitions, and harmonizing them from an international viewpoint, would have been clearly beyond the capacity of even the most talented epidemiologist or linguist.

Professor Toma understood this very well, and he assembled a multidisciplinary team with the skills needed to achieve a successful outcome. Authors with diverse and complementary expertise (education, research, development, etc.) combined their talents to contribute to the development of a relatively new scientific discipline by helping to establish its terminology. The *Glossaire d'Épidémiologie Animale* was created.

The value of this dictionary, until now only available in French, should be enhanced with the English version, the *Dictionary of Veterinary Epidemiology*. We are particularly grateful to Dr. Vaillancourt who supervised the arduous task of translating the original text. He enrolled many contributors to join the French editors in revising the original document and in providing North American and English language perspectives, which produced several additions.

The aims of the *Dictionary of Veterinary Epidemiology* are clearly set out in the introduction: to provide readers with definitions of the main terms used in veterinary epidemiology and to propose a standard nomenclature for veterinary epidemiologists of all countries. This common language will be an important step in the goal to improve the health of animals around the world. The increase in international trade and the signing of the World Trade Organization Agreement on the Application of Sanitary and Phytosanitary Measures, as well as the need to harmonize animal disease diagnoses and control methods, will inevitably result in an increasing number of international agreements underscoring this goal.

These agreements will require clear definitions readily understandable in many languages. In this dictionary, national and international experts will find the most useful definitions to assist preparation of such agreements.

An enthusiastic international team, clear scientific references, a new scientific discipline in the making, these are the keys to the success of this venture. The Dictionary will be warmly welcomed by all those responsible for animal health.

Preface

The French version of the *Dictionary of Veterinary Epidemiology* was published in 1991. It fulfilled the dual need for a pedagogic tool that could also serve as a reference for communication among members of the French-speaking association of veterinary epidemiology (AEEMA: Association pour l'Étude de l'Épidémiologie des Maladies Animales).

Although very useful, it never gained acceptance beyond French-speaking circles, even if it provided a translation for each defined word or expression in English, German, Spanish, Italian, and Portuguese. The definitions were produced by the French editors of the current book, and were only available in French.

This first publication is the core of the English edition. Indeed, in the spring of 1994, Bernard Toma, Barbara Dufour, Jean-Jacques Bénet and Jean-Pierre Vaillancourt met in Paris to discuss the possibility of producing an English version of the dictionary starting with a translation of the French edition. Each definition was then reviewed by English-speaking colleagues and by the original group of French editors. This led to revisions, deletions, and additions to bring together the European and North American perspectives.

The Office International des Epizooties (O.I.E., the World Organization for Animal Health) made this project possible by providing financial assistance. We would like to express our gratitude, in particular, to Dr. Jean Blancou, Director General of the O.I.E., for funding our work and for his constant support of publications in the field of veterinary epidemiology. [The book *Épidémiologie appliquée à la lutte contre les maladies animales transmissibles majeures (Applied Epidemiology: Fighting Major Transmissible Animal Diseases)* was published in 1996 with the support of the O.I.E. and is currently being translated to English.]

This project progressed at a variable pace, depending on the availability of each editor. It met, and had to overcome, several obstacles, in particular, the divergence in concept and in the interpretation of certain words or expressions between French- and English-speaking editors and contributors. The ensuing debates are apparent in this work. Its medium, the English language, universal mode of scientific communication, should assure the accessibility of this multicultural effort to epidemiologists worldwide.

The editors are fully aware of the arbitrary nature of the process that led to the inclusion or exclusion of words and expressions for this dictionary. In addition to epidemiologic terms, some of the terminology used in pathology, statistics, economics, ecology, and preventive medicine were also included. These scientific and medical fields are closely associated with veterinary epidemiology. Their vocabulary, as well as corresponding concepts, are essential to veterinary epidemiology.

For each word or expression defined in this dictionary, the reader may find, in addition to the definition(s), one or several comments and/or examples, synonyms, and a reference to related terms also defined in this book. When synonyms are present, only the most usual term is defined, the other synonyms referring back to the defined expression. Words or expressions in italic with an asterisk in the text are defined in the dictionary.

At the end of this book, the reader will find a list of the principal references used by the editors. This list should be regarded as a source of recommended readings for anyone who wants to go beyond the limited information presented in this dictionary.

Finally, we would like to express our sincere appreciation to our two associate editors, Drs. Philip Kass and Michel Bigras-Poulin, and to the numerous contributors who have assisted us in the production of this book. Many share our vision of increasing the role of epidemiology in solving animal diseases through a better understanding of its terminology by all people involved in animal care. For this we are very grateful.

Dictionary of Veterinary Epidemiology

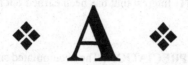

A

ABNORMAL: See **Pathological**

ABSOLUTE ERROR: Absolute value of the difference between the true value and the measured value.

EXAMPLE: True value: 200 g
Measured value: 206 g
Absolute error: 6 g

See also *relative error.*

ACCESSORY RESERVOIR: Reservoir that contributes to the maintenance of a pathogen in nature but is not the primary reservoir for this specific agent.

EXAMPLES: *Brucella abortus* and certain small mammals.
Foxes can be an accessory reservoir for the rabies virus in a region where the primary *reservoir** is the dog.

See also *reservoir.*

ACCOUNTS PAYABLE: Money owed to suppliers.

COMMENT: Accounts payable are classified as a current liability on the *balance sheet.**

EXAMPLE: Money owed on account to a veterinarian.

ACCOUNTS RECEIVABLE: Money owed by customers.

COMMENT: Accounts receivable are classified as a current *asset** on the *balance sheet.**

EXAMPLE: Uncollected receipts from the sale of crops, livestock, or livestock products.

ACCRUAL BASIS ACCOUNTING: Method of accounting based on the concept of matching revenues with expenses, by recording transactions when they occur rather than when payment is made.

COMMENT: Unlike *cash basis accounting,** accrual basis accounting revenues and expenses include changes to inventory, *accounts receivable,** and *accounts payable.**

See also *accounts receivable, accounts payable, cash basis accounting, expense, revenue.*

ACCRUED INTEREST: Interest that has been earned but not yet paid.

See also *interest.*

ACCUMULATED DEPRECIATION: The accumulated sum of depreciation expense of an asset from its date of acquisition to date.

COMMENT: Accumulated depreciation appears on the *balance sheet** together with *noncurrent assets.**

See also *balance sheet, depreciation.*

ACCURACY (OF A TEST OR OF A MEASUREMENT): Degree of agreement between the estimated value (test result or measurement) and the true value.

COMMENT 1: Accuracy is the quality of a test or of a measurement reflecting its *validity** (lack of *bias**) and *reproducibility** or *repeatability** (the tendency to give the same results on repeated measurements).

COMMENT 2: An accurate test always gives valid and repeatable results, but neither validity nor *repeatability** alone ensures accuracy.

COMMENT 3: Accuracy has been used as a synonym for *validity** and *reliability** in some references (Table A1).

COMMENT 4: One should not confuse accuracy and *precision.**

ACTIVE CARRIER: Carrier that provides the support needed for the agent to multiply. In North America: To be considered a carrier, one has to be infected. Therefore, the qualifier "active" is not used.

EXAMPLE: Pig infected with pseudorabies (Aujeszky's disease) virus.

COMMENT: As opposed to *passive carrier.**

See also *carrier.*

ACTUARIAL METHOD: Nonparametric method of estimation of the survival function.

COMMENT 1: The name of this *method** is derived from its utilization by actuaries, specialists in the calculation of *probabilities** applied to insurance, prediction, and *amortization.**

COMMENT 2: It is close to the *Kaplan–Meier method,** the difference being that the survival rates are estimated for time intervals determined a priori and not based on observed dates. In the actuarial method, intervals of time have the same duration ($t1 = t2 = ... = tk$).

TABLE A1. Test evaluation terminology: emphasis put on variability and/or bias depending on the term and the textbook of reference

Terminology	Emphasis (variability [V]/bias [B])	Source
Accuracy	V and B	(2-5,10-14)
Precision	V	(1-3,5-10,12,13)
Validity	B	(1,2,4,5,7,10,13,14)
	V and B	(3,8,12)
Repeatability	V	(3,4,6,8,9,12,13,14)
Reproducibility	V	(1,3-9,12,13)
Consistency	V	(1,7,8,11)
Reliability	V	(1,3,7,8,12-14)
	V and B	(1)
Bias	B	(9-13)

Note: The terminology used to describe test (measurement) qualities is confusing. Definitions from epidemiology textbooks are not consistent (see table above). The definitions provided in this dictionary are based on a consensus from these major texts. The reader should be aware of the variations within epidemiology and that these terms can be used with their common English meaning or their meaning from other specialties (e.g., statistics, social sciences, informatics, economics). **A test can be described by the amount of variability (V) of results on repeated analyses of the same samples and by the amount of systematic deviation or bias (B) from the true state.**

Sources:
1. Feinstein, AR. Clinimetrics, 1987.
2. Fleiss, JL. Statistical Methods for Rates and Proportions, 1981.
3. Fletcher, RH; Fletcher, SW; and Wagner, EH. Clinical Epidemiology: The Essentials, 1988.
4. Kelsey, JL; Thompson, WD; and Evans, AS. Methods in Observational Epidemiology, 1986.
5. Kleinbaum, DG; Kupper, LL; and Morgenstern, H. Epidemiologic Research, 1982.
6. Kraemer, HC. Evaluating Medical Tests: Objective and Quantitative Guidelines, 1992.
7. Kramer, MS. Clinical Epidemiology and Biostatistics, 1988.
8. Last, JM. A Dictionary of Epidemiology, 2nd ed., 1988.
9. Martin, SW; Meek, AL; and Willeberg, P. Veterinary Epidemiology: Principles and Methods, 1987.
10. Rothman, KJ. Modern Epidemiology, 1986.
11. Sackett, DL; Haynes, RB; Guyatt, GH; and Tugwell, P. Clinical Epidemiology: A Basic Science for Clinical Medicine, 1991.
12. Smith, RD. Veterinary Clinical Epidemiology, 2nd ed., 1995.
13. Thrusfield, M. Veterinary Epidemiology, 2nd ed., 1995.
14. Weiss, NS. Clinical Epidemiology: The Study of the Outcome of Illness, 1986.

COMMENT 3: The actuarial method is more frequently used than the *Kaplan–Meier method** in epidemiology. It can be used for events other than death.

EXAMPLE: After inoculating animals with the bovine viral leukosis *agent,** one may want to determine the average period of time prior to seroconversion by testing blood samples on a weekly basis postinoculation. The outcome would therefore be seroconversion and not death.

ACUTE DISEASE: Syn: acute illness Disease of relatively short duration (a few hours to a few days).

EXAMPLE: Influenza.

COMMENT 1: In general, the incubation is also short, with a sudden onset of clinical signs.

COMMENT 2: It can be qualified as peracute (very rapid evolution, often with severe clinical expression and a high *case fatality rate**), acute, or subacute (slower evolution, with less intense clinical signs) according to the duration and intensity of the disease.

COMMENT 3: It is in contrast with *chronic disease.**

ACUTE ILLNESS: See **Acute Disease**

ADJUSTMENT: Set of analytic procedures used to reduce bias by controlling confounding factors.

COMMENT: Adjustment is typically performed by *standardization,* stratification,* or regression.**

See also *bias, confounder, standardization, stratification.*

AETIOLOGICAL FACTOR: See **Etiological Factor**

AETIOLOGY: See **Etiology**

AGE EFFECT: The observed effect when the frequency of a health event or values taken by a quantitative variable changes by age of the animal regardless of time (i.e., year) born (Figure A1).

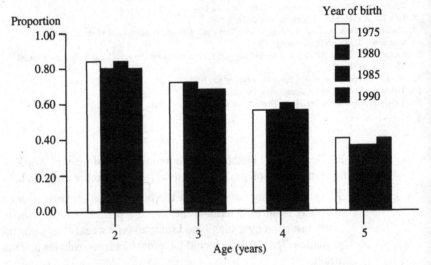

FIGURE A1. A hypothetical example where the *disease* frequency** is higher for younger animals compared with older animals.

COMMENT: The age effect should be viewed as a statistical relationship and not necessarily as a causal one.

• Direct role: An individual's *susceptibility** to a given *pathogen** may differ according to age. Thus, the *mortality rate** for transmissible gastroenteritis is higher in nursing piglets than in growing pigs. The opposite occurs with viral hemorrhagic disease of rabbits for which the mortality rate is lower for the young (< 4 weeks of age) than for the old.

- Indirect role: The age effect is due to the accumulated *risks** over time. Thus, for many *diseases,** the odds of being exposed or infected increases with age (e.g., bovine viral leukosis and feline leukemia virus).

- Role as a *risk marker:** For example, the higher *incidence** of parasitic diseases in 1- to 2-year-old cattle is associated with their first exposure to pasture. Age may also serve as a convenient measurement marker for factors that are less easy to quantify, such as senescence of cell membranes, loss of neurons, etc.

See also *year effect, cohort effect.*

AGENT OF DISEASE: Syn: causal agent, pathogen Biological, chemical, physical, mechanical, social, or behavioral entity for which the presence, the excess, or deprivation influences the occurrence of disease.

EXAMPLES: Presence: foot-and-mouth disease virus.

Excess: ingestion of lead.

Deprivation: vitamin E or C deficiency in the diet.

Presence and/or excess: mechanical agent (bone fracture following a fall); physical agent (burns caused by heat); chemical agent (strychnine intoxication); biological agent (virus, bacteria, yeast, parasites); behavioral agent (pica); social agent (overcrowding leading to an increased rate of violent acts; with animals, overcrowding is a management decision often resulting in an increased rate of cannibalism. Overcrowding can be the result of a primary decision to increase density to increase productivity or the result of secondary circumstances, where animals being held longer because of reduced growth due to disease [e.g., diarrhea] are mixed with animals being added to the group.)

COMMENT 1: A disease could result from the action of a single agent, from several agents each acting separately, or from the *interaction** of at least two different agents.

COMMENT 2: The expressions "agent of disease" and "pathogen" are most often used in reference to biological agents.

AGGRAVATING FACTOR: Factor that worsens an observed pathological phenomenon.

EXAMPLE: In humans, alcoholism could be considered an aggravating factor for different infections.

COMMENT: This expression is seldom used in North America.

ALGORITHM: A procedure used in problem solving and composed of a structured sequence of ordered steps.

EXAMPLE: Algorithm for the calculation of a *mean*:*

• Initialize sum to 0 and number of records to 0.
• Extract data from the records.
• If there are no more records, then mean = sum/(number of records), print mean, stop.
• Add extracted value to sum and increase number of records by 1.
• Go to step 2.

COMMENT 1: These procedures often involve iteration.

COMMENT 2: The etymology of the word comes from the name of the mathematician Al-Khowarismi from Baghdad, who wrote an arithmetic text based on numerical position in the ninth century.

ALPHA ERROR: Syn: type 1 error Error occurring when rejecting the null hypothesis, although it is actually true.

EXAMPLE 1: To assert that the difference between two *means** is significant when it is not in reality.

EXAMPLE 2: To conclude, after recording a statistically significant difference between two percentages calculated on two *samples,** that these samples come from two different *populations,** when, in fact, both samples are from the same population.

COMMENT: The alpha risk corresponds to the probability of committing an alpha error.

ALTERNATIVE HYPOTHESIS (H_1, H_A): The hypothesis that is assumed to be true if the null hypothesis is rejected.

COMMENT: Rejection of the *null hypothesis** does not confirm the veracity of the alternative hypothesis. It merely supports its plausibility.

See also *null hypothesis.*

AMORTIZATION: Repayment of a loan or expense by installments.

COMMENT: Amortization is often used, inappropriately, as a synonym for *depreciation,** which corresponds to a reduction in value of an *asset** through wear and tear.

See also *depreciation.*

ANADEMIC: Human disease, contagious or not, with an epidemic, endemic, or sporadic appearance, and for which all cases have a unique and common origin.

In North America: This word is not used. The expression *point source epidemic** is preferred in reference to an epidemic having a unique and common origin.

EXAMPLES: Foodborne intoxication due to *Clostridium botulinum* or infection due to *Salmonella* or *Staphylococcus.*

Intoxication by tempered oils in Spain in 1978.

Legionnaire disease: *contamination** from the ventilation system.

See also *point source epidemic* (Figure P2).

ANALYSIS OF VARIANCE (ANOVA): Broad statistical method of comparing the statistical variability of the mean of a continuous dependent variable in categories of one or more explanatory variables.

COMMENT 1: There are many kinds of analysis of variance, including one-way, two-way, three (or more)-way, and repeated measures. Analysis of variance can be used for a number of experimental designs, including Latin square, randomized block, and split-plot.

COMMENT 2: Analysis of variance decomposes the variability in data by quantifying an overall group mean, one or more main (intergroup) effects, *interaction** effects (for two-way and higher ANOVA), and intragroup or residual (error) effects.

ANALYTICAL EPIDEMIOLOGY: Division of epidemiology concerned with the etiological evaluation of disease or health states and estimation of putative risk factors directly or indirectly associated with these states.

EXAMPLE: Investigation of the *risk factors** associated with thin sow syndrome.

COMMENT 1: It is one section of observational epidemiology, in which there is no artificial manipulation of the *study** factor.

COMMENT 2: Its prime *objective** is to identify risk factors for the *disease,** estimate their effects on the disease, and suggest possible control strategies.

COMMENT 3: It usually uses elaborate quantitative *methods** to estimate effect measures.

ANALYTICAL STUDY: Observational study designed to evaluate the role of one or several factors in the etiology of a disease.

EXAMPLE: Investigation of *risk factors** associated with enzootic calf pneumonia or porcine reproductive and respiratory syndrome in swine.

COMMENT 1: Ideally, an analytical study should be designed to establish the strength of the *association** between the factor(s) under study and the *disease** of interest. Epidemiologic measures of association, also called effect measures, include the *relative risk,** the *odds ratio,** the *attributable risk,** and the *attributable fraction.**

COMMENT 2: Analytical studies generally follow *descriptive studies,** which are often at the origin of the *hypotheses** to be tested. The a priori generation of one or several hypotheses is essential in order to deduce appropriate conclusions concerning the role of the factor(s) under study. Without preliminary hypotheses, analytical studies are essentially *data dredging,** leading, at best, to the formulation of hypotheses.

COMMENT 3: Various types of study design exist. The principal types are: the *cohort study** (*prospective*), the *case–control study** (*retrospective*), and the *cross-sectional study.**

COMMENT 4: An analytical study requires a reference group for comparison purposes (*cases** versus *controls;** exposed versus nonexposed). This is what differentiates it from a descriptive study.

See also *deduction, cohort study, case–control study, cross-sectional study, relative risk, odds ratio, attributable risk, attributable fraction.*

ANAZOOTIC: Animal disease, contagious or not, with an epidemic, endemic, or sporadic appearance, and for which all cases have a unique and common origin.

In North America: This word is not used. The expression *point source epidemic** is preferred in reference to an epidemic having a unique and common origin.

EXAMPLES: Herd intoxication by polluted drinking water (microbial contamination, chemicals, etc.); bovine spongiform encephalopathy; anthrax.

See also *anademic, point source epidemic.*

ANIMAL HEALTH: State of well-being applied to animals.

Field of knowledge and methodologies designed to prevent disease, preserve health and improve productivity in animal populations through collective actions.

COMMENT: In some countries, the term collective actions refers to programs sponsored by government agencies or producer cooperatives.

ANIMAL-TIME: Unit of measurement combining animals and time, used as the denominator of the incidence density rate.

COMMENT 1: Animal-year is often used. However, other time periods can be considered, such as animal-trimester, animal-month, animal-day, etc. In swine production, preweaning mortality or morbidity rates should be expressed in pig-months. However, with the increasing application of segregated early weaning, pig-weeks could be preferred.

COMMENT 2: Animal-time is analogous to *person-year.**

COMMENT 3: The calculation of animal-time should only include animals at risk of the event of interest, excluding those already affected.

EXAMPLE: A herd of 30 animals uninfected at the initiation of the study is followed for 1 year.

Ten became sick during this time period:

1 on day 6
2 on day 50
2 on day 120
5 on day 240

Two animals were sold on day 60 (withdrawals) and 6 were added to the herd on day 120 (additions). For simplicity, we will assume that none of the additions became sick.

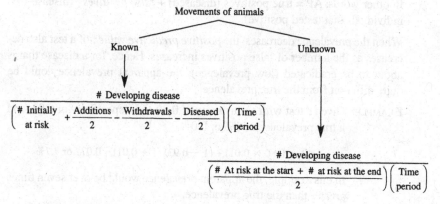

$$Incidence\ density\ rate^* = \frac{10}{(18 \times 1) + \left(1 \times \frac{6}{365}\right) + \left(2 \times \frac{50}{365}\right) + \left(2 \times \frac{120}{365}\right) + \left(5 \times \frac{240}{365}\right) + \left(2 \times \frac{60}{365}\right) + \left(6 \times \frac{245}{365}\right)} = 0.38\ animal\text{-}year$$

COMMENT 4: An exact denominator is not always needed and is often not known. However it can be estimated in two different ways, depending on whether the movements of animals are known or not.

Movements of animals — Known / Unknown

Known:
$$\left(\text{\# Initially at risk} + \frac{\text{Additions}}{2} - \frac{\text{Withdrawals}}{2} - \frac{\text{Diseased}}{2}\right)\left(\text{Time period}\right)$$
with # Developing disease

Unknown:
$$\frac{\text{\# Developing disease}}{\left(\frac{\text{\# At risk at the start} + \text{\# at risk at the end}}{2}\right)\left(\text{Time period}\right)}$$

Note: # at risk at the end should not include diseased animals.

Using the previous example:

$$\frac{10}{(30 + 6/2 - 10/2)\,(1\ year)} = 0.37\ animal\text{-}year = \frac{10}{([30 + 24]/2)\,(1\ year)}$$

ANNUAL PERIODIC VARIATION: See Seasonal Variation

ANNUAL PREVALENCE: Prevalence over a 1-year period, including the point prevalence at the beginning of that period.

See also *prevalence, point prevalence.*

ANNUITY: A series of payments of a fixed amount for a specified number of periods.

EXAMPLE: Mortgage payments or purchasing an *asset** on installment credit, where the principal and *interest** fractions are calculated such that the periodic payments are equal.

ANOVA: See **Analysis of Variance**

APPARENT PREVALENCE (OF A DISEASE OR INFECTION): Estimate of the prevalence based on the means used to identify each case or outbreak of a given disease or infection.

COMMENT: The discrepancy between the apparent and the true *prevalence** is function of the *sensitivity** and the *specificity** of the test used to determine the *disease** or *infection** status.

Assuming that a *random sample** of a given *population** is collected to determine the prevalence of a given *disease** based on a diagnostic test:

Apparent prevalence rate (APR) = (Se $\times$ p) + (1 $-$ Sp) (1 $-$ p)

Where Se = *sensitivity**
Sp = *specificity**
p = true *prevalence rate**

In other words, AP = true positives (diseased) + *false positives** (disease-free individuals that tested positive).

When the prevalence decreases, the *positive predictive value** of a test also decreases as the number of false positives increases. Hence, for a disease that is about to be eradicated (low prevalence), the apparent prevalence could be quite different from the true prevalence.

EXAMPLE: Given a test with a sensitivity of 0.80 and a specificity of 0.93, and a true prevalence of 1% or 0.01.

APR = (0.80 $\times$ 0.01) + (1 $-$ 0.93) (1 $-$ 0.01) = 0.077 or 7.7%

In this example, the apparent prevalence would be over seven times greater than the true prevalence.

APPARENT PREVALENCE RATE: See **Apparent Prevalence**

ARBOVIROSIS: Disease caused by an arbovirus.

EXAMPLES: Equine encephalomyelitis, African swine fever, and yellow fever.

COMMENT: Arbovirosis can go clinically undetected in humans as well as in animals.

ARBOVIRUS: Virus subsisting in nature by means of vertebrate to vertebrate transmission, using hematophagous arthropods as intermediate hosts.

COMMENT 1: To be considered an arbovirus, a virus must be able to multiply in arthropods. This is an integral component of biological transmission (as opposed to mechanical transmission, where virus replication does not occur in the *vector**).

COMMENT 2: Arboviruses are solely defined based on the epidemiologic observation of their biological transmission via arthropods, which differs from the physico-chemical criteria normally used to classify viruses. Hence, arboviruses (close to 500 listed) belong to several families of viruses.

EXAMPLES: Virus of equine encephalomyelitis (Reoviridae family), yellow fever virus (Togaviridae family).

AREA OF ACCEPTANCE: A set or interval of values within which the observation of a calculated statistic test implies the acceptance of the null hypothesis.

COMMENT 1: The *probability** that the value of the *statistical test** is within the area of acceptance, if the *alternative hypothesis** is true, is equal to the *beta error** or 1 − *power.**

COMMENT 2: The *area of rejection** is complementary to the area of acceptance.

See also *beta error, power.*

AREA OF REJECTION: A set or interval of possible values complementary to the area of acceptance.

COMMENT 1: The *probability** that the value of the *statistical test** is within the area of rejection, if the *null hypothesis** is true, is equal to the *alpha error.**

See also *area of acceptance, alpha error.*

ARITHMETIC MEAN: Syn: mean, average The sum of all the *n* observations divided by the number *n*.

For observations $x_1 .... x_n$:

$$\overline{X} = \frac{(x_1 + ... + x_n)}{n}$$

COMMENT 1: The observed mean, or empirical mean, is the mean calculated from a *sample** of observations.

COMMENT 2: Often not appropriately used. If negatively or positively skewed (asymmetrical *distribution**), the mean does not indicate the point of most frequent occurrence. It is also very sensitive to extreme values.

ARMITAGE TEST: A test of the hypothesis that a linear trend exists in terms of risk depending on the level of exposure to a given factor.

COMMENT: This test is more powerful than the more frequently used *chi-square test.**

See also *chi-square test.*

ASCII FILE: Data formatted using a standard coding method for computer representation of numbers, letters, or symbols.

COMMENT 1: The ASCII file is a common format used for transferring data between two different computer programs.

COMMENT 2: ASCII stands for American Standard Code for Information Interchange.

ASSET: An item of value owned by the business.

COMMENT 1: Assets appear on the *balance sheet.* *

COMMENT 2: The traditional method of asset classification according to expected useful life is:

current assets: less than 1 year
intermediate assets: 1 to 10 years
long-term assets: over 10 years

COMMENT 3: An alternative method of asset classification is:

current assets: up to 1 year
noncurrent assets: over 1 year

See also *balance sheet, current assets, noncurrent assets.*

ASSOCIATION: A quantitative connection between the distributions of two or more factors or outcomes.

EXAMPLE: There is an association between consumption of unpasteurized cow's milk and the incidence rate of *Salmonella dublin* infection in susceptible people.

COMMENT 1: An association demonstrates a covariance between *variables,* * but does not necessarily imply that blocking the effect of one variable will directly change the other. For example, in a study relating alcohol consumption to pulmonary neoplasia incidence, despite any apparent association found, blocking any or all effects of alcohol will not change the incidence of pulmonary tumors.

COMMENT 2: Association is a statistical concept that does not necessarily imply a cause–effect relationship.

COMMENT 3: Associations may be described in a number of ways, including the use of covariance, *correlation,* * *odds ratios,* * *statistical tests,* * etc.

ASSOCIATION DUE TO CONFOUNDING: An association between, say, an exposure and an outcome that is noncausal, but instead is explained by the presence of one or more additional variables that are themselves determinants of the outcome and are associated with the exposure.

EXAMPLE: It has been claimed that use of litter prolongs a cat's life expectancy, because cats that live indoors have longer life expectancy and use litter more frequently than cats that live outdoors; however, the cat's living location confounds the apparent association between litter and lifespan.

COMMENT: The degree of confounding can often be assessed by adjusting for confounding factors.

See also *confounder.*

ASYMPTOMATIC CARRIER: See **Healthy Carrier**

ATTACK RATE: Proportion of a population developing an illness during a finite period of time.

COMMENT 1: It is a form of *cumulative incidence** where the *population** is fixed and the exposure has generally occurred during a brief period of time. It is frequently used as a measure of average *risk** during common source *outbreak** investigations.

COMMENT 2: Several forms of attack rate are used:

Crude attack rate: $\dfrac{\text{Number ill}}{\text{Number potentially exposed}}$

Risk factor specific attack rate (e.g., food): $\dfrac{\text{Number exposed and becoming ill}}{\text{Number exposed}}$

Secondary attack rate:

$\dfrac{\text{Number exposed to primary cases during incubation period and becoming ill}}{\text{Total number exposed to primary cases}}$

COMMENT 3: The secondary attack rate translates the degree of *transmission of the disease** from *primary outbreaks.**

See also *Figure A2, rate.*

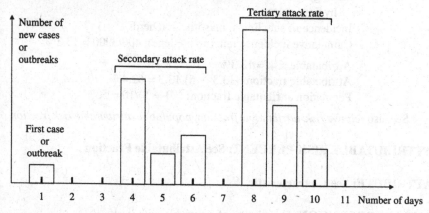

FIGURE A2. Schematic representation of secondary and tertiary attack rates.

ATTRIBUTABLE FRACTION: Syn: etiologic fraction, attributable proportion, attributable risk percent Measure of relative effect associated with exposure to a risk factor.

Attributable fraction = $\dfrac{(\text{incidence in exposed} - \text{incidence in nonexposed})}{\text{incidence in exposed}}$

COMMENT: This calculation provides an *estimate** of how much *disease** can be prevented by eliminating exposure to the *risk factor,** assuming *causality.**

ATTRIBUTABLE PROPORTION: See **Attributable Fraction**

ATTRIBUTABLE RISK: Syn: rate difference A measure of the absolute effect associated with exposure to a risk factor; it represents the difference in risk between individuals exposed to a risk factor and those that have not been exposed.

AR = incidence rate (exposed) − incidence rate (nonexposed)

COMMENT: Attributable risk is an *incidence rate** while *attributable fraction** is a *proportion** (attributable risk over the incidence rate in the exposed group or in the general *population**). Some authors tend to confuse these two different concepts.

EXAMPLE: *Prospective study** on milk hygiene:

Total population: 5000 dairy herds.
*Incidence** (total population) of *subclinical** mastitis: 500 herds.
*Cumulative incidence rate** (total population): 500/5000 = 10%

Among these 5000 herds, 2000 follow predefined rules of milk hygiene.
Incidence of subclinical mastitis: 100 herds
Cumulative incidence rate: 100/2000 = 5%

Among these 5000 herds, 3000 do not follow predefined milk hygiene rules.
Incidence of subclinical mastitis: 400 herds
Cumulative incidence rate (no hygiene): 400/3000 = 13.3%

Attributable risk = 13.3% − 5% = 8.3%
Attributable fraction: (13.3 − 5)/13.3 = 62.4%
Population attributable fraction: (10 − 5)/10 = 50%

See also *relative risk, attributable fraction, population attributable risk fraction*

ATTRIBUTABLE RISK PERCENT: See **Attributable Fraction**

ATTRIBUTE: See **Characteristic**

AUTOCORRELATION: Correlation of a variable with itself.

EXAMPLE: Correlation between consecutive values of a stationary chronological series.

COMMENT 1: It is mostly used to refer to time or spatial correlations.

COMMENT 2: These correlations can represent an analytical problem when they occur in a data set that is analyzed under the assumption of independence between sampled *individuals.**

COMMENT 3: An autocorrelation of order 1 exists between an observation at time t and an observation at time $t − 1$; an autocorrelation of order 2 is said to exist between an observation at time t and an observation at time $t − 2$, and so on.

In practice, the presence of an autocorrelation is assessed after making the series stationary.

AVERAGE: See **Arithmetic Mean**

AVERAGE COST: Total production cost per unit of output.

COMMENT: Due to economies of scale, the average cost should fall as output expands, spreading the *fixed costs** over more units. However, in the short-run, average cost may eventually go up if the increase in output requires additional *expenses,** such as higher maintenance *costs** for equipment. This is shown by producing average and marginal cost functions.

See also *total production cost.*

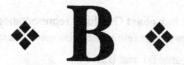

BALANCE SHEET: Accounting report showing the financial position of a business at a given moment in time.

COMMENT 1: The balance sheet is a listing of the items that go into the accounting equation: Assets = Liabilities + Owner Equity.

EXAMPLE:

Assets

Current			
Cash in bank		3,500	
Accounts receivable		8,750	
Inventory		23,500	
Total current assets			35,750
Noncurrent			
Machinery and equipment	35,000		
Less accumulated depreciation		14,000	21,000
Vehicles	10,000		
Less accumulated depreciation		3,000	7,000
Buildings	140,000		
Less accumulated depreciation		45,000	95,000
Land	12,000		12,000
Total noncurrent assets			135,000
Total assets			170,750

Liabilities

Current

Accounts payable	2,200	
Operating loan balance	6,500	
Current portion of noncurrent liabilities	5,500	
Total current liabilities		14,200

Noncurrent

Vehicle loan	7,750	
Mortgage	75,000	
Total noncurrent liabilities		82,750
Total liabilities		96,950
Owners' equity (net worth)		73,800
Total liabilities and net worth		170,750

BAR CHART: See **Bar Diagram**

BAR DIAGRAM: Syn: bar chart Graphical representation in the form of rectangles of the frequency of discrete values obtained by a qualitative variable.

EXAMPLES: See Figures B1 and B2.

COMMENT 1: Rectangles are separated to indicate that each observation can only fall into one category of the *discrete variable.** Frequencies are listed along one axis (if vertical, frequencies appear as columns; if horizontal, frequencies are expressed as a series of horizontal bars). Rectangles have the same width; their height or length corresponding to the frequency of observations for each category (relative frequency or absolute frequency).

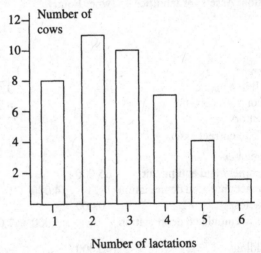

FIGURE B1.   Distribution of lactating cows in a herd according to the number of lactations.

COMMENT 2: Bar diagrams may be used to compare two or more groups (Figure B2)

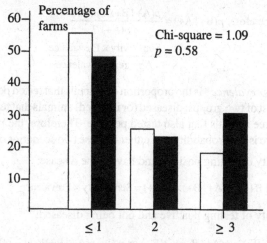

Chi-square = 1.09
$p = 0.58$

Collection of dead birds (times per day)

FIGURE B2. Distribution of farms with laryngotracheitis (open) and without laryngotracheitis (shaded) based on the frequency of daily collection of dead birds.

BAYES' THEOREM: Bayes' theorem provides a means of calculating a *conditional probability.* *

COMMENT 1: Considering two events A and B. Based on the definition of conditional probability, the *probability** of A given B, $p(A|B) = p(A \text{ and } B)/p(B)$; and the probability of B given A, $p(B|A) = p(A \text{ and } B)/p(A)$. Hence, $p(A|B)$ could be rewritten:

$$p(A \mid B) = \frac{p(B \mid A) \times p(A)}{p(B)}$$

This is a simple form of Bayes' theorem. The following example is a practical application.

EXAMPLE: Given test (A) and disease (B): The predictive values of the test can be obtained from the *prevalence** of disease B, the *sensitivity** and the *specificity** of the test by using Bayes' theorem:

Prevalence = probability of disease (B+) = $p(B+)$
Sensitivity = probability of being positive to test A (A+) if diseased = $p(A+|B+)$
Specificity = probability of being negative to test A (A–) if nondiseased (B–) = $p(A-|B-)$

Predictive value of a positive test = $p(B+|A+)$ can be obtained using the information above according to Bayes' theorem:

$$p(B+\mid A+) = \frac{p(A+ \text{ and } B+)}{p(A+)} \text{ and } p(A+\mid B+) = \frac{p(A+ \text{ and } B+)}{p(B+)}$$

Hence, $p(A+ \text{ and } B+) = p(A+\mid B+) \times p(B+)$

$$\text{Therefore, } p(B+ \mid A+) = \frac{p(A+ \mid B+) \times p(B+)}{p(A+)}$$

$$= \frac{\text{Sensitivity} \times \text{Prevalence}}{\text{Apparent prevalence}}$$

The *apparent prevalence** is the proportion of animals that tested positive. These animals consist of two groups: diseased (or infected) animals that tested positive, and disease-free animals that also tested positive. Therefore, the probability of testing positive is the probability that either of these two scenarios occurs.

The probability of testing positive and having the disease:

$$p(A+ \text{ and } B+) = p(A+ \mid B+) \times p(B+) = \text{Sensitivity} \times \text{Prevalence} \qquad [1]$$

The probability of testing positive and not being diseased:

$$p(A+ \text{ and } B-) = p(A+ \mid B-) \times p(B-) \text{ or } = [1 - p(A- \mid B-)] \times [1 - p(B+)]$$
$$= (1 - \text{Specificity}) \times (1 - \text{Prevalence}) \quad [2]$$

$p(A+)$ is the sum of these two probabilities $= [1] + [2]$

Mathematically, this follows from the "law of total probability." Consequently, the predictive value of a positive test:

$$p(B+ \mid A+) = \frac{p(A+ \mid B+) \times p(B+)}{[p(A+ \mid B+) \times p(B+)] + [1 - p(A- \mid B-)] \times [1 - p(B+)]}$$

$$= \frac{\text{Sensitivity} \times \text{Prevalence}}{[\text{Sensitivity} \times \text{Prevalence}] + [(1 - \text{Specificity}) \times (1 - \text{Prevalence})]}$$

which is the formula found under the definition of *positive predictive value.**

COMMENT 2: The applications of this theorem are numerous in *epidemiology.** Bayes' point of view on statistics has led to a new approach called Bayesian statistics.

BEFORE AND AFTER TRIAL: See **Open Trial**

BENEFIT: Anything contributing to an improvement in condition.

COMMENT: Often encountered in the context of *cost–benefit analysis.**

BENEFIT–COST ANALYSIS: See **Cost–Benefit Analysis**

BENEFIT–COST RATIO: See **Cost–Benefit Analysis**

BETA ERROR: Syn: type 2 error Error occurring when accepting the null hypothesis while it is actually incorrect.

EXAMPLE 1: To assert that a difference between two *means** is not significant, although in reality it is.

EXAMPLE 2: To conclude, after recording a non-statistically significant difference, that the results represent two *samples** originating from the same *population,** when, in fact, each sample comes from a different population.

COMMENT: The beta risk corresponds to the probability of committing a beta error.

BETWEEN-GROUP VARIANCE: See Intergroup Variation

BIAS: Systematic error that leads to incorrect quantitative findings; it represents the discrepancy between what is actually being measured and what one actually wants to measure.

COMMENT 1: Should not be confused with *random* error.**

EXAMPLE: In screening body temperatures, use of an electronic thermometer that consistently overestimates the true body temperature by 1 degree would lead to a biased estimate.

COMMENT 2: There are numerous ways authors have proposed to categorize bias into similar groups based on when in the course of a study the bias arises. Such proposed schemes are devised as a matter of convenience and do not have a theoretical foundation.

The following categories of biases are classified by chronological order as they may occur in a study:

1. Selection bias Bias that arises, usually in a *case–control study,** when *individuals** are selected from a pool of potential comparison subjects and the distribution of exposure in these individuals differs from the exposure distribution in the source population of cases and controls.

EXAMPLE: Comparison of canine cases of lung cancer to canine controls with heart disease could lead to a biased estimate of the effect of environmental tobacco smoke on lung cancer if smoke causes heart disease.

2. Censoring bias This bias occurs when differential follow-up across time for subcohorts, and the reason for censoring, is a determinant of the health outcome.

EXAMPLE: In a *randomized trial** to compare the efficacy of an experimental drug to a placebo in inducing disease remission among cancer patients, the experimental drug group experiences more voluntary withdrawal among healthier patients due to the drug's side effects. This group is thus depleted of healthier individuals, and the group's *median** time-to-remission is falsely decreased, making the drug appear to be less efficacious than it actually would be if no censoring occurred.

3. Information (measurement) bias This bias is linked to the process used to obtain measurements, recordings, analyses, etc., and can occur as a result of instrument or operator error. The bias can also result from errors intrinsic to test properties (e.g., *sensitivity** and *specificity** leading to misclassification).

EXAMPLE: Quantification of *Salmonella* colonies in a fecal sample using a culture medium with no Selenite tetrathionate.

4. Confounding bias Bias that arises when a comparison *group** is used that is not comparable with respect to the occurrence of the *health** outcome under study under conditions of nonexposure.

EXAMPLE: In a cohort study of life expectancy of cats that use or do not use litter boxes, confounding can arise because cats that do not use litter boxes may be more likely to live outdoors and have a higher incidence of fatal injuries. In this case, controlling for indoor/outdoor status would mitigate the bias.

5. Specification bias Bias that arises by misspecification of a statistical model.

EXAMPLE: Attempting to fit a straight-line regression to data that are inherently nonlinear.

BIAS (OF A TEST): Quality of a test reflecting its tendency to produce a consistent (directional) deviation from the true state or *gold standard*.

COMMENT: A biased test precludes accurate results (see Table A1).

BILATERAL TEST: See Two-Sided Test

BIMODAL DISTRIBUTION: Distribution having two modes or two regions with a high frequency of observations separated by a region of low frequency (Figures B3 and B4).

COMMENT: A bimodal distribution is often a combination of at least two underlying *groups** of *individuals** or observations (Figure B4).

EXAMPLES: Figures B3 and B4.

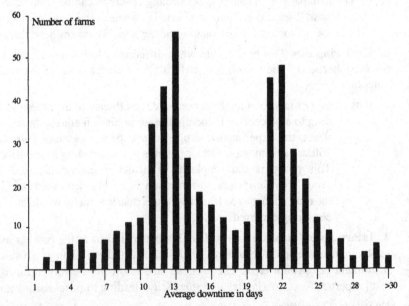

FIGURE B3. Histogram of the distribution of the average downtime between two flocks in 487 chicken farms.

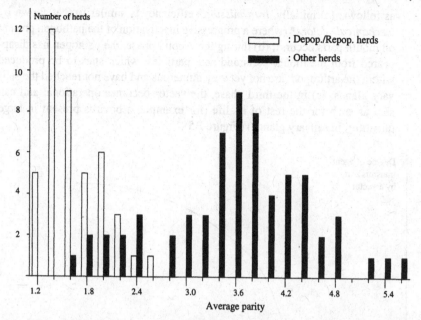

FIGURE B4.   Histogram of the average parity on 106 swine herds in a region depending on their participation in a depopulation–repopulation program over a 2-year period.

BINOMIAL DISTRIBUTION: Distribution of the probability of occurrence of one of two mutually exclusive events in a sample of *n* individuals from a population with a proportion *p* of the event of interest.

COMMENT: This *distribution,** widely used in *epidemiology,** was discovered by Bernouilly and published posthumously in 1713.

EXAMPLE: Number of sick animals among *n* randomly sampled animals.

BIOCENOSIS: The totality of living populations in an ecosystem.

EXAMPLE: All organisms and microorganisms living in a pond.

See also *ecosystem.*

BIOLOGICAL VECTOR: A vector in which the pathogen being transmitted multiplies and/or completes a necessary part of its life cycle.

EXAMPLES: Broad sense: cow and *Brucella abortus.*
              Strict sense: arthropods and arboviroses, rickettsioses...

COMMENT: For an arthropod to fulfill the role of biological vector, there must be an initial phase when the *pathogenic** agent is unlikely to be transmitted. During this phase the *agent** may either multiply (propagative transmission), such that in a few days it increases in number above its original concentration, or accomplish a necessary phase of development (developmental transmission) or undergo a combination of both these processes (cyclopropagative transmission). The success of the vector in transmitting the pathogen develops as follows: (a) initially, *transmission** efficiency is similar to that shown by *mechanical vectors** (where a progressive inactivation of the pathogen present on mouth parts occurs); (b) during the second phase, the pathogen has disappeared from the mouth parts and new particles, which start to be produced within the arthropod, are not yet very numerous and have not reached the salivary glands; (c) in the third phase, the vector becomes operational and can stay as such for the rest of its life (for example, arbovirus present in large quantities in salivary glands) (Figure B5).

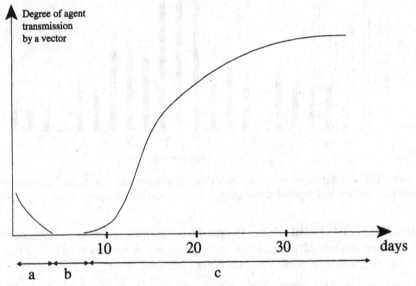

FIGURE B5. Schematic representation of pathogen (virus) transmission by a biological vector (arthropod) over time.

BIOSECURITY: Health plan or measures designed to protect a population from transmissible infectious agents.

EXAMPLES: Restricted access to barns, shower-in/shower-out facilities, footbath, disposal of animals that died on the farm, washing and disinfection of facilities, rodent and insect control measures, etc.

COMMENT: Term commonly used to embody all measures that can or should be taken to prevent viruses, bacteria, fungi, protozoa, parasites, *disease** carriers** (rodents, insects, wild birds, people, etc.) from entering and endangering the *health** status of a *population.**

BIOTOPE: Portion of the environment where all chemical and physical factors remain appreciably constant or undergo periodic variations.

EXAMPLES: A pond, a cave.

COMMENT: The biotope is constituted of nonliving elements and vegetation. With animals (the *biocenosis**), it forms the *ecosystem.**

BIRTH RATE:

$$\frac{\text{Number of individuals born}}{\text{Average number of individuals in the population}} \text{ during a given time period}$$

COMMENT 1: Like most *rates** calculated in veterinary medicine, the birth rate is a *proportion** relevant to a given period of time (often calculated on an annual basis). It is usually multiplied by 100 (giving a percentage) or 1000 or 10,000, depending on the species or the animal production. It is considered a crude birth rate if the entire population is included in the denominator, a refined birth rate if only the females are included, and a true birth rate if only the females of reproductive age are part of the denominator.

COMMENT 2: The birth rate is often interpreted as equivalent to the live birth rate (numerator limited to individuals born alive).

COMMENT 3: Do not confuse with *fecundity** and *pregnancy rates.**

See also *rate, fecundity rate, pregnancy rate.*

BLIND STUDY:
Randomized trial in which the observer is unaware of the treatment group to which subjects have been allocated.

EXAMPLE: Clinical trial in which two sets of bottles, one containing drug A and one containing drug B, are labeled using a numerical code.

COMMENT 1: There are three levels of blinding:

- Simple-blinding (only subjects under observation are unaware of the treatment group they belong to).
- Double-blinding (both subjects and observers are unaware of the treatment groups).
- Triple-blinding (statistical analysis is also performed "blind," where the affiliation of a given subject to a treatment group is revealed only after the analysis is complete).

COMMENT 2: Blinding is aimed at ensuring that neither the subjects, the observers nor any other participants influence the response or outcome in ways that would promote *bias.**

See also *randomized trial.*

BOND:
A long-term debt instrument.

BOOK VALUE:
The value of an asset, determined by subtracting its accumulated depreciation from its acquisition cost.

COMMENT: An alternative method of valuation to *market value.**

See also *asset, accumulated depreciation, market value.*

BREAKEVEN ANALYSIS:
Analysis of the level of sales at which a project would just break even.

COMMENT: An analytical technique for studying relationships among *fixed costs,** *variable costs,** and *profits.** The breakeven point represents the volume of sales at which total cost is equal to total revenues, i.e., profits equal zero.

See also *fixed costs, variable costs, profits.*

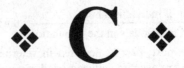

❖ C ❖

CANONICAL CORRELATION ANALYSIS: Analysis of the relationships between two groups of variables.

EXAMPLE: Study of the relationship between a group of *variables** used to characterize milk quality in a dairy operation and a second group of variables describing *herd* health management** on that farm.

CANONICAL CORRELATION COEFFICIENT: Coefficient measuring the degree of linear relationship between two sets of variables measured on the same sample of individuals.

COMMENT: It is a *multivariate** equivalent of the simple *correlation** and should be distinguished from the *multiple correlation coefficient.**

EXAMPLE: Correlation between a first set of *variables** composed of weight and height and a second set composed of diet composition in proteins and carbohydrates.

CAPITAL: Money or wealth used in the operation of any business.

COMMENT 1: A business uses capital in two main ways. Investment capital is used to purchase land, buildings, machinery, equipment, and other durable inputs, the use of which represents the *fixed costs** of production. Operating capital is used to support the purchase of variable inputs such as labor, feed, and energy costs.

COMMENT 2: The main source of capital in any business is *equity** funds. Equity capital is supplied by the owners (or shareholders) of the business. Equity capital is also referred to as "risk capital" because, in the event of liquidation of the business, the holders of equity funds are last in line for proceeds after all other debts have been settled.

COMMENT 3: Most business owners borrow debt capital against the security of the equity capital in the business. Provision of debt funds by financial institutions or individuals conveys no ownership interest in the business. Consequently, debt funds are provided at a cash cost in the form of interest, and hold first claim in the event of liquidation of the business.

CAPITAL ASSET: An asset with a life of more than 1 year that is not bought and sold in the ordinary course of business.

EXAMPLES: Farm buildings, farm tractors, combine harvesters, breeding livestock.

CAPITAL BUDGETING: The process of comparing investment opportunities in assets or projects expected to last more than 1 year.

COMMENT: Cash flows from competing projects or *investments** are compared using *net present value,* *internal rate of return,* and/or *payback period** as decision criteria.

See also *investment, net present value, internal rate of return, payback period.*

CAPITAL EXPENSE: The amount paid, or debt incurred, for the acquisition of a capital asset.

EXAMPLES: Purchase of farm buildings, breeding livestock, etc.

See also *capital asset.*

CAPITALIZATION: A procedure used in the appraisal of real estate, based on the present value of the income stream in perpetuity.

EXAMPLE: The formula for determining the income or earnings value of real estate (a farm for this example):

$$V = \frac{(R - E - L - I)}{r}$$

Where V = value
R = total cash farm receipts
E = total cash farm expenses
L = the value of the operator's and unpaid family labor
I = interest on non-real estate capital
r = capitalization rate

CAPITALIZATION RATE: See Discount Rate

CAPTURE–RECAPTURE: A method used to estimate the density of an animal population on a specific territory.

EXAMPLE: This *method** is frequently used by ecologists, who suggested it, to estimate wildlife density, for example, the density of mice in a field.

COMMENT 1: This method is based on marking and releasing a random sample of animals (M) captured on a designated territory populated by P individuals (unknown parameter of interest). A second random capture campaign is then conducted (p individuals are captured, including m marked ones). The estimate of density is provided by:

$P/M = p/m$, therefore, P' (estimate of P) $= pM/m$

Population density: P'/surface of territory

COMMENT 2: This method assumes that the *population** is constant over the period during which the estimation process takes place. It also assumes that the risk of recapture is the same as that of capture and that this risk is homogeneous over the territory. This last assumption can be alleviated by using certain rules during sampling.

CARRIER: Individual that harbors a specific pathogen or potential pathogen in the absence of discernible clinical signs, but that may serve as a source of this agent.

COMMENT 1: In France, *epidemiologists** classify carriers as either active (infected) or passive (mechanical carrier state, without multiplication of the *pathogen**). In English, the word carrier is restricted to *cases** where *infection** or *infestation** occurs. Therefore, the adjectives active and passive are not used.

COMMENT 2: The carrier state may be transient or chronic.

EXAMPLES: Transient carrier state as with influenza in swine and poultry; chronic carrier state as with herpes virus disease.

COMMENT 3: Different types of carriers are recognized depending on the stage of disease (healthy or asymptomatic if no disease; incubatory, latent and chronic) (Figure C1).

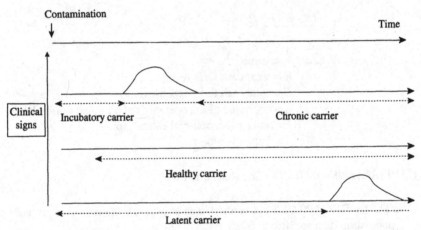

FIGURE C1. Schematic representation of the different types of carrier relative to the period when clinical signs are present.

COMMENT 4: A carrier may transmit an agent, but it is usually not necessary for the perpetuation of this agent. This is in contrast with an animal *reservoir,** whose presence is often essential for the subsistence of the agent.

COMMENT 5: In genetics, a carrier is a heterozygote that has both a normal and an abnormal gene that is not expressed, but that may be detectable by laboratory tests.

See also *healthy carrier, incubatory carrier, convalescent carrier.*

CASE: Individual identified as having the characteristics of a condition under investigation.

EXAMPLES: Dog with hip dysplasia based on clinical signs and radiographic findings.

An abortion due to brucellosis in cattle.

A pig seropositive to *Actinobacillus pleuropneumoniae* serotype 1.

A turkey condemned for "dark flesh" based on visual observation of the breast muscle mass at slaughter and the absence of any other gross lesions.

COMMENT 1: The epidemiologic definition of a case may differ from the usual one in *pathology** or medicine. For example, in the context of an epidemiologic *study,** turkey carcasses condemned for "dark flesh" (see example above) may only be considered as cases based on the absence of gross lesions and on a colorimetric assessment of the breast muscles using a spectrocolorimeter.

COMMENT 2: An *outbreak** may include from one (a cat diagnosed with Aujeszky's disease in an urban environment) to several thousand cases (influenza in a flock of chickens).

In *population medicine,** a herd or flock affected with a disease may be considered as one case. Here the unit of interest is the herd or flock and not the individual animal. Likewise, in a *case–control study,** one could define a case as being a herd or flock where a particular condition is present.

CASE–CONTROL STUDY: Syn: case–referent study Analytical study, retrospective in nature, which consists of comparing a diseased group (cases) to a nondiseased group (controls), based on the collection of information on prior exposure to one or more risk factor(s) (see *cohort study** and Figure C7).

COMMENT 1: A case–control study is particularly suited when the *disease** is rare or when the interval between exposure to the *risk factor** and the appearance of clinical signs is long.

COMMENT 2: The *ratio** of *cases** to controls can be fixed by the investigator (for example, four controls for each case). For a given *sample size** and study *cost,** this feature usually makes the analysis more statistically efficient than in other study designs.

COMMENT 3: Selection of case and control groups is crucial to the *validity** of the *study.** In many case–control studies, the case definition specifies the *health** problem that needs to be addressed, and the choice of controls guides the analytical approach that needs to be taken for the analysis.

COMMENT 4: Case–control studies are very susceptible to most forms of *bias.** Common reasons for the introduction of biases include the noncomparability of the case and control populations (the controls must be representative of the same *population** from which the cases arise) and the noncomparability in the assessment of exposure (when there is a potential recall/report bias among cases, controls should be chosen that will produce a similar misclassification error).

COMMENT 5: The magnitude of the *association* * between a risk factor and the outcome is determined by the *odds ratio.* *

See also *cohort study, nested case–control studies, odds ratio.*

CASE FATALITY RATE:

$$\frac{\text{Number of deaths during a given time period}}{\text{Number of diseased individuals in a population during the same time period}}$$

EXAMPLE: The case fatality rate for calves in a herd was 25% between March and June (of 40 sick calves, 10 died).

COMMENT: Case fatality rate should be differentiated from *mortality rate* * in which the denominator differs. A case fatality rate is, in fact, a *risk* rate.* *

CASE FINDING: Screening of a specific section of a population, designed to identify sick or infected individuals or groups in the context of a disease control or eradication program.

EXAMPLE: *Traceback* * investigation and *screening* * of all herds within a 5-km radius of swine herds found positive for pseudorabies (Aujeszky's disease).

COMMENT: Case finding is a strategic form of screening targeted at groups or individuals suspected to be at high *risk* * of being infected or diseased because of their potential association (e.g., physical proximity) with other known infected or diseased individuals or groups. This approach is an integral part of many disease control or *eradication* * programs.

See also *screening.*

CASE–REFERENT STUDY: See **Case–Control Study**

CASH BASIS ACCOUNTING: Method of accounting where transactions are recorded when payment is made, rather than when a transaction occurs.

COMMENT 1: *Revenues* * and *expenses* * may not necessarily match due to delays between transaction dates and the time when payments are made.

See also *accrual basis accounting, expense, revenue.*

CASH FLOW STATEMENT: Accounting report showing cash flows (receipts, disbursements, and net cash) for a business over a specified period.

COMMENT: Provides information about cash: where it came from and how it was spent for operating, investing, and financing activities during the period specified.

CATEGORICAL VARIABLE: See **Qualitative Variable**

CAUSAL AGENT: See **Agent**

CAUSAL ASSOCIATION: Syn: causal relationship Association between a variable X (exposures, events, or causal factor) whose variations precede and determine the status of another variable Y (disease or production outcome). $X \rightarrow Y$.

COMMENT 1: Each *disease** or production outcome is usually the result of multiple events.

COMMENT 2: Determining a causal association is a decision based on weighing all available evidence. This includes field-based and laboratory-based findings. Of all information, that obtained via rigorous *experiments** is often the strongest.

COMMENT 3: A significant *statistical association** between two events is not sufficient to establish the existence of a *cause** to effect relationship between these two events (Figure C2). Indeed, several conditions must be taken into account in the assessment of the relationship between a factor and a specific outcome:

• the time sequence (the exposure to the presumed *causal factor** precedes the appearance of the outcome);
• the *consistency** and the *repeatability** of the *association** (the exposure-outcome relation has to be found in different *populations** and under different conditions);
• the strength of the statistical association (the stronger the statistical relationship between a factor and the outcome of interest, the less likely is the observed association the result of a third unknown factor acting as a *confounder**);
• the existence of a dose–response relationship;
• the plausibility based on current knowledge (biological plausibility, scientific merit).

These conditions can be found in *Evans'** and *Hill's postulates.** Hence, in order to determine the status of a *variable,** the *epidemiologist** needs to consider the requirements listed above when designing and executing a *protocol.**

See also *indirect association, Evans' postulates, Hill's postulates.*

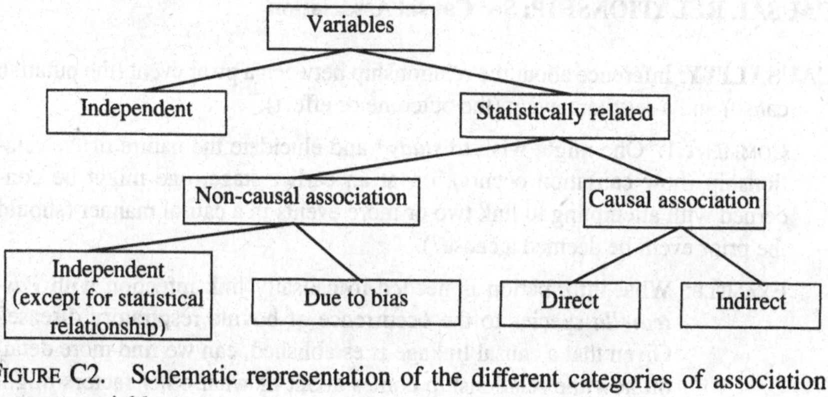

FIGURE C2. Schematic representation of the different categories of association between variables.

CAUSAL FACTOR: Syn: **etiological factor** An event or exposure that has been shown, scientifically, to produce a specific effect (health or disease outcome).

COMMENT 1: A risk factor becomes a causal factor when the corresponding pathological phenomenon is present and has been shown to be triggered by this factor.

COMMENT 2: Ideally, the scientific proof comprises experimental and observational elements.

COMMENT 3: Do not confuse causal factor and *risk factor** (Table C1).

TABLE C1. **Different degrees of certainty of causality using bovine tuberculosis as an example**

Event	Degree of certainty	Type of factor
Mycobacterium bovis	Maximal	Cause
Purchase of infected cattle		
Purchase of cattle from an infected herd		Causal factors
Purchase of cattle from unknown source		
Purchase of disease-free cattle that have been in transit at an auction		Risk factors

EXAMPLE 1: The use of a poorly fitting milking machine (exposure) was the causal factor of mastitis (disease) observed at a dairy farm.

EXAMPLE 2: It has been shown experimentally that rabbits exposed to tobacco smoke (causal factor) developed lung cancer (disease).

See also *causal association, causality, cause, risk factor.*

CAUSAL RELATIONSHIP: See **Causal Association**

CAUSALITY: Inference about the relationship between a prior event (the putative cause) and a resultant event (the outcome or effect).

COMMENT 1: One might wish to *study** and elucidate the nature of the relationship (how causation occurs), or, at an earlier stage, one might be concerned with attempting to link two or more events in a causal manner (should the prior event be deemed a cause?).

EXAMPLE: What information is needed to causally link infection with *Pasteurella* species to the occurrence of bovine respiratory disease? Given that a causal linkage is established, can we find more detail on how the relationship comes about or what other factors might influence this relationship?

COMMENT 2: The actual demonstration of a causal link requires a controlled *experiment;* * *observational studies* * cannot be used to conclusively demonstrate causation. A perfect experiment can demonstrate that the outcome was a result of the *cause,* * whereas a perfect observational study can only demonstrate that the outcome differs when the suspected cause differs (e.g., is present versus absent). Nevertheless, consideration of and fulfillment of a certain number of accepted criteria for causation (for example, temporal relationship, consonance, consistency, strength of *association,* * and *specificity*) can lead to the accumulation of evidence sufficient to produce quasi-certainty in causally linking the two events. In most instances, causal inferences based on results of observational studies should refer to suspected causes as *risk factors* * as opposed to causes.

See also *Hill's postulates, Evans' postulates.*

CAUSE: A variable or factor whose responsibility in bringing about an effect has been clearly demonstrated.

COMMENT 1: Often one's view of causation depends on the context; for example, if the context is one of classifying causes of *syndromes* * as in microbiology versus identifying causes of a syndrome for purposes of therapeutic decisions in *individuals* * versus conceptualizing causes for purposes of *prevention* * in *populations.* * The needs are different in each of these contexts, as are the important causes.

COMMENT 2: One can distinguish different categories of relationships between causes and their *effects.* * Two common concepts about relationships include first, the concepts of necessary and sufficient causes, and second, the concepts of direct and indirect causes.

A cause is said to be "necessary" if the corresponding effect is observed only following this cause (the outcome-effect is never seen following the absence of the cause). A cause is said to be "sufficient" when it always produces the effect (if the cause is present the effect will always be present—with due allowance for *latency*). Any single cause can be necessary, sufficient, both, or neither.

Four possible causal relationships for putative cause *X* are as follows:

• *X* is necessary and sufficient to produce *Y*.

EXAMPLE: Productive infection with the rabies virus will always produce clinical rabies in canines. No other agent produces rabies.

• *X* is necessary but not sufficient to produce *Y*. This implies that one or more additional factors are needed to render the factor *X* sufficient. In a technical sense, this represents interaction between the cause and the other factor(s) because the cause has no effect on its own but produces the effect when the other factor(s) is present.

EXAMPLE: Many microorganisms are necessary for etiologically defined syndromes (*E. coli* for colibacillosis), but often they are insufficient to produce the syndrome. These microorganisms often are not necessary for a more general manifestational syndrome (e.g., *E. coli* is not necessary for diarrhea). The other factors could include lowered host resistance, lack of specific antibody, etc.

- *X* is not necessary but is sufficient.

EXAMPLE: There is no single cause of bovine respiratory disease, but a large number of *Pasteurella haemolytica* in the pulmonary tissue is sufficient to produce the illness.

- *X* is not necessary and is not sufficient.

EXAMPLE: Most manifestational syndromes do not have a single necessary cause, nor a cause that by itself is sufficient to produce the disease. There are several so-called "multifactorial (or multietiological) syndromes" in which a number of factors participate. Some of these factors are living agents, others relate to factors of management, breed, genetics, and so forth. In general, the larger the number of causal factors present in an individual, the more likely that a sufficient cause will be created that will result in the disease. Usually, the risk of the disease is increased proportionally to the number of causal factors present, although one needs to bear in mind the effect of scale of *measurement** on *inferences** about how factors combine to produce the effect. If the disease (or effect) is observed in the absence of all the known causal factors, this signals the presence of unknown factors that can form a sufficient cause (perhaps by combining with some or all of the known causes) for the outcome.

The second way of conceptualizing causes is as direct and indirect. Direct causes have no known other causes between them and the effect, and both cause and effect must be measured at the same level of organization. All other causal relationships are indirect. This approach is most completely formalized in path (or structural equations) modeling where one identifies and quantifies the direct and indirect causal pathways. It extends into specific classifications where causes are deemed, as examples, to be simple antecedents, explanatory antecedents, or intervening variables. Direct causes are often the basis for classification purposes (naming the *disease** or *agent**), but indirect causes may be more subject to manipulation and thus more important for disease control purposes.

CENSORED DATA: See **Life Table**

CENSORING BIAS: See **Bias**

CENTRAL TENDENCY PARAMETERS: A numerical descriptive measure that indicates the center of occurrence of a population for a given variable.

COMMENT 1: There are three frequently used central tendency parameters: the *mean,** the *mode,** and the *median.**

COMMENT 2: Central tendency parameters are normally estimated from a *sample** of observations. Ideally, the *sampling** should be *random.**

COMMENT 3: In a unimodal distribution representing a group of individuals, there is one central tendency. If this distribution is symmetrical, the mean, the mode and the median have the same value.

See also *sample mean, median, mode.*

CENTRAL VALUE OF A GROUP: The middle value of a class, i.e., within equal distance of the inferior and superior limits of the class.

EXAMPLE:

Limits	Central Values
15 cm to less than 20 cm	17.5 cm
20 cm to less than 25 cm	22.5 cm

See also *class.*

CHAIN OF INFECTION: Syn: infectious disease cycle, chain of transmission
Set of parameters implicated in the transmission of an infectious agent (Figure C3).

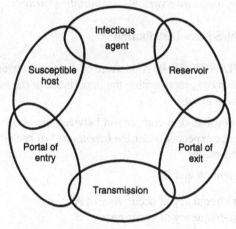

FIGURE C3. Representation of the various links (*parameters**) of the chain of infection.

COMMENT: These parameters include:

• the source of *infection,** where the *pathogen** is found in *virulent** material;
• modes of transmission (direct, indirect, by *vectors**);
• a susceptible *host:** *individual** without *immune** protection or whose immune system is compromised due to a concomitant problem.

CHAIN OF TRANSMISSION: See Chain of Infection

CHARACTERISTIC: Syn: attribute, host factor, host determinant Inherent trait of an individual.

EXAMPLES: Species, breed, genotype, phenotype, age, sex, reproductive status, behavior, size.

COMMENT 1: The characteristics of *individuals** should be included in the description of the *natural history of a disease.**

COMMENT 2: In general, the characteristics of an individual are *qualitative variables** that cannot be expressed in numeric terms. Age and size are notable exceptions.

COMMENT 3: In most cases, an individual will fit in only one category of a particular characteristic or attribute. For example, sex: male, female, hermaphrodite. This classification should allow each individual of a *population** to be classified into one category.

COMMENT 4: Advances in genetics and biotechnology (i.e., production of transgenic animals, genotypic characterization, etc.) may allow for, or require, a more refined categorization of individuals depending on the attribute and the disease being investigated. For example, transgenic *Salmonella*-resistant poultry, *E. coli*–resistant pigs, body conformation changes within a given breed having a potential impact on some musculoskeletal and skin conditions, etc.

See also *variable, qualitative variable, quantitative variable.*

CHI 2 LAW: See Chi-Square Distribution

CHI-SQUARE DISTANCE ($D\chi^2$): A measure of distance between the observed frequency of two events, representing the importance of the associated occurrence between these events.

COMMENT 1: It consists of a comparison between the observed coincidence and the coincidence expected under the *hypothesis** of probabilistic independence between the events.

Assuming two events A and B:

f_A = absolute frequency of occurrence of A
f_B = absolute frequency of occurrence of B
$f_{EXP(AB)}$ = expected coincidence AB
$f_{OBS(AB)}$ = observed coincidence AB
n = total number of observations

The absolute frequency of occurrence of events A and B and their observed coincidence occurrences can be tabulated in a 2×2 table:

	A	$\bar{A}$	
B	34	12	$f_B = 46$
$\bar{B}$	28	56	$f_{\bar{B}} = 84$
	$f_A = 62$	$f_{\bar{A}} = 68$	$n = 130$

$f_{EXP(AB)} = (f_A/n)\,(f_B/n) \times n = (62/130) \times (46/130) \times 130 = 21.9$
$f_{OBS(AB)} = 34$

$D\chi^2 = (f_{OBS(AB)} - f_{EXP(AB)})^2/f_{EXP(AB)} = (34 - 21.9)^2/21.9 = 6.7$

The same calculation would be repeated for the other three cells in this *contingency table** as part of the *chi-square test.**

COMMENT 2: The chi-square distance between two variables consists of the sum of the chi-square distances for each cell of the contingency table.

See also *chi-square test.*

CHI-SQUARE DISTRIBUTION: Syn: CHI 2 law Probability distribution of a random variable that is the sum of squares of n independent and standard normal variables.

COMMENT 1: A standard normal variable has a *mean** of 0 and a *variance** of 1.

COMMENT 2: Many *statistical tests** require the calculation of *statistics** that follow a χ^2 distribution under the *null hypothesis.** The most common test is the χ^2 test of independence.

COMMENT 3: The χ^2 distribution is a nonsymmetrical *distribution.** It also varies in shape depending on the degrees of freedom. Hence, one should specify that a given distribution follows a χ^2 distribution with n degrees of freedom.

Among the other mathematical properties of the χ^2 distribution, one should note that the *mean** and *variance** are k and $2k$, respectively; the *modal** value is $k-2$ for values of $k \geq 2$ and is zero for $k = 1$; chi-square values are between zero and infinity, as they are the sum of values that have been squared; and the sum of two or more independent chi-square variables also follows a χ^2 distribution.

CHI-SQUARE TEST: Test of independence between two categorical variables.

COMMENT 1: The hypothesis is that the *chi-square distance** between the variables is null. This implies that there is no difference between the observed coincidences and those predicted under the hypothesis of probabilistic independence.

COMMENT 2: The test is interpreted by comparing the calculated *chi-square distance** with the *chi-square distribution** values having $(r-1)$ times $(c-1)$ *degrees of freedom** (r = row; c = column).

See also *chi-square distance, degree of freedom.*

CHRONIC CARRIER: Individual remaining in a carrier state for a long period of time after convalescence, sometimes until death.

EXAMPLES: Pigs that recovered from pseudorabies (Aujeszky's disease); cattle following bovine infectious rhinotracheitis.

See also *carrier.*

CHRONIC DISEASE: Syn: chronic illness Disease of relatively long duration (several weeks to several years).

EXAMPLE: Tuberculosis.

COMMENT 1: In general, the incubation period may be long, but this is variable.

COMMENT 2: It is in contrast to *acute disease.**

CHRONIC ILLNESS: See **Chronic Disease**

CHRONOLOGICAL SERIES: See **Time Series**

CIRCADIAN: Exhibiting a periodicity of approximately 24 hours.

COMMENT: To be differentiated from *nyctohemeral.* *

CLASS: A subset of individuals that are regrouped based on a classification rule.

EXAMPLE: Classification of dairy farms based on the number of dairy cows. From 1 to 19; 20 to 39; 40 to 59, etc.

COMMENT 1: There are many kinds of classes because there are several potential classifications. For example, (1) classification can be based on a single continuous *variable* * obtained from various *individuals.* * In that case, the *range* * of values of the variable is separated in intervals that are the classes' intervals and that are limited by upper and lower limits (class boundaries); (2) classification can also be constructed by a classification or ordination *algorithm,* * which is based on a measure of distance or a measure of similarity between the individuals to which it is applied.

COMMENT 2: These classes are more or less, depending on the technique used, dependent upon the sample of individuals considered to construct the classification.

COMMENT 3: In data analysis, it is useful to classify observed values in classes for which the number and limits are defined by the observer.

COMMENT 4: The class limits must be defined in such a way that classes are mutually exclusive.

If we consider the following classes: 10–15; 15–20; 20–25 cm, recording errors could occur for individuals with a reading of 15 cm because they could be placed in two adjacent classes. The convention is always to include in a class the inferior limit and to exclude its superior limit, which would give:

> class 1: 10 to less than 15 cm
> class 2: 15 to less than 20 cm
> class 3: 20 to less than 25 cm.

CLASSIFICATION: Assignment of individuals into mutually exclusive categories (classes) on the basis of shared qualities or characteristics.

COMMENT 1: The classification scheme can be postulated before or after a *study* * begins, and should encompass no more *classes* * than necessary for the purposes of the study *objectives* * as well as including enough to include all subjects.

COMMENT 2: Methods of classification that attempt to create homogeneity within categories and heterogeneity across categories can be based on intuition, biologic knowledge, data distributions, or multivariate statistical methods (e.g., *discriminant analysis* *).

See also *discriminant analysis, multifactorial analysis.*

CLASSIFICATION OF DISEASES: Distribution of diseases in groups according to common characteristics.

COMMENT 1: There are several international disease classifications: one of them, published and revised regularly by the World Health Organization (WHO), concerns human diseases; another, published by the Office International des Epizooties (OIE) and updated regularly, focuses on transmissible animal diseases, and features two lists: list A (diseases that have the potential for very serious and rapid spread, irrespective of national borders and are of major importance in international trade) and list B (diseases of importance within countries and which are also of significance in international trade). Classification of animal diseases into several groups has also been undertaken by the Commission of the European Union.

COMMENT 2: In practice, a common classification scheme is based on etiological categories:

1. Genetic
2. Physical and mechanical
3. Chemical and toxic
4. Psychosomatic
5. Nutritional deficiency, excess, or imbalance
6. Metabolic
7. Autoimmune, immune, and allergic
8. Neoplastic
9. Infectious
    a) virus
    b) bacteria, mycoplasma, etc.
    c) fungus and yeast
    d) parasitic (insects, helminths, protozoa)
10. Aging
11. Unknown and other

CLINICAL EPIDEMIOLOGY: Application of epidemiologic principles and biometric methods to the study of diseases in order to improve medical decision-making, namely in the areas of diagnosis, prognostic appraisal, and treatment.

EXAMPLE: Evaluation of results obtained following the treatment of a particular disease using two distinct therapeutic protocols (See *trial**).

COMMENT 1: Veterinary clinical epidemiology focuses on questions directly relevant to the practice of veterinary medicine at the individual and herd/flock levels (See *health management**).

COMMENT 2: Sackett et al. (1991) consider clinical epidemiology to be a "basic science for clinical medicine." However, the idea itself of clinical epidemiology as a distinct entity within epidemiology is not unanimously accepted in the scientific community.

CLINICAL INFECTION: Infection associated with clinical signs; infectious disease.

COMMENT: As opposed to *subclinical infection.* * However, because a clinical infection is essentially an *infectious disease,* * the latter expression is more commonly used.

CLINICAL TRIAL: See Trial

CLOSED INFECTION: Syn: encapsulated infection Infection of an individual by a microorganism that is circumscribed to an internal organ or tissue and that is not excreted.

This expression is seldom used in English.

EXAMPLES: Visceral abscess, cellulitis, osteomyelitis, etc.

COMMENT: A closed infection is a non-*contagious** condition that may only be transmitted from an infected individual to a susceptible individual via unusual circumstances, such as accidental inoculation.

CLOSED QUESTION: Syn: multiple-choice question Question offering a limited number of options to the respondent.

EXAMPLE 1: How many cows do you have in your herd?
 (Please circle the appropriate choice)

   1. Less than 10
   2. Between 10 and 19
   3. Between 20 and 29
   4. Over 29

EXAMPLE 2: Who catches birds on your farm prior to shipping?
 (You may select more than one option)

   1. Your own employees
   2. Local people are hired for this job
   3. A crew provided by the processor
   4. Varies with the flock

COMMENT 1: One or several options may be selected depending on the question. It is important for all choices to be mutually exclusive. It is preferable to use a different font for the question and the proposed answers.

COMMENT 2: Closed questions are more popular than *open-ended questions** because choices are forced, they are easy to code and, consequently, they are easier to analyze. A major advantage is that underreporting of an event listed as a possible answer is less likely since the respondent is prompted.

COMMENT 3: Closed questions may result in poor precision as in example 1 where the exact number of animals is not obtained. Valuable information may also be missed and the order of choices may affect the respondent's answer, mainly for personal (face-to-face) and phone interviews.

COMMENT 4: There is a practical limit to the number of choices that can be offered. While up to 10 choices for a single question could be considered in mail questionnaires, it is difficult to offer more than five options by phone or during personal interviews. When this is the case, the respondent is more likely to choose the first or the last option because they are easier to remember.

COMMENT 5: Closed questions can be designed as rating or intensity scales.

CLOSED QUESTIONNAIRE: Document comprised exclusively of closed questions. See also *closed question.*

CLUSTER: (1) Group of study units (e.g., individuals, pens) used as a sampling unit in cluster sampling; it is then part of the study protocol and data should be analyzed accordingly. (2) A regrouping of individuals obtained through cluster analysis or based on a decision by the observer.

EXAMPLE: A farm may be considered a cluster of animals. It is an important concept in veterinary epidemiology.

COMMENT 1: This concept is usually associated with a level of organization existing in the population under study whether it is used a priori (definition 1) or a posteriori (definition 2).

EXAMPLE: In a survey on bovine viral leukosis, herds were randomly *sampled,** and in each *herd,** all animals older than 1 year were serologically tested. Hence, each herd constituted a cluster, which was the *sampling** unit (randomly chosen) while each animal corresponded to the *statistical unit** (unit under study).

COMMENT 2: To be differentiated from *stratum** (Figure C4).

See also *stratum, clustering, cluster sampling, disease cluster.*

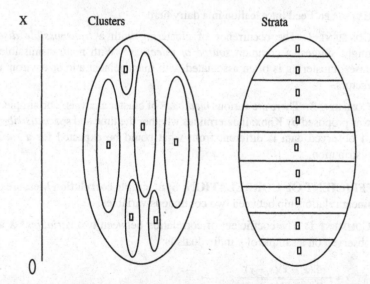

FIGURE C4. Schematic representation of clusters and strata included in a sampling protocol. Note that individual values may vary greatly within a cluster (the small rectangle represents the mean), while they are similar within a stratum (depending on the range defining each stratum).

CLUSTER SAMPLE: A sample in which each of the sampling units is an assemblage of individuals.

EXAMPLE: In a *study** of the *prevalence** of feline leukemia virus infection in a major city, certain city blocks are selected, and all cats on those city blocks are studied.

COMMENT: Cluster samples are not to be confused with a *herd sample.** In the former, clusters within *herds** can be sampled, while in the latter, entire herds are by definition the *sample units** (also referred to as *sampling** units).

CLUSTER SAMPLING: Sampling in which random selection is performed on groups (clusters), rather than on individual animals.

EXAMPLE: Random selection of *herds,** within which all of the animals will be entered into the *study.**

COMMENT 1: Cluster sampling should be distinguished from *stratified sampling.**

COMMENT 2: In cluster sampling, *precision** is improved when each cluster is more heterogeneous. Such clusters, with high intracluster *variance,** are said to be efficient. Very homogeneous clusters, with low intracluster variance, lead to inefficient sampling. Conversely, in stratified sampling, *stratification** is based on *characteristics** associated with the *variable** under study and consequently with low intrastratum variance.

CLUSTERING: Concentration of cases in space and/or time.

EXAMPLE: Feed intoxication in a dairy herd.

COMMENT 1: The occurrence of clustering with a *transmissible disease** might suggest a common *source of infection.** With nontransmissible diseases, clustering is often associated with management and/or environmental factors.

COMMENT 2: There are various *methods** of cluster analysis. The simplest one was proposed by Knox: it determines whether the time and space *distribution** of observed data is different from what could be expected for a *random** distribution.

COEFFICIENT OF CORRELATION: Syn: **simple correlation** Measure of the linear relationship between two continuous variables.

COMMENT 1: The coefficient of correlation between two *variables** X and Y observed on a sample of n individuals is:

$$r = \frac{\Sigma(x_i - \bar{x})(y_i - \bar{y})}{\sqrt{\Sigma(x_i - \bar{x})^2(y_i - \bar{y})^2}}$$

where $\bar{x}$ and $\bar{y}$ are the *arithmetic means** calculated on n observations from the sample, x_i and y_i are observed values of X and Y on the individual i (i varies from 1 to n).

EXAMPLE: Adjusted correlation between weight and height controlling for age.

COMMENT 2: The existence of a correlation, even a strong one, is not synonymous with a cause–effect relationship between the two variables.

COMMENT 3: The coefficient of correlation varies between −1 and +1. The sign indicates the direction of the relationship. Positive indicates that variations are in the same direction and negative indicates that they are in opposite directions (i.e., when one variable increases the other decreases). A value of 0 indicates independence between the variables (see Figure C10).

COEFFICIENT OF VARIATION: Ratio between the standard error and the mean.

COMMENT 1: The coefficient of variation is often expressed as a percentage.

COMMENT 2: This statistic should be used with caution as it is highly dependent on the value of the *mean.* * If the mean is small, close to 0, then the coefficient of variation can be misleading.

COHORT: Broad sense: A group of individuals that experienced a similar event, usually during the same time period.

EXAMPLE: All foxes born during the spring of 1997 in the Fontainebleau forest.

COMMENT: A *generation** is a special type of cohort defined by the event "born during the same time period." However, all individuals in a cohort do not have to enter the observation period at the same time. They could have been selected based on another time event (such as calving date or conception date for dairy cows) and studied at different moments.

Epidemiologic sense: A group of individuals sharing similar exposure characteristics (for example, age, sex, vaccination status), and followed or traced over a defined period of time in order to detect a specific outcome.

EXAMPLE: In a herd, all cows that calved in 1996 enter the cohort at the calving date, and are observed over their lactation periods.

COMMENT 1: The term cohort has a broader meaning than the term *generation*: all generations are cohorts, but a cohort can consist of individuals from different generations. The cohort illustrated in Figure C5 is composed of individuals belonging to different *generations** but entering the study at the same time.

COMMENT 2: A cohort is qualified as "fixed" if no entries are permitted into the study after the onset of the observation period. However, losses can occur during the observation period (nonparticipation, migration, *lost to follow-up,* * attrition, death).

See also *cohort study, prospective study, generation.*

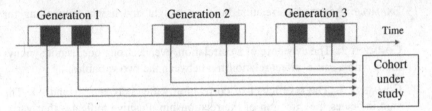

FIGURE C5. Difference between a cohort and a generation.

COHORT EFFECT: Syn: generation effect Variation in the frequency of health status in a cohort by time (e.g., year) of birth regardless of age of the animals.

COMMENT 1: A cohort effect occurs when animals in a particular *cohort* group** are exposed to unique environmental or management conditions and, as a result, the *study** outcome is modified.

EXAMPLE: Figure C6.

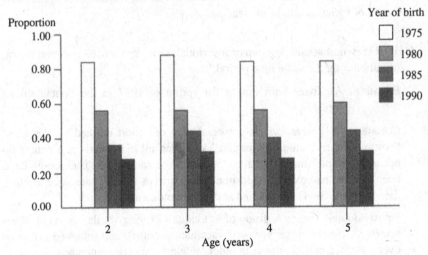

FIGURE C6. Hypothetical example where disease frequency is lower for animals born in recent years regardless of their age.

See also *confounder, effect modification.*

COHORT LIFE TABLE: See Life Table

COHORT STUDY: An observational study in which two or more groups within a population are defined according to their exposure or nonexposure (or degree of exposure) to a risk factor of interest and followed through time to determine the frequency of occurrence of the outcome of interest (Figure C7).

COMMENT 1: The *groups** should be free of the outcome of interest at the start of the *study.**

COMMENT 2: Cohort studies are usually carried out prospectively but in selected instances; when very good *historical data** are available, cohort studies may be carried out retrospectively.

COMMENT 3: Cohort studies are most useful for relatively common *diseases** that have a short period between the exposure to the *risk factor** and the occurrence of the clinical signs.

COMMENT 4: Cohort studies allow direct determination of the *relative risk** of a disease.

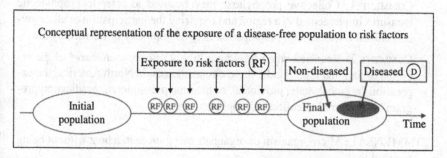

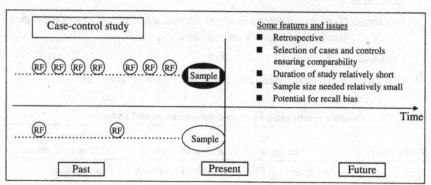

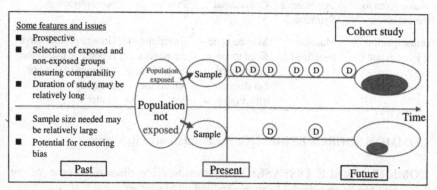

FIGURE C7.   Schematic representation of differences between case–control (retrospective) and cohort (prospective) studies.

COLLECTIVE PROPHYLAXIS: In France: prophylactic measures agreed upon and implemented by the individuals responsible for the health of a given group of animals.

This expression is not used in English. In North America, one would be referring to the implementation of a herd health program or to the application of a disease prevention program (comment 2).

EXAMPLES: In most developed countries, collective prophylaxis is implemented to prevent bovine tuberculosis and brucellosis.

COMMENT 1: Collective prophylaxis may be used to refer to prophylactic measures implemented in a region and requiring the participation of all or several animal owners. Such participation may be voluntary or decreed by law.

COMMENT 2: Required when fighting a highly *infectious disease** at the regional or national level. Under these circumstances, in North America, the expression "regional, state, provincial, or national prevention or eradication program" is preferred to collective prophylaxis.

COMMENSAL: Microorganism or organism living on or in a host without being harmful to it.

EXAMPLE: Numerous bacteria living at the surface of mucosa or in the digestive tract of animals and humans.

COMMENT 1: As opposed to *parasite.**

COMMENT 2: To be differentiated from *saprophyte** (Table C2).

TABLE C2. **Possible relationships between an organism and its *host***

Relationship	The organism lives in or on the host			The organism lives in the environment
Type	Symbiosis	Commensalism	Parasitism	Saprophytism
Name given to the organism	Symbiote or Symbiont	Commensal	Parasite	Saprophyte
Impact on the organism and the host	Mutually beneficial	May be beneficial to the commensal, but does not affect the host	Beneficial to the parasite, but adversely affects the host	Growth of saprophyte is possible due to the presence of dead or decaying organic matter

COMMON SOURCE EPIDEMIC: See **Point Source Epidemic**

COMMUNICABLE DISEASE: Syn: transmissible disease Disease whose agent can be transferred from one individual to another.

COMMENT 1: This term is opposed to *noncommunicable* or nontransmissible *disease.**

COMMENT 2: All *infections** and *infestations** are communicable diseases.

COMMENT 3: A disease can be transmissible (communicable disease) but not *contagious** if it requires a *vector** for its *transmission** (for example, Tabanidae for equine infectious anemia and *Culicoides* for African horse sickness).

COMMENT 4: Genetic diseases (hemophilia, daltonism, etc.) are also vertically transmitted diseases, i.e., they can be transferred from parent to offspring.

See also Figures C8 and C9 (*contagious disease*).

COMMUNICABLE PERIOD: Syn: period of communicability Period during which an infected individual may be the source of contagion.

EXAMPLE: For a rabid dog, the communicable period extends from 10 days before the onset of clinical signs until death.

COMMENT: This period varies greatly depending on the *disease.** Knowledge of the communicable period is very useful for the implementation of effective prophylactic measures.

See also *contagion, period of infectiousness*, Figure G1 (*generation time*).

COMORBIDITY: Morbidity linked to a disease that coexists with the disease of interest in a study or an experimentation.

EXAMPLES: Diarrhea due to colibacillosis in piglets affected with coccidiosis.

Airsacculitis, a respiratory condition, may be present in chickens affected with cellulitis. Both diseases are often associated with *Escherichia coli*. In the context of an *observational study** on cellulitis designed to assess the impact of this disease on productivity, one should take into account a comorbid condition such as airsacculitis.

COMMENT: The effect of comorbid conditions should be considered when evaluating the validity of *randomized* controlled *trials.**

COMPARABILITY: Quality of samples that allows for a valid comparison.

EXAMPLE: The *random** allocation of subjects of a *population** in two subpopulations is an ideal *method** to ensure the comparability between the two subpopulations.

COMMENT 1: Comparability is obtained if the populations or *samples** to be compared are constituted without *bias.** This underlines the importance of identifying potential biases in order to control them.

COMMENT 2: Comparability is achieved a priori given a proper *study** design (for example, random allocation of groups, *matching**), and given an appropriate execution of the research *protocol** (*follow-up* leading to a high *response rate*,* collection of *data** without bias).

COMMENT 3: Comparability is essential for explanatory studies, if one expects to reach valid conclusions.

COMMENT 4: Comparability of two *groups** or samples does not indicate that the two are similar in every way. It simply implies that they are worthy of comparison given the specific *objective(s)** of the study. For example, in a *case–control study** on mammary neoplasia in dogs designed to investigate environmental *risk factors,** one would expect diseased dogs to be comparable to *controls** for *characteristics** such as sex, age, and breed.

COMMENT 5: In *observational studies,** it is not possible to control exposure factors. Therefore, it is not feasible to form the subpopulations in a way that will guarantee the degree of comparability obtained with *experimental studies.** For example, one subpopulation may not be exposed because of conditions that prevent such exposure (i.e., animals raised on concrete floors are not likely to be infected by certain parasites). These conditions may relate to the animals themselves (age, sex, breed, genetic lines) or to their *environment** or management. Consequently, to prevent the introduction of major flaws or biases in the study design, one must pay close attention to the selection process for each subpopulation.

See also *random, analytical study, experimental study, observational study.*

COMPARISON OF MEANS WITH KNOWN VARIANCES: See Z-Test

COMPETING CAUSE: Causes of health outcomes that preclude each other from occurring.

EXAMPLE: Fatal myocardial infarction is a competing cause of death because it precludes other causes.

COMPLETE POPULATION STUDY: Study in which the whole population under consideration is included.

This terminology is not used in North America.

COMMENT 1: The totality of the *population** is included in the *study,** as opposed to studies with *sampling.**

COMMENT 2: When an entire population is included in a study, some investigators may refer to the sampling as a census.

COMPOSITE VARIABLE: Syn: compounded variable Variable supporting the global fluctuations of several related variables during data analysis.

EXAMPLE: The composite variable "working of the milking machine" could be created as a categorical *variable** combining the effects of the following variables: suction level, pulse ratio, suction reserve, and vacuum regulator.

COMMENT 1: To be differentiated from *index** variable.

COMMENT 2: The farm effect, the unexplained effect attributed to "the farm" in a *multivariate analysis** on an animal production issue, is another example of the combination of several effects ascribed to one variable.

COMMENT 3: These variables can be created during the data-entry stage of a *study** in order to better capture a *phenomenon** from elementary information.

COMPOUND GROWTH: Increase of a number at a given annual rate applied to the sum of this number plus the growth of previous years.

EXAMPLE: Given an initial number of 1000 at an annual rate of 10%.

Year	Beginning of year	Compound annual growth	End of year
1	1,000	100	1,100
2	1,100	110	1,210
3	1,210	121	1,331
4	1,331	133	1,464

COMMENT 1: In practice, almost all forms of annual increases are calculated on a compound basis. For example, unless artificially regulated, *populations** grow in a compound manner.

COMMENT 2: As opposed to *simple growth.**

COMPOUND INTEREST: Interest calculated by applying the percentage rate to the initial amount plus the accumulated interest.

COMMENT: In contrast, *simple interest** is calculated only on the invested *capital.**

See also *interest rate, simple interest.*

COMPOUNDED VARIABLE: See **Composite Variable**

COMPOUNDING: The arithmetic process of determining the final value of a payment or series of payments when compound interest is applied.

COMMENT 1: Also known as *compound growth.** For example, *populations** typically exhibit compound growth.

COMMENT 2: It is the reverse of *discounting.**

COMMENT 3: Tables and various *software** packages are readily available to obtain the *future value** of a current investment (*present value**) depending on *interest rate** and time.

See also *present value, future value.*

COMPUTER SIMULATION MODEL: An algorithm written in a computer language.

COMMENT 1: Simulation models can be deterministic or probabilistic. The Monte Carlo method is a class of stochastic computer simulation.

COMMENT 2: The computer is used because it can easily execute the algorithm, which allows for the dynamic *study** of the outcome under various conditions.

CONDITIONAL PROBABILITY: Probability of occurrence of an event, given that another event has occurred.

COMMENT: It is a measure of the occurrence of the event relative to a subset of the possible occurrences of the event.

EXAMPLE: The epidemiologic *sensitivity** and *specificity** of a test are conditional probabilities.

CONFIDENCE INTERVAL: Range of values within which one is reasonably sure that, given a specified error level, the true value of the population variable lies.

EXAMPLE: The true *population** central tendency for the weight of *individuals** in a given population is between 420 and 480 g at an error level of 5%.

COMMENT 1: It is estimated from the results of a *sample.** It expresses the uncertainty associated with *sampling variation.**

COMMENT 2: The boundaries of a confidence interval are the confidence limits.

COMMENT 3: Population statistics should always be expressed with their confidence interval when obtained from a sample.

CONFOUNDER: Syn: confounding factor A factor that leads to a distortion in the effect estimate between another variable (e.g., an exposure) and an outcome (e.g., disease).

EXAMPLE: Age is a frequent confounder of measures of exposure-disease relationships because it is often a determinant of health outcomes. In a study of the relation between milk production in dairy cows and the incidence of mastitis, age is a potential confounder because mastitis occurs more often at certain ages and also influences a cow's milk production.

COMMENT 1: There are three necessary (but not sufficient) criteria for a factor to be a confounder. First, it must be an independent (e.g., in the absence of exposure) determinant of the outcome. Second, it must be associated with the exposure. Third, its distribution must not be determined by the exposure variable (this is often taken to mean that the confounder is not on the causal pathway between exposure and outcome).

COMMENT 2: Ignoring the presence of confounders can lead to biased effect estimates between exposures and outcomes.

COMMENT 3: The presence of a confounder leads to a confounded effect estimate. Note that it is not required for an investigator to specify what factors are confounders in order for confounding to be present.

COMMENT 4: Confounding can be analytically controlled through a number of means, including *stratification,** calculation of standardized mortality ratios, and regression.

COMMENT 5: Do not confuse confounder (or confounding factor) with *interaction** factor.

See also *bias, stratification, adjustment.*

CONFOUNDING BIAS: See Bias

CONFOUNDING FACTOR: See **Confounder**

CONGENITAL DISEASE: Disease existing at birth and whose origin occurs during intrauterine life.

EXAMPLES: Brucellosis in a calf born from an infected mother; listeriosis in newborns.

COMMENT: A disease that is transmitted from the mother to the fetus during the gestation is congenital, but not hereditary (examples: toxoplasmosis, listeriosis, etc.).

See also *hereditary disease, vertical transmission.*

CONSISTENCY (OF A TEST): Measure of the closeness of agreement between values obtained from repeated measurements performed on samples or individuals under specific conditions.

COMMENT 1: This notion can include the concept of *reproducibility** (e.g., repeated measurements by different clinicians or laboratories) and *repeatability** (e.g., repeated measurements taken by the same operator).

COMMENT 2: A consistent test gives repeatable results but does not ensure *accuracy** (see Table A1).

CONTACT: Nature of the spatial relationship between two organisms or individuals in the context of the transmission of infection.

COMMENT 1: Contact is a mode of *transmission** of *infection.**

COMMENT 2: Contact may also refer to a susceptible individual (person or animal) who has been in a relationship with an infected being or a contaminated environment such as to be at *risk** of becoming infected.

See also *direct contact, indirect contact.*

CONTACT RATE: $\dfrac{\text{Number of individuals that have been in contact with a source of pathogens during a given time period}}{\text{Population at risk during this period}}$

EXAMPLE: One-half of the calves in a barn were in the same pen with a sick calf during the month of March. Therefore, the contact rate for calves on this farm was 50% in March.

COMMENT 1: All *individuals** exposed to a source of *infection** do not necessarily come down with the *disease;** this depends on their *susceptibility.**

COMMENT 2: Some authors use "contact rate," in the context of mathematical modeling, to refer to the average number of contacts that each individual of a *population** has had with others individuals of the population during a given time period.

See also *rate.*

CONTAGION: Transmission of a microorganism to a healthy subject by indirect or direct contact with an infected subject.

EXAMPLES: Contagion by direct contact (rabies by bite); contagion by indirect contact (foot-and-mouth disease, transmission by wind [airborne condition]); contagion by indirect and direct contacts (brucellosis, by contact with the female having aborted and by the external environment soiled by aborted material).

COMMENT 1: Because of the mode of transmission (contact), contagious diseases may be defined as a subset of *communicable diseases** (See Figure C8, *contagious disease**).

COMMENT 2: Contagion only applies to living beings whereas *contamination** applies to *fomites** as well.

See also *contagious disease.**

CONTAGIOSITY: The quality of being contagious.

Propensity of a microorganism or a disease to spread more or less effectively within a susceptible population by indirect or direct contact with infected individuals.

EXAMPLES: Foot-and-mouth disease is a condition with high contagiosity. Enzootic bovine leukosis is a disease with low contagiosity.

COMMENT 1: Contagiosity is determined by several factors (the duration of the incubation period, the concentration of the pathogen and its resistance in the environment, etc.).

COMMENT 2: The notion of contagiosity can apply to individuals, to diseases, or to microorganisms.

COMMENT 3: Do not confuse with *infectiousness.**

CONTAGIOUS: (1) Transmitted by indirect or direct contact with an infected subject. (2) Capable of transmitting disease.

EXAMPLES: (1) Contagious disease.
(2) Contagious animal.

COMMENT: In a broad sense, contagious means that it is easily communicated (communicable). For example, laughter is said to be contagious.

CONTAGIOUS DISEASE: Disease transmitted by the transfer of a pathogen from one infected host to another either by direct or indirect contact (Latin, *contagium* = contact).

EXAMPLES: Rabies, scabies, etc.

COMMENT 1: A disease is transmissible but noncontagious when the pathogen must go through a *vector** (Figures C8 and C9) or when it is a genetic defect.

EXAMPLE: Eastern equine encephalomyelitis.

COMMENT 2: Contagious diseases are infectious or parasitic.

<table>
<tr><td colspan="2" align="center">**Communicable diseases**</td></tr>
<tr>
<td>

Noninfectious and non-
contagious diseases

    e.g., Infestations exclusively
        transmitted by vectors
        (filariasis, etc.)
        Genetic defects, etc.

</td>
<td>

Contagious
diseases

    e.g., Scabies, fascioliasis,
        strongyloidiasis

</td>
</tr>
<tr>
<td>

Infectious
diseases

    e.g., Arboviroses

</td>
<td>

Infectious & contagious
diseases

    e.g., Rabies, brucellosis

</td>
</tr>
</table>

FIGURE C8. Diagram showing the relationship between the concepts of communicable (transmissible), infectious, and contagious diseases.

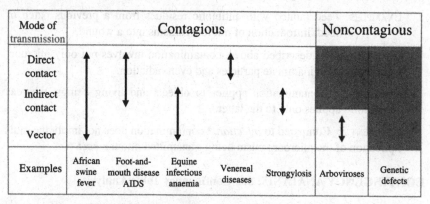

FIGURE C9. Schematic representation of the different categories of contagious and noncontagious communicable diseases.

CONTAGIUM: Organic material that causes contagion.

In North America: Word not commonly used and its definition differs from the above: Refers to any infectious agents causing disease.

COMMENT: In France, contagium comprises the microorganisms themselves as well as the organic matter in which they can be found: saliva (rabies, foot-and-mouth disease), urine (leptospirosis), fecal matter (canine parvovirus, salmonellosis), products of expectoration (Aujeszky's disease, tuberculosis), placenta (brucellosis), etc. Often known as virulent material.

See also *contagion, source of infection.*

CONTAMINATED: To be the object of a contamination.

EXAMPLE: A person or animal is said to be contaminated if bitten by a rabid dog.

COMMENT 1: Contaminated comes from the verb contaminate and, as for *contamination,* * it applies to objects, preparations, and living beings.

COMMENT 2: In general, all animals of a group that were exposed to a *pathogen* * are considered contaminated until it is possible to differentiate between contaminated and noncontaminated individuals. When this is not possible, the original assumption prevails (all animals should be treated as if they were contaminated). This reasoning also applies to objects.

EXAMPLES: All cattle, sheep, goats, and swine on a farm where a case of foot-and-mouth disease has been recorded.

All aspects of an environment where a toxic chemical spill has occurred.

See also *contamination.*

CONTAMINATION: Presence or transfer of a microorganism or substance in or on an object, in a preparation, in or on a living being.

EXAMPLES: Feed tainted with antibiotic residues from a previous batch of feed; introduction of microorganisms into a wound.

COMMENT 1: As described above, contamination involves not only microorganisms but also inanimate particles and even radiation.

COMMENT 2: Contamination applies to objects and living beings, whereas *contagion* * applies only to the latter.

COMMENT 3: Compared to *infection,* * contamination does not imply the multiplication of the microorganism being transmitted into the *host.* *

CONTINGENCY ANALYSIS: See **Contingency Table Analysis**

CONTINGENCY TABLE: Statistical table representing the distribution of at least two qualitative variables.

EXAMPLE: The most basic contingency table cross-classifies two dichotomous *variables,* * e.g., presence or absence of disease and exposure/nonexposure to a *risk factor.* * If n individuals are observed, the following contingency table is obtained:

	Disease present	Disease absent	Total
Exposed	a	b	a + b
Nonexposed	c	d	c + d
Total	a + c	b + d	n

If a third variable is included (e.g., sex):

	Disease present	Disease absent	Total
Male			
Exposed	a_1	b_1	$a_1 + b_1$
Nonexposed	c_1	d_1	$c_1 + d_1$
Female			
Exposed	a_2	b_2	$a_2 + b_2$
Nonexposed	c_2	d_2	$c_2 + d_2$
Total	$a + c$	$b + d$	n

COMMENT 1: Contingency tables with several qualitative variables are also known as multidimensional tables. They allow a group of individuals to be considered by simultaneously considering several of their attributes or *characteristics** (with two or more categories or levels per characteristic).

COMMENT 2: A contingency table can be reformatted into a *disjoint dataset.**

See also *contingency table analysis.*

CONTINGENCY TABLE ANALYSIS: Syn: contingency analysis Statistical method that studies the relationship between categories of two qualitative variables represented by a table with cross-classified data.

EXAMPLE: A study of foot lesions in dairy cattle (12 categories) and their sequelae (lameness, recovery, and culling). In this case, a 12×3 contingency table can be constructed and analyzed.

COMMENT 1: A variety of statistical methods can be used for categorical data analysis; some of the more common include *chi-square tests,** *Fisher's exact test,** *likelihood ratio tests,** permutation tests, and log-linear models.

COMMENT 2: Not to be confused with *multifactorial analysis,** which is used to test the relationship between more than two *qualitative variables.**

CONTRIBUTED CAPITAL: Capital that the owners have contributed to the business.

See also *capital.*

CONTROL GROUP: Group of subjects used for comparison.

COMMENT 1: In a case–control study, selection of controls from the population is based on their nondiseased or unaffected status in terms of the health condition considered. However, control animals may be affected by other conditions (e.g., *hospital controls**).

COMMENT 2: In an experimental design, control group refers generally to a group of subjects not exposed to the treatment being investigated (a therapeutic drug, a prophylactic biologic such as a vaccine, or an entire program composed of many individual treatments such as a preconditioning program for beef calves). However, controls could be a group of individuals receiving a different medication (often the one considered the *gold standard** on the market).

EXAMPLES: In a field trial, one group of nonvaccinated animals (controls) is used for comparison with one group of vaccinated animals for the evaluation of immunization on the incidence of respiratory disease.

A group of cattle put on the prophylactic treatment most commonly used in the industry. This group would serve as control in a trial designed to evaluate the advantages of a new product over the current treatment.

See also *case–control study, experiment, hospital control.*

CONTROL OF A DISEASE: Syn: disease control Reduction of the prevalence of a disease to a level where it is no longer considered a major health and/or economic problem.

COMMENT 1: *Disease** control is compatible with the existence of a limited number of *cases** or *outbreaks.** Contrary to *eradication,** control does not imply the disappearance of the disease and of its causal agent(s). The primary *objective** is to contain the disease by significantly limiting, if not stopping, its spread to susceptible individuals.

EXAMPLE: In France, in 1997, bovine tuberculosis was considered under control. However, its eradication has not yet been achieved.

COMMENT 2: Many disease control strategies result in permanent or long-term changes, such as routine vaccination, converting facilities from multi-age to all-in/all-out rearing, etc.

COMMENT 3: The level of *prevalence** considered acceptable to declare a disease under control varies depending on the disease: swine fever (low); bovine tuberculosis (higher).

CONVALESCENT CARRIER: Individual remaining in a carrier state as it recovers from the disease and for a variable period of time afterward depending on the individual and the infectious agent.

COMMENT: The carrier state may be limited to the convalescent period or go beyond (postconvalescence). When it lasts for a long time, the individual is said to be a *chronic carrier.**

CONVENIENCE SAMPLE: See Haphazard Sample

COOPERATIVE TRIAL: See Multicenter Trial

CORRELATION: A measure of a tendency for two or more variables to be associated.

EXAMPLES: Amounts of sodium and chloride in serum are related in mammals. Height is related to weight in most animals.

COMMENT 1: The degree of correlation indicates how common the variation is among individuals in a sample for a given set of variables. Variables are considered correlated whether the communality of variation is in a similar or opposed direction (Figure C10).

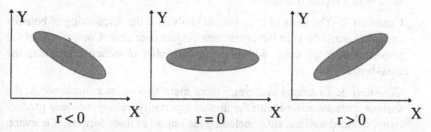

$r < 0$ $r = 0$ $r > 0$

FIGURE C10. Schematic representation of the correlation between two variables X and Y. Three different schema are presented, corresponding to different coefficients of correlation (r). The shaded areas depict the distribution of (x_i, y_i) observations for these two random variables. A graphical evaluation is paramount for the interpretation of a coefficient of correlation. It allows detection of a nonlinear relationship, if present, which cannot be assessed by the coefficient alone.

COMMENT 2: When one of the variables is not completely random (e.g., administration of different doses of a drug to an individual and assessment of a blood parameter), the random variable (blood parameter) is said to be regressed on the fixed variable (drug dosage).

COMMENT 3: Correlation does not necessarily imply *causality*.*

See also *coefficient of correlation, regression analysis, causality.*

COST: Amount, generally expressed in currency, necessary for the acquisition or production of a good or a service.

EXAMPLE: A tractor has a sale price that constitutes a cost for the producer that desires to acquire it. After the purchase, an *expense** is recorded. On the balance sheet, a 10th of the purchase price will be recorded each year during 10 years for *depreciation.**

COMMENT: Some authors do not make a distinction between costs and expenses. Others consider that costs have solely a monetary value whereas expenses have a more accounting aspect (for example, amortization, which is nonmonetary, is an expense).

COST–BENEFIT ANALYSIS: Syn: benefit–cost analysis The appraisal of a project encompassing all social and financial costs and benefits, which determines its profitability, including the possibility of net losses.

COMMENT 1: For some authors, cost–benefit analysis is a technique applied when attempting to evaluate the social *costs** and social *benefits** of investment projects. Investment appraisal methods, which are essentially based on financial considerations, are used for individual business decisions, such as capital investments. However, in the context of disease intervention or control programs at the farm (individual business) or state level, financial and social considerations may be included in the analysis. In this case, one would refer to the cost–benefit analysis of implementing a control program on a particular farm or in a region (Comment 3).

COMMENT 2: The basis of cost–benefit analysis is the discounting of benefits and costs attributable to the investment project over time. Comparison of the *present value** of costs with the present value of benefits provides the cost–benefit ratio.

COMMENT 3: In animal *diseases,** three main factors are considered: A, the various costs associated with the disease (mortality, culling, reduced productivity, reduced welfare, etc.), including the impact of trade barriers, if relevant; B, the cost of implementing a control program; C, benefits resulting from the implementation of the program (lower mortality, improved productivity, improved welfare, etc.).

The cost–benefit ratio is then A/(C – B). Hence, the lower the ratio, the more interesting or valuable the program. A high benefit–cost ratio [(C – B)/A] would be the equivalent. In fact, the latter ratio is normally the one reported (a benefit–cost ratio of 3 is easier to interpret than a cost–benefit ratio of 0.33).

COST–EFFECTIVENESS RATIO: The ratio between the cost of a program and its quantifiable and nonquantifiable benefits.

COMMENT 1: Cost–effectiveness analysis overcomes some of the difficulties involved in putting monetary value on all benefits of a disease control program.

COMMENT 2: The cost–effectiveness ratio may be calculated as follows:

$$\text{Cost–effectiveness ratio} = \frac{\text{Total cost of program}}{\text{Losses avoided by implementing program}}$$

or

$$\text{Cost–effectiveness ratio} = \frac{\text{Total cost of program}}{\text{Epidemiologic benefits of program}}$$

COMMENT 3: In practice, the numerator is often the *cost** part of the benefit–cost analysis. The estimation of the value of the denominator may be strictly political. In many instances, the purpose of the analysis may be to determine how the desired result may be achieved at minimum cost.

COMMENT 4: Do not confuse the cost–effectiveness ratio with the *benefit–cost ratio,** which is strictly a financial calculation.

See also *cost–benefit analysis.*

COX'S MODEL: Syn: Cox's regression, proportional hazard model, proportional risk model Semiparametric model used to study the relative impact of different cohorts on the survival and hazard functions.

COMMENT 1: This *method** uses the conditional *survival function** and a family of *models** referred to as the class of Lehmann's Alternatives.

COMMENT 2: The survival function is expressed in two terms, one depending on time and the other not depending on it. The second term allows one to introduce the presumed *risk factor** associated with death or the pathological occurrence under study.

COMMENT 3: This method assumes that the *instantaneous incidences** are multiplicative and remain unchanged over time.

COMMENT 4: The method was proposed by the English statistician D.R. Cox in 1972.

See also *survival function, survival model.*

COX'S REGRESSION: See Cox's Model

CROSSOVER TRIAL: Trial in which each subject is submitted successively to two interventions or treatments under investigation.

COMMENT 1: Each subject is its own *control.** This is labeled a crossover trial because two groups are constituted: one receiving A then B, the other receiving B then A, the treatment order being *randomly* allocated. The objective of this procedure is to avoid a possible *bias** resulting from the timing of the interventions.

EXAMPLE: In a *randomized* controlled clinical *trial** to evaluate the drug clomipramine as a treatment for canine compulsive disorder, an AB–BA balanced crossover design was used. Dogs were randomized to treatment sequence (clomipramine–placebo; placebo–clomipramine) in blocks of two with a washout period between treatments (period of time needed to make sure that the potential effect of the drug is not carried over to the next assessment of each animal). The outcome was measured on the last day of each treatment and statistical analysis tested whether treatment contrast (level of behavior on drug – level of behavior on placebo) was different from zero.

COMMENT 2: The crossover design is suitable for chronic conditions that will not be changed permanently by either treatment. Indeed, the condition should revert to baseline during the washout period. The advantage of this design is that it eliminates intersubject variability (on the assumption that intersubject variability is greater than intrasubject variability). This was the key for the example presented above, as the human–animal bond and owner circumstances were very different between owners, which meant that the *environment** of each dog was unique.

COMMENT 3: It is critical to have some knowledge about the length of an adequate washout period for the interventions being evaluated. Testing for carryover is possible, but this statistical procedure is not powerful. Therefore, if no information exists regarding this period, one should seriously consider other *study** designs.

COMMENT 4: The crossover design is useful if not too many subjects are available (e.g., trial of treatment for rare *disease**) because power can be high with a relatively small *sample size.** The main disadvantages are the potential carryover effect and if individuals drop out during the *trial.** The AB–BA design also has limitations because the *model** is overparameterized and cannot account for all of the effects (period, order, etc.).

CROSS-PRODUCT RATIO: See Odds Ratio

CROSS-SECTIONAL STUDY: Syn: prevalence study A study in which the data on the factor(s) and the outcome(s) of interest in the population being studied are recorded at the same time.

EXAMPLE: Serological *sampling** to estimate the *herd* prevalence** of *infection** with Aujeszky's disease virus in pigs in a region and to determine if the prevalence depends on *risk factors,** such as type of housing.

COMMENT 1: A cross-sectional study is usually carried out over a short time period in order to obtain a "snapshot" of the *population** under consideration.

COMMENT 2: If the outcome of interest is a disease, then it is the prevalence of the disease that is determined rather than the *incidence.**

COMMENT 3: The main disadvantage of cross-sectional studies is that it is impossible to determine whether the factor of interest or the outcome of interest came first in the subjects being studied. Consequently, it is difficult to distinguish between the *cause** and the effect.

CRUDE INDEX: See Index

CRUDE MEASURE: Quantification of an object or a phenomenon without any adjustment.

EXAMPLE: Number of specks on a fly speck card used to assess the fly *population** in a barn without adjusting for ambient temperature.

See also *index, crude rate.*

CRUDE RATE: Rate corresponding to the frequency of an event within a population over a given time period.

EXAMPLE: Five *herds** out of 325 became infected with bovine viral leukosis in a state over a 6-month period. The crude rate was 1.5% for this period.

COMMENT: As opposed to standardized *rate.** In the example above, age would be a *characteristic** worth adjusting for in a comparison between two states.

See also *rate.*

CULLING: Disposal of live animals by sending them to a slaughter plant, as part of a strategy to renew the herd.

COMMENT 1: Reasons for culling are multiple (e.g., age, low productivity, chronic disease, undesirable conformation). The number of animals culled in a herd is most often equal to the number of animals that entered the herd during the same period of time (replacement heifers and purchases).

COMMENT 2: Reproductive and growing-finishing animals culled from a herd are sent to an abattoir. However, in poultry operations, they are sent to the slaughter plant when the entire flock is culled (breeders and egg-layers); whereas individual culled birds are euthanized at the farm (see examples).

COMMENT 3: Culling is usually expressed as a proportion of the number of animals present in the herd/flock over a period of time, which is often 1 year. The time period may vary depending on the type of production. It is a *risk** *rate,** referred to as *culling rate.**

COMMENT 4: To differentiate from *removal.**

EXAMPLES: In a herd of 25 cattle, three were culled for low productivity last year. But removal was five; indeed, in addition to the cullings, a cow was sold, and another one died.

In a flock of 10,000 broiler chickens, 45 birds were culled during the production period. These are usually poor-doing birds culled for slow growth rate or for welfare reasons.

CULLING RATE:

$$\frac{\text{Number of culled animals}}{\text{Average number of animals in the herd}} \text{ during a given period of time}$$

COMMENT 1: The period of time is often 1 year in dairy and swine production. The length of the period of interest may vary depending on the circumstances. In dairy production, it could be the equivalent of one lactation period. In growing facilities, it is normally the production period (6 weeks in broiler chickens, 4 to 6 months in swine, etc.).

COMMENT 2: The culling rate is usually expressed as a percentage.

COMMENT 3: The denominator varies with the type of production. For example, when the culling rate refers to reproductive animals, a dynamic *population** with *individuals** being added and removed, the average number in the *herd** over the time period is used as the denominator. In contrast, an all-in/all-out grow-finish facility has a more stable population with only removals (culls and deaths) throughout the production cycle. Hence, in practice, the denominator is normally the initial number of animals placed at the beginning of the growing period.

See also *culling.*

CUMULATIVE FREQUENCY: The sum of the number of occurrences of values falling within two or more contiguous class intervals for a given variable.

EXAMPLE: See Table C3 (*cumulative relative frequency**).

COMMENT: Seldom used on its own in veterinary epidemiology. It is often presented in publications as a step toward the calculation of the cumulative relative frequency.

See also *frequency, cumulative relative frequency.*

CUMULATIVE INCIDENCE: The proportion of a closed population at risk (i.e., no immigration) that experiences a health event during a defined period of time.

COMMENT 1: As the time period increases, the cumulative incidence is a monotonically nondecreasing measure.

COMMENT 2: The cumulative incidence is equivalent to the probability of developing a health event when no censoring occurs within the time period.

EXAMPLE: Figure C11.

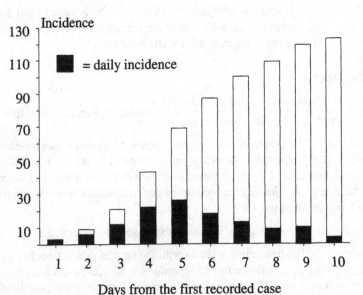

Days from the first recorded case

FIGURE C11. Cumulative incidence of porcine pleuropneumonia in a 1200 pig growing facility during the first 10 days of the outbreak.

CUMULATIVE INCIDENCE RATE:

$$\frac{\text{Sum of the incidence for successive periods}}{\text{Population at risk during these periods}}$$

COMMENT: The evolution of the cumulative incidence rate in a *population** can be represented with a graph (see Figure C14, *cumulative mortality rate**).

See also *incidence, cumulative mortality rate*.

CUMULATIVE MORTALITY: Sum of the mortality for successive periods.

COMMENT: The evolution of the cumulative mortality can be represented by a bar or a line chart (Figures C11 and C12).

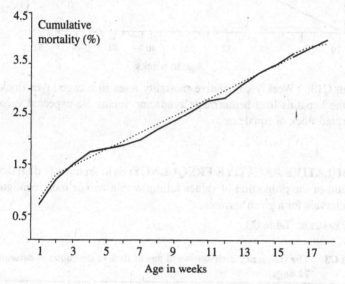

FIGURE C12. Cumulative mortality expected (·········) and observed (———) in a DEKALB-LINK pullet flock in 1998.

CUMULATIVE MORTALITY RATE:

$$\frac{\text{Sum of deaths occurring during successive periods}}{\text{Population at risk during these periods}}$$

COMMENT 1: In practice, the cumulative mortality rate is often a simple *proportion** calculated as the number of deaths during a particular period (or a series of periods) over the number of individuals at *risk** in the *population** at the beginning of that period (or series).

COMMENT 2: The evolution of the cumulative mortality rate is often represented by a graph. It is rarely used unless comparative (expected) values are available (Figure C13).

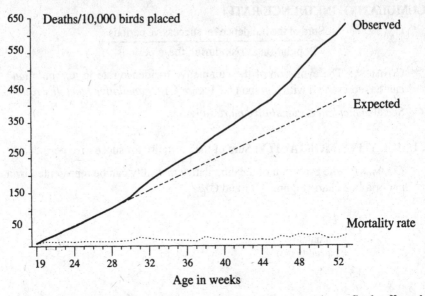

FIGURE C13. Weekly cumulative mortality rates in a cage-layer flock affected with the hepatitis-liver-hemorrhage syndrome versus the expected values for an unaffected flock of equal size.

CUMULATIVE RELATIVE FREQUENCY: Syn: frequency distribution The sum of the proportion of values falling within two or more contiguous class intervals for a given variable.

EXAMPLE: Table C3.

TABLE C3. The frequency distribution of age at time of diagnosis of osteosarcoma in 72 dogs

Class interval (age in years)	Frequency	Cumulative frequency		Relative frequency (%)		Cumulative relative frequency (%)	
< 2	12		12	(12/72) × 100	16.7		16.7
2 to < 4	2	(12 + 2)	14	(2/72) × 100	2.8	(16.7 + 2.8)	19.5
4 to < 6	3	(14 + 3)	17	(3/72) × 100	4.2	(19.5 + 4.2)	23.7
6 to < 8	12	(17 + 12)	29	(12/72) × 100	16.7	(23.7 + 16.7)	40.4
8 to < 10	14	(29 + 14)	43	(14/72) × 100	19.4	(40.4 + 19.4)	59.8
10 to < 12	16	(43 + 16)	59	(16/72) × 100	22.2	(59.8 + 22.2)	82.0
12 to < 14	9	(59 + 9)	68	(9/72) × 100	12.5	(82.0 + 12.5)	94.5
≥ 14	4	(68 + 4)	72	(4/72) × 100	5.5	(94.5 + 5.5)	100

COMMENT 1: As for the *relative frequency,** the cumulative relative frequency may be expressed as a *proportion** with values ranging from 0 to 1 or, more likely, as a percentage.

COMMENT 2: Note that relative frequency information may be misleading if data on the relative distribution of the population are not available. In other words, a high relative frequency for a particular condition in a specific interval may just reflect the relative frequency of the population per se.

CUMULATIVE SURVIVAL RATE: Syn: survival rate in a population The proportion of survivors in a group studied over a period of time:

$$\frac{\text{number of survivors of a disease at the end of a given time period}}{\text{number of subjects present at the beginning of the period}}$$

COMMENT 1: The time period usually corresponds to the duration of the episode of the pathological event.

EXAMPLE: Following an *outbreak** of colibacillosis in a group of 100 calves, there were 20 deaths. Therefore, the cumulative survival rate in the *population** is 0.8 or 80% for the period under consideration.

COMMENT 2: Calculation of survival rate assumes there are no additions or removals (censoring) from the population except from the outcome of interest.

COMMENT 3: The survival rate is equivalent to 1 minus the *cumulative mortality rate.**

CURRENT ASSETS: Assets that will normally be consumed by the business or converted into cash within 1 year.

EXAMPLES: Cash on hand, *accounts receivable,** prepaid expenses, livestock feed, and crops or livestock held for sale are examples of current assets.

See also *accounts receivable.*

CURRENT LIABILITIES: Liabilities that will normally be repaid within 1 year.

CURRENT RATIO: Current assets divided by current liabilities.

COMMENT: A measure of *liquidity.**

See also *balance sheet, current assets, current liabilities.*

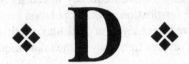

❖ D ❖

DATA ANALYSIS: Mathematical/statistical conversion of data from a crude to an interpretable form.

COMMENT: In a broad sense, the analysis of data includes both descriptive and inferential statistical methods. A more restrictive usage would apply only to descriptive multivariate statistical methods (Table D1).

TABLE D1. **Examples of methods of data analysis**

	Type	Examples	
Descriptive statistics	Univariate	Mean; variance; mode; median; histogram; kurtosis.	
	Multivariate	*Factorial methods* Principal component analysis Contingency table analysis Discriminant analysis	Restrictive sense of data analysis
		Classification methods Hierarchical classification	
Inferential statistics	Univariate	Comparison between two means or two proportions; chi-square.	
	Multivariate	Multiple linear regression; logistic regression.	

DATA BANK: The accumulation of data into a repository, possibly in a computer system, usually for research or monitoring purposes.

EXAMPLE: Daily collection and accumulation of 10 blood parameters on experimental animals.

COMMENT: To be differentiated from a *database,** which is always organized in a computer system.

DATABASE: Syn: Data base A collection of data organized into a specific format and stored in a computer system, allowing for data manipulation (retrieval, aggregation, and use in calculations of numerical data) and dissemination.

EXAMPLES: Medline is a bibliographical database.

VMDP is a database consisting of organized, coded, patient-specific data collected from North American veterinary teaching hospitals.

COMMENT 1: A database management system (DBMS) is the *software** that allows for the effective storage, retrieval, and updating of data.

COMMENT 2: To be differentiated from *data bank,** which may lack a DBMS.

DATA DREDGING: Analysis conducted usually on a large number of variables without having any prestated hypotheses underlying the design of the protocol, and performed to detect significant differences.

COMMENT: Conclusions based on these *studies** are usually suspicious and/or unacceptable, unless they are limited to generating *hypotheses.**

DATA PROCESSING: Set of statistical procedures used for data analysis usually using computer programs.

COMMENT: This expression is also used by various types of organizations (industrial, business, governments, etc.) and usually refers to specific computer-based functions within these organizations, such as the storage of data and the production of reports for the organization's employees, its customers or suppliers, etc. The following is a list of typical applications: financial accounting, *cost** and management accounting, market research and sales forecasting, order processing, investment analysis, financial modeling, production planning and control, payroll, personnel records.

See also *data analysis.*

DEAD-END HOST: Species or individuals hosting a pathogen that do not permit transmission of that pathogen under normal circumstances.

EXAMPLES: Humans infected with hydatid cysts (*Echinococcus* spp.); horses that have transmissible equine encephalopathy in an environment free of arthropods.

COMMENT 1: Note that the designation "dead-end host" only applies to one host–agent combination; the same host may be a *definitive, intermediate* or *transport host** for a different *pathogenic** agent.

COMMENT 2: To be a true dead-end host, an organism must not excrete the pathogen or permit transmission through vectors.

COMMENT 3: A species or an individual can lose the dead-end host status in unusual circumstances. For example, humans are dead-end hosts for hydatid cysts because human remains are normally buried or burned and therefore are not available to be eaten by canines. However, if human remains are allowed to be eaten by dogs, the cestode is fully capable of infecting these dogs.

See also *infectivity.*

DEATH RATE: See Mortality Rate

DEBT TO ASSET RATIO: Total debt divided by total assets.

COMMENT: Also known as debt ratio.

DECISION TREE: Syn: decision tree analysis Diagram presenting, in chronological order, the alternative actions available to the decision maker as well as the options occurring by chance.

COMMENT 1: The decision tree is among the most frequently used techniques of decision analysis. It helps visualize the different possible options (application of a diagnostic procedure, different intervention methods, etc.). Choices that are controlled by the decision maker (such as whether or not to treat) are known as decision or choice nodes and are represented by squares (Figure D1). Events not under the direct control of the decision maker (such as response to treatment) are represented by circles and are known as chance nodes. Each node is connected to the next event by a line or branch. The branches following each decision node must encompass all possibilities and these must be mutually exclusive.

COMMENT 2: The decision tree is completed by *probabilities** assigned to events that may occur at each chance node. These probabilities may be determined based on published results, experimental data or an expert opinion. They must always add up to 100% for each node. The expected outcome is entered at the far right of the tree branches. This approach allows the determination of the best outcome according to certain decision criteria and assuming that the decision tree is valid.

EXAMPLE:

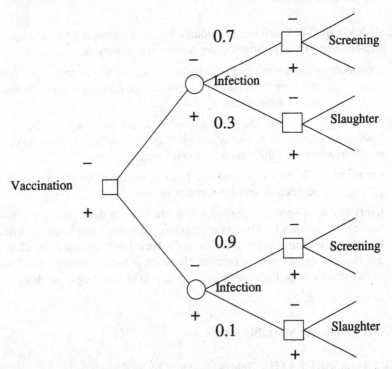

FIGURE D1. Decision tree for the management of pseudorabies (Aujeszky's disease) at the herd level.

DECISION TREE ANALYSIS: See Decision Tree

DEDUCTION: Reasoning based on hypotheses and rules of logic that allow one to conclude on the truthfulness of a statement.

EXAMPLE: The observation of a *statistical association** (conditional on appropriate conditions of observation) between a proposed *risk factor** and a pathological event allows one to deduce that it is indeed a risk factor.

COMMENT 1: The scientific method is a cyclic process of *induction** and deduction (Figure I4, *inference**). In the induction phase, initial observations (e.g., many turkey farms with a high fly population density have broken with coronavirus disease) suggest a conceptual *hypothesis** (flies are a vector in the transmission of coronavirus in turkeys). The phase of deduction begins with the elaboration of a *study** design (research *protocol**) based on the formulation of the operational hypothesis (actual hypothesis being tested: fly population density is associated with the incidence of turkey coronavirus in the field). The protocol must include a priori decision criteria based on expected results in order to determine whether the operational hypothesis should be accepted or rejected; following the implementation of the protocol (data collection), the analysis and interpretation of the findings are driven by the characteristics of the protocol. If these findings concur with the expected results (taking *measurement errors** into consideration), the study is said to support the hypothesis. The *validity** of the conclusions depends on the quality of the study design.

COMMENT 2: Given only one set of observations, one cannot at the same time formulate a hypothesis and evaluate the validity of this hypothesis using *statistical tests.** A second set of data is needed to test the hypothesis inferred by the first set of observations, using *analytical epidemiology,** for example.

COMMENT 3: Claude Bernard has epitomized these different steps: "The facts suggest the idea, the idea leads to the experimentation, the experimentation judges the idea."

See also *analytical epidemiology, experimental epidemiology, experiment.*

DEFENSIVE PROPHYLAXIS: Translation of a French expression referring to prophylaxis applied in an environment where the disease does not exist.

This term is not used in English. Equivalent: prevention program in a disease-free area.

COMMENT 1: Can be sanitary (e.g., *quarantine** and control of movements of animals or animal products to prevent introduction of *exotic diseases**) or medical (e.g., vaccination against foot-and-mouth disease in the absence of disease in France from 1982 to 1990; Danish subsidization of vaccination of swine in Northern Germany against pseudorabies (Aujeszky's disease) to reduce the *risk** of spread to Denmark).

COMMENT 2: It is an application of *primary prevention.**

DEFINITIVE HOST: Syn: **final host, main host, primary host** A term in parasitology to indicate a host in which a parasite undergoes sexual reproduction.

EXAMPLES: Ruminants and equines for the giant liver flukes; canines for hydatid echinococcosis; small ruminants and chamois for the protostrongylid nematodes.

COMMENT: The concepts of definitive (main), paratenic (*transport**), and *intermediate hosts**relate to parasitology. Note that a particular host species can be a definitive host for one group of parasites, an intermediate host for a second group of parasites and a transport host for others. For bacteria and viruses, one normally speaks of usual hosts and occasional hosts. For vulpine rabies, the usual host would be the fox and an occasional host, the badger or the deer.

DEGREE OF FREEDOM: Statistical concept linked to the number of independent individuals (*n*) in the sample under study, and referring to the number of independent items of information available to estimate unknown parameters.

EXAMPLE: When the *variance** is calculated from *n* independent observations, the number of degrees of freedom is equal to *n* - 1 (because there are only *n* - 1 independent deviations from the *mean**).

COMMENT: Degrees of freedom are used differently in univariate and multivariate statistics.

DEPENDENT VARIABLE: Syn: **outcome, response variable, manifestational variable (rarely used)** Variable that is affected by other variables, and that is the focus of the analysis.

COMMENT 1: Variability of the results recorded for the dependent variable is partly explained by the variability recorded for the *independent variables.**

EXAMPLE: Dependent variable: bovine respiratory disease.
Independent variables: time in transit; feeding of corn silage or a high percentage of grain; aggregation of cattle from many sources; use of respiratory vaccines on entry.

COMMENT 2: *Disease** status is often a dependent variable. However, it could also be an independent variable. For example, in an investigation of factors affecting growth performances in cattle, disease status would be considered one of the *variables** of interest.

See also *variable, independent variable*.

DEPOPULATION: Disease control method in which the whole animal population is sacrificed; this includes diseased and infected or contaminated animals, as well as those that have not yet been in contact with the pathogen.

EXAMPLE 1: In France, this method was used for controlling foot-and-mouth disease (FMD).

COMMENT 1: This costly approach is used for highly contagious diseases (e.g., FMD) or for herd and flocks affected with an endemic condition characterized by a high infection rate (e.g., tuberculosis, brucellosis).

EXAMPLE 2: Depopulation as part of a depopulation/repopulation scheme designed to increase productivity by eliminating endemic diseases and boosting genetic quality.

COMMENT 2: Depopulation in the context of Example 2 may be used as a health management strategy in swine production. In contrast to Example 1, depopulation is not regulated by any government agencies and diseases are often not the main reason for this course of action. In some depopulation/repopulation programs in the United States, managers of farrowing units have actually produced more piglets during the year of depopulation/repopulation than in previous years with the same herd size.

See also *selective slaughter, eradication.*

DEPRECIATION: Spreading the acquisition cost of an asset over its useful life at a rate that approximates its use and eventual obsolescence.

COMMENT 1: Even though an asset may have a wear-out life of 20 years, the owner may plan to replace it after 10 years due to obsolescence.

COMMENT 2: There are at least three commonly used methods for calculating depreciation.

COMMENT 3: Straight line depreciation is calculated as:

$$\text{Annual depreciation} = \frac{(\text{Purchase cost} - \text{Salvage value})}{\text{Years of useful life}}$$

COMMENT 4: The declining balance method uses a fixed rate of depreciation each year:

$$\text{Depreciation in a specific year} = (\text{Rate} \times \text{Value at start of year})$$

DESCRIPTIVE APPROACH: Method that seeks to qualitatively and/or quantitatively describe one or more observations.

EXAMPLE: A study that aims to estimate the incidence rate of bovine leukosis virus infection among dairy herds in a province or state.

COMMENT 1: The term "approach" is intended to refer more to the thought processes of the *epidemiologist** than the data itself. Several approaches have been postulated that are available to investigators; besides descriptive, there are also *explanatory** and *pragmatic approaches** to *health** studies.

COMMENT 2: Note that a study resulting from a descriptive approach can still contain statistical measures. For example, means, *standard deviations,** incidence rates,** incidence *proportions,** etc., are frequently used to describe health events in *cohorts** or *populations.**

DESCRIPTIVE EPIDEMIOLOGY: Division of epidemiology concerned with description of the characteristics and the evolution in time and space of health phenomena in a population.

EXAMPLE: Descriptive epidemiology of rabies in France in 1991: species affected, *incidence,** and geographical distribution.

COMMENT 1: It is one section of *observational epidemiology,** in which there is no artificial manipulation of the study factor.

COMMENT 2: Estimate of *disease** occurrences and *trends** are parts of descriptive epidemiology.

COMMENT 3: Descriptive epidemiology generates etiologic *hypotheses** and suggests the rationale for new *studies.**

DESCRIPTIVE STATISTICS: A group of statistical methods used to depict and quantitatively summarize the data collected on a sample taken from a population.

COMMENT 1: To be differentiated from inferential statistics (used for *hypothesis** testing).

COMMENT 2: The numbers used to express the summarized information may be included in other forms of representation such as tables, graphics, and verbal or written common language communications.

COMMENT 3: This is an efficient way to communicate the information depicting the *population** of interest. The description can be *univariate* (*mean,** *variance,** *histograms,** etc.) or *multivariate** (scatter plots, main component analysis, factorial analysis, etc.) depending on the information needed.

DESCRIPTIVE STUDY: Observational study whose objective is to describe the characteristics, the time and the spatial distributions of a health condition in a population.

EXAMPLES: Study of the incidence of fasciolosis in France in 1997.

Comparative study of the seasonal and geographical incidence of *Escherichia coli* O157:H7 human infection reported in 49 counties of Ontario between 1990 and 1995.

COMMENT 1: Descriptive studies are not designed to test hypotheses, but they may be used to generate some, or to assess a situation in the field and to provide the rationale for further studies or interventions.

COMMENT 2: The host, time and environmental/geographical factors are the three major axes for which the effect of a disease should be described. In veterinary epidemiology, the effect of disease on productivity is also often considered.

See also Figure O1, *observational study;* Figure S7, *study.*

DETECTION LIMIT: Syn: minimum detectable level, laboratory sensitivity of a test The concentration or prevalence threshold below which a test or surveillance process is unable to identify positive samples or individuals.

EXAMPLE: The concentration of an antimicrobial in milk below which a residue test is unable to identify the compound's presence. Current on-farm milk residue tests for beta-lactam antimicrobics show a detection limit of 5 parts per billion.

COMMENT 1: Detection limit is categorical, as opposed to *sensitivity,** which is a continuous term. Below the detection limit, sensitivity will be 0.0; above the detection limit, sensitivity will assume a positive value. Laboratory workers often use the term sensitivity as synonymous to detection limit.

COMMENT 2: Up to a certain point, the sensitivity of a *test** increases as the detection limit decreases. For example, an enzyme-linked immunosorbent assay (ELISA) that is applied to bulk milk and that has a detection capacity allowing one infected cow to be detected among 200 non*infected** ones, will be more sensitive than a test having a detection capacity of 1 in 10. However, if most of the *herds** in a region have fewer than 100 cows, a test with a detection capacity of 1 in 1000 would not have a better sensitivity.

If a disease is known to spread rapidly within infected herds, most of them would either be exempt of *infection** or would be heavily infected. In this case, an ELISA with very good detection capacity on bulk milk, would not necessarily offer a significant advantage, in terms of sensitivity, over a test with a higher detection limit.

DETERMINANT CAUSE: Syn: cause, determining factor, determining cause, determinant of a disease Usually refers to the proximate or direct cause of a disease, but has also been used as a synonym for cause or causal factor.

EXAMPLE: *Erysipelothrix rhusiopathiae* is the determinant of swine erysipelas (in this example the organism is a necessary cause; without this agent, whatever the other causal factors of swine erysipelas are, the disease cannot occur).

See also *causality, cause.*

DETERMINANT OF A DISEASE: See **Determinant Cause**

DETERMINING CAUSE: See **Determinant Cause**

DETERMINING FACTOR: See **Determinant Cause**

DETERMINISTIC MODEL: A model whose existence and behavior are completely determined by a given set of conditions and in which a random number generator does not intervene.

COMMENT: A given set of parameters will always provide the same response.

EXAMPLES:

1. $y = ax + b$

2. $y = a + bx + cx_2... + zx_m$

e.g., $\log_e SCC = 0.1 \, (TWOMM) + 0.077 \, (MILKL) - 0.022 \, (TEATEFD) - 0.312 \, (TEATE) + \beta_5 \, (SIRE)$

Where SCC = Somatic cell count in first lactation Norwegian cattle
TWOMM = Two-minute milk
MILKL = Milk leakage between milkings
TEATEFD = Teat-end-to-floor distance
TEATE = Teat-end shape
SIRE = Identification of sire
β_5 = Represents several regression coefficients obtained for dummy variables created to represent the different sires included in the study.
(from T. Slettbakk, A. Jorstad, T.B. Farver, and D. Hird, 1990).

3. The Reed-Frost model

DIAGNOSIS: Identification of a disease or other specific health status of an individual or group of individuals (herd, flock) showing clinical signs.

EXAMPLES: Clinical diagnosis of pneumonia; etiological diagnosis of tuberculosis.

Clinical diagnosis of enteritis; etiological diagnosis of salmonellosis.

Clinical diagnosis of the "thin sow syndrome" in a herd based primarily on the proportion of thin sows observed in the herd and on the reproductive performances (herd level) associated with this syndrome.

COMMENT 1: The diagnosis should relate to the clinical approach that is based on the semiology (clinical signs) and the use of complementary examination and laboratory procedures; the diagnosis itself should remain under the interpretation of the clinician after assimilation of all the available information.

COMMENT 2: Four different strategies of clinical diagnosis are often recognized: (1) pattern recognition (the instantaneous realization that the animal's (or herd's) presentation corresponds to a previously learned *disease** pattern); (2) multiple-branching or arborization strategy (*decision tree** approach mainly used by technical assistants); (3) exhaustion approach (collection of all possible data followed by a search for the diagnosis); (4) hypothetico-deductive strategy (based on an initial working *hypothesis** (arrived at from early clues) producing a manageable list of potential diagnoses, followed by the assessment of clinical and paraclinical procedures selected to narrow this list). Clinicians may use a combination of these four strategies, although the fourth one, hypothetico-deductive, is the most logical and widely used diagnostic approach.

COMMENT 3: Diagnosis differs from *screening**. See Comment 4 under the definition of screening.

See also *screening*.

DIRECT CONTACT: Relationship between two subjects when one touches the other or is in its immediate vicinity.

EXAMPLES: Coitus, nursing, biting, promiscuity in a free stall.

COMMENT 1: As opposed to *indirect contact.**

COMMENT 2: Represents one of the two modes of *contagion,** the second being indirect contact.

See also *contagion.*

DIRECT COST: See **Variable Costs**

DIRECT TRANSMISSION: Passage of a pathogen from one individual to another by close physical contact/proximity between individuals or by common use of an enclosed airspace (for aerosol/droplet transmission).

EXAMPLE: Transmission of rabies by a bite, of respiratory viruses via droplets suspended in the air by coughing.

COMMENT: As opposed to *indirect transmission.** In direct transmission the *agent** is transmitted without the involvement of any intermediate biological or mechanical agent. Transmission by aerosols is generally regarded as direct because pathogens utilizing this means of spread generally do not survive for long in this form and close proximity of diseased and *susceptible* individuals** is normally required.

DISCOUNT RATE: Syn: capitalization rate The interest rate used in the discounting process.

COMMENT: For the economic calculation, one can use either the *interest rate** of the financial market or the discount rate recommended by the plan, taking into account the general economic context (such as *inflation**).

See also *discounting, interest rate.*

DISCOUNT TABLE: Table providing discounting coefficients for various discounting rates (generally from 2% to 50%) depending on time (1 to 50 years).

See also *discounting.*

DISCOUNTING: The process of calculating the present value of a series of future cash flows.

COMMENT 1: Discounting is the reverse of *compounding.**

COMMENT 2: Discounting considers the economist's preference for the present. For example, $100 received today is preferable to $100 received in 1 year's time because the money could be invested to earn interest during the intervening year.

COMMENT 3: The discounting calculation is:

$$\text{Present Value} = \frac{C1}{(1+r)} + \frac{C2}{(1+r)^2} + \frac{C3}{(1+r)^3} + \ldots + \frac{Cn}{(1+r)^n}$$

Where Ci = sum to be received at the end of each year
r = discount rate

EXAMPLE: Assuming a discount rate of 7%, what is the present value of $100 to be paid now, followed by three annual payments of $100 each?

$$PV = 100 + 100/(1 + 0.07) + 100/(1 + 0.07)^2 + 100/(1 + 0.07)^3$$
$$PV = 100 + 100/1.07 + 100/1.14 + 100/1.23$$
$$PV = 100 + 93.46 + 87.72 + 81.30$$
$$PV = \$362.48$$

COMMENT 4: Discounting to present value is one criterion upon which to base investment decisions. Present values of a series of alternative investment options with different time horizons can easily be compared.

See also *capitalization, interest, internal rate of return, net present value.*

DISCRIMINANT ANALYSIS: Mathematical maximization procedure used either to describe differences between groups on two or more dependent variables or to classify individuals into groups on the basis of multiple explanatory variables.

COMMENT 1: The function that classifies *individuals** into *groups** by linearly combining the values of different *variables** is called the discriminant function.

COMMENT 2: Use of discriminant analysis to classify individuals into diseased and nondiseased subgroups on the basis of their levels of *independent variables** (a priori classification) has diminished since the 1970s and has been supplanted in large part by *logistic regression.** One of the reasons discriminant analysis is less used is that it assumes *populations** are *multivariate** normal on the explanatory variables in the discriminant function, an assumption that is suspect when the variables are categorical.

COMMENT 3: There are several methods of discriminant analysis: factorial discriminant analysis (achieved following a *principal components analysis** or a factorial analysis), multiple linear regression, logistic regression, and linear discriminant analysis of Fisher.

DISCRETE DATA: See **Discrete Variable**

DISCRETE VARIABLE: Syn: **discrete data** Quantitative characteristic of a population whose data fall naturally, or can be arbitrarily arranged, into groups or sets of values.

EXAMPLES: Number of *cases** of a *disease;** number of liveborns per litter.

COMMENT 1: Values are often whole numbers with a definite distance between them. For example, number of lactations: 1, 2, 3, 4, etc. The distance between each value is 1.

COMMENT 2: Continuous data can be expressed as discrete data. For example, weight (in kg) can be recorded or transformed to fit in a limited number of categories: < 1, 1 to 1.5, 1.51 to 2, > 2.

COMMENT 3: The adjective discrete is only applied to *measurements.** Values of qualitative variables vary in kind but not degree, and, hence, are not measurements. For example, the *variable** "sex" can be categorized as male, castrated male, female, spayed female, and, although one could label the categories as 1, 2, 3, 4, these values are only codes and have no quantitative interpretation.

DISEASE: Syn: sickness, illness Noncompensated perturbation of one or several functions of an organism.

Pathological condition occurring in a susceptible population.

EXAMPLE: Rabies in the raccoon *population** of southern Ontario.

COMMENT 1: This concept can be used to describe the *health** status of a single individual or a whole population.

COMMENT 2: A disease is expressed by *symptoms,** clinical signs and/or by a decrease in production. An infection or an infestation may not translate in any perceptible symptoms or reduction in productivity (subclinical infection). However, the limit between the state of disease and health is sometimes difficult to define (example: absence of symptoms but reduced productivity).

COMMENT 3: Depending on the individual, the same disease can appear with variable intensity in a susceptible population; from *subclinical infection** to death of the individual.

COMMENT 4: The magnitude of a disease in a population can be assessed using different *rates:* mortality rate,* morbidity rate,* case fatality rate.**

DISEASE CLUSTER: Aggregation of individuals with identical health events in space and/or time.

EXAMPLES: *Individuals** in an *outbreak** of gastroenteritis from food intoxication.

A higher-than-expected number of cancer cases in a defined geographic region during a finite period of time.

COMMENT 1: This expression is typically used to describe unusual health events, the concentration of which would be expected to be unlikely if they were etiologically unrelated.

COMMENT 2: There are various methods for the analysis of space/time clustering. The simplest method has been proposed by Knox: it determines whether the time and space distribution of observed data is different from what could be expected for a random distribution.

DISEASE CONTROL: See Control of a Disease

DISEASE CYCLE: Syn: stages of disease Different stages in the course of a disease, from contact with the pathogen to recovery.

COMMENT 1: Knowledge of the disease cycle is important in *population medicine.** Indeed, determining the time progression of *disease** within an *individual** or *group** is an essential component in the development of disease control strategies.

COMMENT 2: The disease cycle may be divided into different phases, some of which may overlap:

Phase 1: Exposure; the initial act of being infected or being subjected to an *infectious** agent; entrance of infectious agent into or on an individual;

Phase 2: Incubation period; the period of time between exposure to the pathogen and the onset of clinical signs (e.g., 24 to 48 hours for infectious bronchitis in chickens);

Phase 3: Prodromal period; period of transition between health and disease characterized by the initial (often nonspecific) clinical signs;

Phase 4: Clinical disease; the period of time in the disease cycle when the clinical signs normally observed with the disease of interest are preeminent;

Phase 5: Regression period: reduction of the clinical signs of disease; response based on natural or acquired *resistance** to disease;

Phase 6: Convalescent or recovery period. This period corresponds to the progressive restoration of the integrity of the morphological and physiological functions of affected organs or tissues. Note that a disease may permanently disable an individual (e.g., atrophic rhinitis) or a group (in terms of production performances);

Phase 7: *Carrier** period (carrier state); a period of time when an individual harbors an infectious agent or parasite, and is capable of transmitting the agent to other individuals but does not show clinical signs of disease; carriers are subclinically infected. Note that the carrier state occurs as early as during the incubation period (*incubatory carrier**). This is very disease dependent.

See also *disease, carrier.*

DISJOINT DATASET: A dataset containing one line per individual with one entry per category for all variables, but where the categories of each variable are the components of.a disjoint set.

COMMENT 1: These tables are generally used in *multifactorial analysis.**

EXAMPLE: *n* individuals are checked for the presence of a *disease** and exposure to some *risk factor.** The following table is obtained in which each level is coded according to presence or absence of the disease/exposure:

| Individual | Disease | | Risk factor | |
number	Disease present	Disease absent	Exposed	Nonexposed
1	0	1	1	0
2	1	0	0	1
3	0	1	0	1
4	1	0	1	0
—	—	—	—	—
—	—	—	—	—
—	—	—	—	—
Total	m+	m–	e+	e–

m+ = number diseased; m- = number nondiseased; e+ = number exposed; e- = number nonexposed.

COMMENT 2: The presence of each category of each *variable** is coded with 1 when present and 0 when absent (= "disjunctive"). Since categories of a variable are exhaustive and exclusive by definition, the sum of codes of levels by individual and by variable is always equal to 1 (= "complete").

COMMENT 3: The sum of each column corresponds to the number of times one has observed the corresponding level. For the same example, the sum of the "disease present" column (m+) will be equal to the number of diseased individuals among all observed individuals.

COMMENT 4: A disjoint dataset can easily be transformed into a *contingency table.**

COMMENT 5: When preparing a dataset to be analyzed using a computer *software,** it is typical to record only one column per variable. Indeed, in the example above, the information in the "disease present" and the "exposed" columns would be sufficient to perform the analysis.

See also *multifactorial analysis*.

DISPERSION: A measure of the variation existing between the individuals of a sample or of a population.

EXAMPLE: *Variance** and *standard deviation** are two measures of dispersion commonly used in unimodal frequency distributions.

DISPERSION PARAMETERS: A numerical descriptive measure depicting the distribution of values from a population for a given variable.

COMMENT 1: The *variance** and the *standard deviation** are the most widely used dispersion parameters. They are measures of variability.

COMMENT 2: Dispersion parameters are normally estimated from a *sample** of observations. Ideally, the *sampling** should be *random.**

DISTANCE: A geometrical measure of the length of travel to go from one individual to another.

COMMENT 1: It is a function of the differences between values of variables used to describe the two *individuals*.* These variables also define the dimensional space in which these individuals exist for the purpose of the *study*.*

EXAMPLE: Distance between two swine herds based on their productivity results.

COMMENT 2: The usual measure of distance between two objects is the Euclidean measure.

COMMENT 3: The notion of distance between individuals is essential in data analysis (multifactorial). There are many possible calculations of distance. Most of these are used in *cluster analysis*,* *classification*,* and ordination. Multivariate density functions are dependent on the measure of distance used. A well-known method in *multivariate analysis*,* is the Mahalanobis distance.

DISTRIBUTION: Representation of the probability of observing a specific value or class of values for a variable measured on a given population.

COMMENT 1: It is a measure of the density of the *population** along the spectrum of possible values. It is expressed as a density function. The Gaussian or normal density function (normal distribution) is used for several *variables** with a symmetrical distribution. Many other types of distributions exist in *statistics:** *log normal distribution,** *chi-square distribution,** Poisson distribution, etc.

COMMENT 2: There are essentially three types of geographical distributions: random, uniform, and cluster.

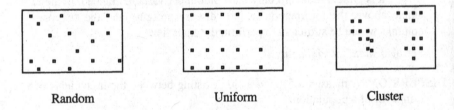

Random   Uniform   Cluster

In the particular area of spatial or temporal distribution, the frequency of observation or the density is defined with respect to spatial or temporal location. The coefficient "K" of Neyman, characterizes the three types of geographical distribution mentioned above.

EXAMPLES: Random distribution of nests in a region.
Uniform distribution of bacterial colonies in a homogeneous media.
Cluster distribution of ticks on some anatomical regions of cattle.

DUMMY VARIABLE: See **Indicator Variable**

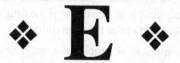

❖ E ❖

EARNINGS: See **Profit**

ECOLOGY: Study of the environment and of the interrelationships between organisms and their environment.

EXAMPLES: Ecology of the fox; ecology of *Salmonella*; human ecology.

COMMENT 1: The ecology of microorganisms includes two study levels, the level dealing with organisms that host them and the *environment** where these organisms live.

COMMENT 2: Application of the term "ecology" to the study of what some consider nonnatural systems (as in human ecology) is controversial.

ECOPATHOLOGY: In France: Study of pathology in relation to the environment.

In North America: Not used. The term *epidemiology** is preferred in reference to the examples listed below.

EXAMPLES: Study of the relationship between environmental conditions (altitude, temperature, exposure, latitude, etc.) and the density and degree of activity of vectors in the context of investigations on leishmaniasis.

The infertility of dairy cows studied in relation to nutritional and herd management factors (heat detection by the producer, age at first insemination, etc.).

ECOSYSTEM: A natural unit which includes all the biological and physical components of a given area, and the relationships linking them together.

EXAMPLES: A pool, a forest, an individual (for a necessary parasite) represent three different ecosystems.

COMMENT 1: Odum defined an ecosystem as "... any unit that includes all of the organisms in a given area interacting with the flow of physical environment so that a flow of energy leads to a clearly defined trophic structure, biotic diversity, and material cycles within the system."

COMMENT 2: Ecosystems may be defined at different spatial scales and include *biotopes** and *biocenoses.**

EFFECTIVENESS: The ability of a practice, product, or program to achieve its goals under noncontrolled, "in-field" situations.

EXAMPLES: The goal of a *clinical trial** evaluating the effectiveness of a new anticancer drug is to determine if the drug's outcomes are acceptable when used under field conditions.

The effectiveness of a tuberculin test is normally less than its *efficacy** because of the variability of its application under field conditions, i.e., storage conditions of the tuberculin, technique of injection (strictly intradermal), reading and interpretation of test results.

COMMENT: In order to correctly assess the effectiveness of a *test** or of a program, it must be conducted by the *individuals** who will be expected to use it in practice.

See also *efficacy, efficiency*.

EFFECT MODIFICATION: Changes in the magnitude of an effect measure (between a risk factor and an outcome) that are a function of a third variable, the effect modifier (i.e., this factor modifies the effect of the risk factor).

EXAMPLE: In a *study** of the relationship between hypocalcemia prepartum and dystocia in dairy cows, lactation number is an effect modifier because hypocalcemia occurs more often in older cows and dystocia in younger cows.

COMMENT 1: A factor could be both an effect modifier and a *confounder.** When this occurs, confounding is secondary because the effect of the *risk factor** depends on specific values of the factor considered to be an effect modifier.

COMMENT 2: Confounding is a *validity** issue, whereas effect modification is a *precision** issue. Therefore, effect modification is measured by interaction terms. An interaction term must be biologically meaningful.

See also *confounding*.

EFFICACY: The ability of a practice, product, or program to achieve its goals under experimental or otherwise "best-case" situations.

EXAMPLES: The goal of a laboratory efficacy *trial** testing a new anticancer drug is to determine if the drug can be used successfully to treat the disease.

Serology applied to individuals offers the highest efficacy compared to all other *screening** methods used to detect *herds** infected with bovine viral leukosis.

See also *effectiveness, efficiency*.

EFFICIENCY: A measure comparing outcome to input; it can be represented as the cost to achieve some nonmonetary outcome or a ratio of a program's costs and returns, or any other means of associating outcome and inputs.

EXAMPLE: The *evaluation** of a clinical *trial** testing a new anticancer drug determines that the *average cost** per cure is twice that of the current therapy, making it an inefficient therapeutic choice.

COMMENT: Efficiency can be measured in monetary terms or in nonmonetary terms. For instance, milk production per labor hour is an efficiency measure, as is the number of *cases** discovered per *traceback,** or the number of cases treated per day. Normally, efficiency is anchored on a monetary basis through comparing some mix of outcome, outcome costs, or outcome benefits to inputs, input costs, or *opportunity costs.**

See also *efficacy, effectiveness.*

ELIGIBLE POPULATION: Fraction of the source population possessing the inclusion criteria.

EXAMPLE: Herds of more than five cows included in the *source population.**

COMMENT: It corresponds to the *sampling frame.**

See also *population* (Figure P3), *sampling frame, source population, target population* (Figure T1).

ELIGIBILITY CRITERIA: Syn: inclusion criteria Set of rules used to determine which units (individuals, pens, herds, etc.) are included or excluded from a study.

EXAMPLES: In a *study** of the *prevalence** of equine ehrlichiosis, in which prevalence is defined by the presence of circulating serum antibodies, vaccinated *individuals** would be excluded.

In a retrospective study on preweaning mortality in swine, litters included in the project were selected based on the following criteria: (1) They were from herds of over 60 sows; (2) the herds had been on a computerized recording system for at least 1 year; (3) an internal consistency evaluation of preweaning data revealed a percentage of agreement at the herd level in excess of 90.

COMMENT: Criteria should be specified prior to beginning a study, and must be reconciled with the study *objectives.**

ELIMINATION OF A DISEASE: Disappearance of all clinical cases of a specific disease in an area.

COMMENT 1: Elimination normally differs from *eradication.** Elimination concerns only clinical cases, while eradication includes the disappearance of the pathogen from clinical and nonclinical *cases.** In the case of noninfectious conditions, such as nutritional deficiencies, elimination is equivalent to eradication.

COMMENT 2: The area or location may be a geographical region or a commercial organization present in one or several locations (i.e., an integrated food animal company).

EMPIRICAL SAMPLE: See Haphazard Sample

ENABLING FACTOR: See Predisposing Factor

ENCAPSULATED INFECTION: See Closed Infection

ENDEMIC DISEASE: Disease clinically expressed or not, constantly present in a population in a given region (Figure E1).

EXAMPLES: In humans: Malaria in tropical areas.

In animals: Bovine tuberculosis.

COMMENT: Endemic is preferred to enzootic, when referring to animal diseases, to express the concept defined above.

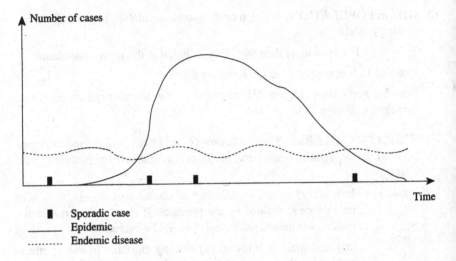

FIGURE E1. Graphic representation of the differences among epidemic, endemic, and sporadic diseases.

ENDEMO-EPIDEMIC: That has endemic and sometimes epidemic characteristics.

EXAMPLES: In humans: Cholera and yellow fever can sometimes take on an epidemic appearance in regions where they are normally endemic.

In animals: Venezuelan equine encephalitis is endemic in South America, but epidemics can occur as in Colombia and Venezuela in 1995.

COMMENT: Endemo-epidemic is preferred to enzoo-epizootic, when referring to animal diseases, to express the concept defined above.

ENDOGENOUS FACTOR: See **Intrinsic Factor**

ENDOGENOUS INFECTION: Infection due to the reactivation of a microorganism already present in an individual whose defense mechanisms are often weakened.

EXAMPLE: Infection by bacteria of the intestinal flora.

COMMENT 1: These microorganisms are *opportunist agents.* *

COMMENT 2: As opposed to *exogenous infection.* *

ENTRY: Observation logged in a recording system.

    EXAMPLE: Number of piglets born alive to sow X.

    COMMENT: This term applies to computerized as well as noncomputerized record-keeping systems.

ENVIRONMENT: Set of natural, social and/or cultural conditions in which organisms live.

    EXAMPLES: Natural environment (a pond for a frog); artificial environment (industrial swine farm for pigs).

    COMMENT: Everything that is external to the individual *host.**

ENVIRONMENTAL FACTOR: See **Extrinsic Factor**

ENVIRONMENTAL HEALTH: Organized set of multidisciplinary activities aimed at the study and interpretation of associations found between diseases and environmental hazards.

    COMMENT 1: These hazards include biological, chemical, physical, familial, occupational, and socioeconomic factors, as well as psychological stressors and other circumstances that affect the likelihood of *disease** occurrence. Much overlap exists between these various categories of factors. For example, a family includes a variety of biological, social, and environmental factors. However, it is useful to differentiate one category from another because of the different *methods** used to study them.

    COMMENT 2: Differences in disease occurrence among genetically similar *populations** are likely to reflect environmental influences.

    COMMENT 3: Environmental health encompasses *occupational health,** which is a domain of intervention in *public health.**

    COMMENT 4: This term is sometimes used in a more literal sense to describe the state of sustainability of an *ecosystem.**

ENZOO-EPIZOOTIC: See **Endemo-Epidemic**

ENZOOTIC DISEASE: See **Endemic Disease**

EPIDEMIC: Syn: **disease epidemic** Occurrence of a disease or any other health-related event affecting a number of individuals in clear excess of what would be expected for a specific region and period of time.

For some authors: Disease suddenly affecting a large number of individuals in a given region.

    EXAMPLES: Salmonellosis affected the elderly community of Owen Sounds in Ontario, Canada, in 1993, resulting in several hundred reported cases, including seven deaths.

    In the Niagara Peninsula (Ontario) in 1994, 38 *outbreaks** (flocks) of infectious laryngotracheitis (ILT) were recorded over a

4-month period in broiler chickens. Although outbreaks of ILT have been reported in this area in the past, only up to three ILT flocks are expected per month in this region during the Spring, which corresponds to the peak season for this disease.

COMMENT 1: The number of *cases** constituting an epidemic varies depending on the *agent,** the region (size and type of *population,** including its *immune** status) and the period of the year. This number can be relatively small. For example, three cases of rabies in humans in a county or district in North America would certainly qualify as an epidemic. However, some authors may prefer the word outbreak for this situation. It is important to note the difference between these two definitions when reviewing the international scientific literature.

COMMENT 2: The word epidemic often conveys the notion of rapid *spread of disease.** This word can be used in reference to human or animal populations.

See also *epidemic threshold, outbreak.*

EPIDEMIC THRESHOLD: Baseline population incidence from which we can determine the occurrence of an epidemic.

COMMENT: For an endemic with fluctuating *incidence,** it is difficult to define the level of incidence at which the *endemic** becomes an *epidemic.** For humans, Serfling proposed calculating the expected incidence from data recorded during many years of an endemic. Using this method, the epidemic threshold is obtained by adding 1.65 times the standard error to the expected incidence. If current incidence is greater than the epidemic threshold during three previous consecutive weeks, it is considered to be an epidemic (Figure E2).

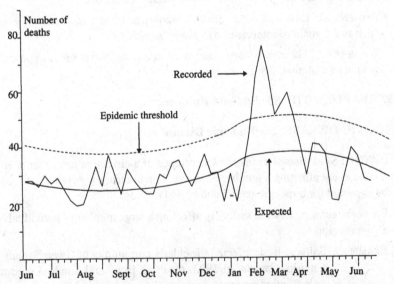

FIGURE E2. Schematic representation of the expected weekly mortality incidence, the recorded incidence, and the epidemic threshold (calculated according to Serfling) for a population affected by a disease that went from endemic to epidemic.

EPIDEMIOLOGIC SURVEILLANCE: Syn: surveillance Ongoing systematic and continuous collection, analysis, and interpretation of health data (often designed to detect the appearance of specific diseases), allowing epidemiologists to follow in time and space the health status and some of the risk factors associated with diseases for a given population, for use in the planning, implementation, and evaluation of disease control measures.

EXAMPLES: Systematic recording by mandatory reporting of *cases** of *notifiable diseases,** such as brucellosis abortions, foot-and-mouth disease, or systematic tuberculin testing of cattle; follow-up of fascioliasis infestation in some slaughterhouses.

COMMENT 1: Epidemiologic surveillance is descriptive in nature.

COMMENT 2: Surveillance may be designed to cover different objectives, such as: to estimate the relative importance of a disease in a *population at risk;** to detect *outbreaks** or *epidemics;** to document and understand the *natural history of a disease** or any other health event; to monitor changes in *infectious** agents; to detect changes in *health management** programs; to identify research needs and provide preliminary information for such research; and to evaluate or help in the planning of control strategies. It may also be useful for political, social, or economic decision making.

COMMENT 3: It is usually limited to a few diseases or pathologies, based on economic and/or medical criteria. Of particular interest are new or *exotic diseases** that may be of economic or *public health** importance.

COMMENT 4: Data recording must be standardized and homogeneous, in particular if observations and recordings are obtained from several distinct locations.

COMMENT 5: Many authors use epidemiologic surveillance interchangeably with *monitoring.** Indeed, they have in common the routine and ongoing collection of data.

See also *monitoring.*

EPIDEMIOLOGIC SURVEY: See Survey

EPIDEMIOLOGIC UNIT: An individual animal living alone or a group of animals living together under observation for a particular health event.

COMMENT 1: A key issue in selecting an epidemiologic unit is if relevant covariate information is available on and known to vary between *individuals,** or if covariate information is identical for all animals in an aggregation.

COMMENT 2: Depending on the animal species, *herd** condition, or housing, the epidemiologic unit can be represented by individuals living separately (e.g., house cats) or by groups of individuals (e.g., herds).

COMMENT 3: In some cases the epidemiologic unit may be obvious, such as domestic animals living in herds separated by space. However, it is more difficult to define the unit for wildlife (mammals, birds) or fish.

COMMENT 4: From an *infectious disease** epidemiology standpoint, a herd is often characterized as a *group** of animals for which the *risk** of *trans-*

*mission** of a pathogen within the group is higher than among animals from other groups.

COMMENT 5: Two groups of animals belonging to the same owner, but without any other link between them, constitute two epidemiologic units (e.g., two herds), whereas two (or many) groups of animals belonging to two (or many) owners, but living together, constitute one epidemiologic unit.

COMMENT 6: When production conditions result in frequent mixing (free-range poultry in a village, groups of animals in nomadic tribes), the entire group of animals should be considered as one epidemiologic unit.

EPIDEMIOLOGIST: A person practicing the science of epidemiology.

See also *epidemiology.*

EPIDEMIOLOGY: Study of the health status of populations.

COMMENT 1: Epidemiology may also be defined in a more restricted way as the *study** of *disease** and its *causes** in a *population.** In either context disease and *health** are used in a broad sense to include not only the traditionally defined *syndromes,** but also a lack of productivity or the presence of abnormal behavior as "disease" syndromes.

COMMENT 2: There are many more specific and elaborate definitions for the term epidemiology. Most authors of veterinary texts have coined their own term, but all are consistent with the above definition.

COMMENT 3: The populations studied in epidemiology can be human, animal, vegetable, or microbial. Indeed, the etymology of the word (epidemia) denotes everything living (human or other "things") in a country or area. In the past there has been a differentiation between the study of health states in people (epidemiology) and the study of health states in animals (the more general term *epizootiology,** or more specific terms such as *epornitic** for diseases of birds and epiichthyology for diseases of fish.). Since the general approaches and methods are very similar, and because of a desire to foster "one medicine" (the definition of *pathology** is not dependent on the species being studied), it is recommended to discontinue use of the term epizootiology. Clearly this positions humans as other animals, but this should be acceptable from a biological perspective.

COMMENT 4: Epidemiology functions as a diagnostic discipline in populations, in a manner similar to pathology (in its broadest diagnostic laboratory sense) and clinical medicine (in *individuals**). The *epidemiologist** aims to identify factors that have an effect on the health status of populations.

COMMENT 5: From a methodological viewpoint, one can distinguish three fundamental activities in epidemiology: *descriptive,** *analytic,** and *experimental.** *Theoretical epidemiology,** including the development and use of models (often computer based), is a more recent area of effort for epidemiologists.

COMMENT 6: The particular characteristics of the general "study methods" of epidemiology make it a valuable tool for the solution of problems ("problem solving"). The practical nature (usually) of the problem studied makes economics a strong ally of epidemiology for the management of health in populations.

EPIDEMIOVIGILANCE: Surveillance program targeted at exotic diseases (diseases that do not occur in the country of interest).

COMMENT: This expression is of French origin. It is not used in English at this time.

See also *epidemiologic surveillance.*

EPIDEMIZATION: Outset of an epidemic disease in a given population, from an endemic disease or from sporadic cases.

EXAMPLE: Human plague can shift from sporadic *cases** or *endemic disease** stage (usually with transmission from rodents to humans by the rat flea) to an *epidemic disease** (with airborne interperson *transmission** during pulmonary plague).

COMMENT 1: The term epidemization (created by Baltazard, a French plague specialist) is only applied to the passage from a "sporadic cases" form or an endemic form to an epidemic form, and not to the beginning of an epidemic resulting from the introduction into a country of a pathogen spreading rapidly in an entirely susceptible *population.**

COMMENT 2: Epidemization happens when some components of the transmission system of a disease (pathogen, *vector,** *host,** *environment**) are modified: appearance of a new antigenic variant (human influenza), introduction of a large number of receptive hosts or vectors in an endemic region (hemorrhagic fevers).

EPIZOOTIC: Epidemic in animals.

COMMENT: While still frequently used, this animal-specific terminology does not add anything biologically meaningful to the concept of *epidemic** (see comment 3, *epidemiology**). Therefore, it is recommended to use the word epidemic instead of epizootic.

See also *epidemic.*

EPIZOOTIC THRESHOLD: Epidemic threshold in an animal context (see definition of epidemic threshold).

COMMENT: The use of *epidemic** is preferred to *epizootic,** even in an animal context.

EPIZOOTIOLOGY: Archaic term used to refer to epidemiology applied to animal populations.

See also *epidemiology.*

EPORNITIC: Term occasionally used in English publications to designate an epidemic in a population of birds.

COMMENT: The term epornitic is still used in the English literature. However, its usage is no longer recommended. The word *epidemic** is proposed as a more universal expression.

EPSEM: See **Equal Probability of Selection Method**

EQUAL PROBABILITY OF SELECTION METHOD (EPSEM): Sampling performed in such a way that all units of a population have the same probability of selection.

COMMENT: A *simple random sample** uses the equal probability of selection method. However, in other sampling designs this method may only hold within *strata** or *clusters.**

EQUITY: See **Net Worth**

ERADICATE: To make (a disease) disappear.

See also *eradication of a disease.*

ERADICATION OF A DISEASE: Total elimination of a disease due to the removal of its cause.

COMMENT 1: To be differentiated from *elimination of a disease.**

COMMENT 2: Necessary conditions to declare disease eradication include elimination of both the clinical *cases** of a disease and of the pathogen, thus making future cases impossible (Latin: *eradicatio* = to uproot).

COMMENT 3: The disappearance of the clinical cases due to a vaccine that leaves *subclinical infections** does not qualify as eradication.

COMMENT 4: In human medicine, an exceptional eradication example based on *prophylaxis** is illustrated by smallpox.

COMMENT 5: The expression "total eradication" is redundant, and the expression "partial eradication" is an oxymoron.

COMMENT 6: Some authors use eradication in a global sense (i.e., disappearance of the *cause** from the planet); others use it to refer to removal of the agent from a country, a group of countries or a continent. There are very few candidate diseases for eradication in a global sense.

ERROR: A false or mistaken result or decision.

EXAMPLES: When taking the temperature of animals included in a *study,** the investigator forgets to reset the thermometer before measuring one of the *individuals.**

Making the wrong *diagnosis** is considered a medical decision error.

Accepting the *null hypothesis** in *statistics** when it is actually false.

COMMENT 1: There are many kinds of errors: misclassification, *measurement errors,** sampling errors (*sampling variation**), hypothesis testing errors, interpretation errors, errors following a decision, etc.

COMMENT 2: An error can be *random,** systematic (*bias**) or both.

COMMENT 3: In statistics, three types of error may be associated with hypothesis testing: *alpha** (of type I), *beta** (of type II), and *gamma** (of type III) (Figure E3).

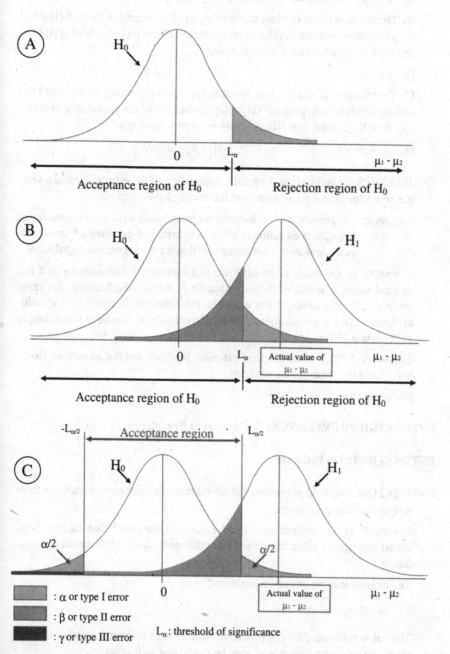

FIGURE E3. Schematic representation of the three types of errors for the comparison of two means μ_1 and μ_2.

A: Distribution of the random variable $(\mu_1 - \mu_2)$ according to the null hypothesis (H_0). Representation of the probability of a type I (α) error for a one-sided test.

$H_0 : \mu_1 - \mu_2 = 0$ Alternative hypothesis $H_1 : \mu_1 - \mu_2 > 0$

B: Distribution of the random variable $(\mu_1 - \mu_2)$ according to the null (H_0) and the alternative hypothesis (H_1). Representation of the probability of type I (α) and type II (β) errors for a one-sided test.

$H_0 : \mu_1 - \mu_2 = 0$ $\qquad\qquad H_1 : \mu_1 - \mu_2 > 0$

C: Distribution of the random variable $(\mu_1 - \mu_2)$ according to the null (H_0) and the alternative hypothesis (H_1). Representation of the probability of type I (α), type II (β), and type III (γ) errors for a two-sided test.

$H_0 : \mu_1 - \mu_2 = 0$ $\qquad\qquad H_1 : \mu_1 - \mu_2 \neq 0$

ESTIMATE: Syn: estimation A specific application of the estimator from a sample characterizing a population, and the result of this exercise.

EXAMPLE: The *proportion** of diseased subjects, based on a *random sample** of animals, is an estimate of the proportion of the *disease** in the animal *population,* * assuming that this is a homogeneous population.

COMMENT 1: Do not confuse estimate and *estimator.** The estimate is a numerical value, whereas while the estimator is the *variable** taking this value given a particular *sample.** For example, the estimator "weight" (of individuals from a given population) may take different values: "estimate 1" for sample 1, "estimate 2" for sample 2, etc.

COMMENT 2: The most frequent estimate methods are the *maximum likelihood** and the least-square methods.

See also *estimator.*

ESTIMATED PREVALENCE: See Apparent Prevalence

ESTIMATION: See Estimate

ESTIMATOR: Function permitting the estimation of an unknown parameter from a sample of the population.

COMMENT 1: The estimator is itself a *random variable** that takes values, called *estimates,* * when calculated from different *samples** of the same *population.* *

The estimator of an unknown *variance** s^2 is:

$$s^2 = \Sigma(x_j - m)^2/(n - 1)$$

The value calculated from a particular sample is an estimate. Another estimator of the unknown variance s^2 may be calculated as follows:

$$s^2 = \Sigma(x_j - m)^2/n$$

but this is of inferior quality compared to the first one.

Note: One should keep in mind that the estimator of the variance s^2 could be biased, meaning that there could be a systematic error as compared to the true value s^2.

COMMENT 2: A parameter may have several estimators (i.e., the variance example above) that do not necessarily have the same statistical characteristics.

COMMENT 3: An estimator should be unbiased and with minimal variance.

ETIOLOGIC FACTOR: See Etiological Factor

ETIOLOGIC FRACTION: See Attributable Fraction

ETIOLOGICAL FACTOR: Syn: aetiological factor, etiologic factor, causal factor

COMMENT: *Causal factor** is more widely used than etiological factor in the veterinary epidemiology literature.

ETIOLOGY: Other spelling: aetiology The study of causes of pathological conditions.

COMMENT: Etiology is often used (mainly in conversation) as synonymous with *cause,** such as in "the etiology of this *disease** is a virus." This practice is not recommended. In written communications, most authors make use of this word as a subheading for the section of articles or book chapters dealing with *causality.**

See also *causality, cause.*

EVALUATION:
1. The act of determining or fixing the value of something.
2. The act of rating, interpreting.

COMMENT: This word may evoke the notion of approximation or relativity, in particular in the following areas:

• Estimation of a quantity without precise measurement.
• Estimation of a price.
• Estimation of the value of a test.
• A judgment.

Epidemiologic *studies,** in particular *intervention studies,** rarely offer the opportunity to measure with *precision** (except for *experimental studies** or certain clinical *trials**). Therefore, the word evaluation is well suited to several activities in *epidemiology.**

EVALUATIVE EPIDEMIOLOGY: Expression used in some francophone countries to designate the domain of epidemiology concerned with the study of methods associated with a health program (or an intervention) and their impact.

This expression is not used in English.

EXAMPLES: Field evaluation of a vaccine; evaluation of a teat dip method for mastitis prevention in dairy cows.

COMMENT 1: The evaluation has for *objectives** to determine the potential *efficacy,* * the true efficacy, or *efficiency** of *methods.* * It requires *intervention studies** [i.e., *experimental studies,* * trials,* * observational (analytical) studies**].

COMMENT 2: It corresponds, in part, to activities in North America regrouped under "program and policy" that evaluate the extent to which public health goals are achieved; determine potential problems and the impact of interventions (including the potential impact of new policies that have not yet been implemented); compare the *costs** and *benefits** of interventions and suggest appropriate changes in the current health policies or functioning programs.

EVALUATIVE STUDY: Epidemiologic study having for objective to evaluate consequences and impacts associated with the implementation of a health program.

COMMENT 1: *Intervention studies** have a priori an explanatory structure (ideally with an experimental or quasi-experimental method) as opposed to evaluative studies which have a more *descriptive approach.* *

COMMENT 2: Evaluative studies can also be used, under certain conditions, in an explanatory perspective, connecting results measured and the intervention implemented. In this case the distinction between the intervention study and the evaluative study comes from the use of observational methods as opposed to experimental or quasi-experimental methods.

COMMENT 3: Evaluative studies are usually performed to provide a basis for decision making associated with the operation of a health program.

EVANS'S POSTULATES: Criteria for causation presented in 1976 by Alfred Evans as a unified concept of causality.

1. *Prevalence** of the *disease** should be significantly higher in those exposed to the putative cause than in controls not so exposed.[a]
2. *Exposure* to the putative cause should be present more commonly in those with the disease than in controls without the disease when all risk factors are held constant.
3. *Incidence** of the disease should be significantly higher in those exposed to the putative cause than in those not so exposed, as shown in prospective studies.
4. *Temporally,* the disease should *follow* exposure to the putative agent with a distribution of incubation periods on a bell shaped curve.
5. A *spectrum* of host responses should follow exposure to the putative agent along a logical biologic gradient from mild to severe.
6. A *measurable host response* following exposure to the putative cause should *regularly appear* in those lacking this before exposure (i.e., antibody, cancer cells) or should *increase* in magnitude if present before exposure; this pattern should not occur in persons so exposed.

7. *Experimental reproduction* of the disease should occur in higher incidence in animals or man appropriately exposed to the putative cause than in those not so exposed; this exposure may be deliberate in volunteers, experimentally induced in the laboratory, or demonstrated in a controlled regulation of natural exposure.
8. *Elimination or modification* of the putative cause or of the vector carrying it should decrease the incidence of the disease (control of polluted water or smoke or removal of the specific agent).
9. *Prevention or modification* of the host's response on exposure to the putative cause should decrease or eliminate the disease (immunization, drug to lower cholesterol, specific lymphocyte transfer factor in cancer).
10. The whole thing should make *biologic and epidemiologic sense.*

*The putative cause may exist in the external environment or in a defect in host response.

(From Evans, A.S. 1976. Causation and disease: the Henle-Koch postulates revisited. Yale J. Biol. Med. 49: 175-195.)

EX-ANTE ANALYSIS: Syn: project appraisal Evaluation of a project's overall merit prior to commencement.

This expression is not used in North America. "Project appraisal" is preferred.

COMMENT 1: Focuses on the expected costs and benefits of a project, and is generally used to assist in making a decision on project funding.

COMMENT 2: As opposed to *ex-post analysis.**

EXISTING CASE: See Prevalent Case

EXOGENOUS FACTOR: See Extrinsic Factor

EXOGENOUS INFECTION: Infection caused by a microorganism that has gained entrance from the environment.

COMMENT: As opposed to *endogenous infection.**

EXOTIC DISEASE: In a broad sense: transmissible disease that is not present in the country or region of interest.

In a more restricted sense (European and North American perspective): serious transmissible disease usually present in tropical areas.

COMMENT 1: In a broad sense, almost all *communicable diseases** could qualify as exotic because one can find an unaffected region or country for any given *disease.** Indeed, the exotic connotation is relative to the country of interest, because each disease is indigenous to countries where it occurs and exotic where it does not.

EXAMPLES: Bovine tuberculosis and brucellosis for Denmark; fox rabies for Britain.

COMMENT 2: In the more restricted sense, the term "exotic" is reserved for diseases that may trigger important *health** problems (for humans, animals, or plants) or serious economic *losses.** Normally, the detection of an exotic disease in a temperate zone would prompt a disease *eradication** program.

EXAMPLES: African horse sickness, yellow fever, other arboviral diseases, rinderpest.

EXPECTATION OF LIFE: See **Life Expectancy**

EXPECTED RETURN: The mean of possible returns weighted by their probability of occurrence.

EXPECTED VALUE OF A VARIABLE: See **Mathematical Expectation**

EXPENDITURE: Accounting statement describing all cash outflows from a business.

COMMENT 1: *Expenses** are often viewed as a subset of expenditures that are tax deductible. However, these two terms are sometimes used interchangeably.

COMMENT 2: The word expenditure is seldom used in economics compared to *cost.**

See also *expense, cost.*

EXPENSE: A cash outflow that is tax deductible.

EXAMPLE: If the interest portion of a loan repayment is tax deductible, then it is considered an expense.

COMMENT 1: While expenditures include all cash outflows, expenses refer to only those that are tax deductible.

COMMENT 2: As principal payments on loans are not tax deductible, they are termed *expenditures,** not expenses.

See also *expenditure.*

EXPERIMENT: Syn: experimental study A study in which the investigator can alter the course of events by manipulating the study factors under controlled conditions, with randomized allocation of the subjects.

EXAMPLE: A vaccine trial performed on a given day, in a laboratory, on a group of animals.

COMMENT 1: An experiment is a logical approach to *hypothesis** testing.

COMMENT 2: An experiment can be laboratory- or field-based (for example, clinical *trial,** community intervention, field trial).

COMMENT 3: Typically, one group of subjects is given an experimental or new treatment (new drug, vaccine, surgery procedure, etc.) and other groups are given either no treatment, a placebo, or the standard treatment. The comparison group is often called the control group or "controls." Groups are composed with respect to initial comparability criteria (*random** allocation of subjects in treatment or control groups) and final *comparability** (environmental and observational conditions rigorously identical). Designs where subjects are not allocated at random are called quasi-experiments.

EXPERIMENTAL EPIDEMIOLOGY: A study of a causal factor or an intervention measure in an experimental setting (all factors are controlled, study of the variation produced by one study factor alone) and using epidemiologic methods.

EXAMPLE: Field trial of a vaccine against fox rabies.

COMMENT 1: Experimental epidemiology can be performed in a laboratory or in the field on a limited *population.** It should always precede the use of an intervention on the whole population.

COMMENT 2: The studied population is always in its usual environment, whereas, in conventional experimentation, environmental conditions are artificial and manipulated according to the situation.

See also *experiment, observational study, study* (Figure S7).

EXPERIMENTAL STUDY: See **Experiment**

EXPLANATORY APPROACH: Method that seeks to relate occurrence of health events to explanatory factors.

EXAMPLE: A *randomized* clinical *trial** is used to explain differences in the distributions of health outcomes between two or more *groups** as a function of one or more explanatory factors.

COMMENT: Note that an explanatory approach is used for virtually all analytical epidemiologic *studies.**

EXPLANATORY VARIABLE: See **Independent Variable**

EXPOSED POPULATION: See **Population Exposed**

EX-POST ANALYSIS: Syn: project evaluation Comparison of a project's performance following its completion with the expected performance prior to its inception.

This expression is not used in North America. "Project evaluation" is preferred.

COMMENT: As opposed to *ex-ante analysis.**

EXTERNALITIES: Costs and benefits accruing to entities outside those directly involved in an investment project under consideration.

EXAMPLE: The consumer's *risk** of drinking antibiotic-tainted milk and the processor's benefit of purchasing milk with lower somatic cell counts are externalities to a dairy farm business where a decision has been made to invest in a mastitis control program.

COMMENT: When the impact is positive, one may refer to the expression "external economy." For example, the professional training undertaken by a firm profits other firms when workers change employment.

When the impact is negative, one may refer to the expression "external diseconomy." For example, the pollution created by a swine farm.

Of course, it is not unusual to observe both positive and negative effects resulting from a single investment or activity (see example above).

See also *benefit, cost, internalities.*

EXTERNALITY: See Externalities

EXTRAPOLATION: Transposition of conclusions based on a set of observations to another population, another situation, or to conditions not yet observed.

EXAMPLE: Utilization of the results of a *study** conducted in another region, or another country, presenting sufficiently similar environmental conditions to estimate a priori the possible value of the *variable(s)** under consideration.

COMMENT 1: Statistical *inference** is a form of extrapolation.

COMMENT 2: The ability to extrapolate results from a study sample to the general *population** is directly linked to the *sampling strategy** used in the study.

EXTRINSIC FACTOR: Syn: exogenous factor, environmental factor Factor that is external to, or not a component of, an individual.

EXAMPLES: Ambient temperature, weather conditions, farm facilities, *herd** management.

COMMENT: As opposed to *intrinsic factor.**

EXTRINSIC INCUBATION: The time interval between the infection of an arthropod vector and the moment when the vector becomes capable of transmitting the infection to a new host.

EXAMPLE: For *Anopheles* mosquitos, the extrinsic incubation period for the transmission of malaria is approximately 10 days.

COMMENT 1: This interval varies with the agent and the vector.

COMMENT 2: The extrinsic incubation in the vector is separate from the intrinsic incubation of the disease in the definitive host.

COMMENT 3: Because the ability of the vector to become infected depends on the size of its (blood) meal and the timing of that meal in relation to the peak bacteremia or viremia, the disease interval is not the sum of the extrinsic and intrinsic incubation periods.

See also *generation time.**

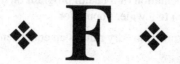

❖ **F** ❖

FACE-TO-FACE INTERVIEW: See **Questionnaire**

FACTORIAL ANALYSIS: See **Contingency Table Analysis**

FALSE NEGATIVE: Unit (individual or herd) classified as diseased by the best available means (i.e., *gold standard**) and classified as nondiseased by a diagnostic or screening test.

EXAMPLE: No metastases are observed on thoracic radiographs (test: negative) but multiple metastatic tumors found in lungs at necropsy (gold standard: positive).

COMMENT: The false negative rate is the proportion of diseased units, as classified by the gold standard, that are classified as not diseased by the diagnostic or screening test.

False negative rate = C/A + C = 1 – *Sensitivity**

Gold Standard

		+	–
Test	+	A	B
	–	C	D

FALSE POSITIVE: Unit (individual or herd) classified as nondiseased by the best available means (i.e., *gold standard**) and classified as diseased by a diagnostic or screening test.

EXAMPLE: Apparent metastases are observed on thoracic radiographs (test: positive) but no metastatic tumors are found in the lungs at necropsy (gold standard: negative).

COMMENT: The false positive rate is the proportion of nondiseased units, as classified by the gold standard, that are classified as diseased by the diagnostic or screening test.

False positive rate = B/B + D = 1 – *Specificity**

Gold Standard

		+	–
Test	+	A	B
	–	C	D

FEASIBILITY STUDY: Preliminary study evaluating the practicability of a procedure or a program and the factors capable of influencing either one.

EXAMPLE: Implementation of a health program on a sample before its generalization to a wider population.

COMMENT: The expression "dry run" is an equivalent, and popular, nonscientific expression.

See also *pilot study.*

FECUNDITY RATE:

$$\frac{\text{Number of individuals born}}{\text{Number of reproductive females in production}} \text{ during a given period of time}$$

COMMENT 1: The numerator: individuals born alive + stillborns = total born. The denominator: all females bred.
Both numerator and denominator should be part of the same production *cohort** (breeding group).

COMMENT 2: This expression, seldom used in North America, has the merit of integrating the notion of prolificacy into a *ratio.**

See also *ratio, rate.*

FINAL HOST: See Definitive Host

FINAL STUDY POPULATION: Fraction of the sample that underwent the application of the expected protocol and on which expected observations were effectively collected.

EXAMPLE: 1760 of the 1892 farms included in the *study population.**

COMMENT: Essentially, this is what is left of the *sampled population** after exclusion of all *cases* that have been rejected or *lost to follow-up** throughout the *study.**

See also *population* (Figure P3).

FINANCIAL HISTORY OF A BUSINESS: See Balance Sheet, Income Statement, Cash Flow Statement

FINANCIAL STATEMENT: A formal accounting statement that includes a balance sheet, income statement, statement of retained earnings, and cash flow statement.

COMMENT: The four statements listed above provide a continual financial history of a business.

See also *balance sheet, income statement, cash flow statement.*

FIRST QUARTILE: In a given series, the value of the variable that is higher than 25% of all values but lower than 75% of them.

EXAMPLE: Weights of newborn piglets from a litter of 12 (in kg):

1.1, 1.4, 1.5, 1.6, 1.6, 1.7, 1.4, 1.9, 1.8, 1.7, 1.5, 1.6

Mean: 1.5667
1st Quartile: 1.425
Median:* 1.6
3rd Quartile:* 1.7

COMMENT 1: The values for the quartiles do not necessarily correspond to values found in the dataset (such as in the example above for the first quartile).

COMMENT 2: The second quartile corresponds to the median.

FISHER'S EXACT TEST: Test of independence based on hypergeometric probability distribution.

COMMENT 1: It is used to test the independence between two dichotomous categorical variables. As for the *chi-square test,* * the observed occurrence of each category of each variable is considered fixed. Under this constraint, the probability corresponding to the observed contingency table is calculated using the hypergeometric formula. The probability of occurrence of all other possible tables under the same constraint is also calculated. Hence, the value of the Fisher test is the sum of each of the probabilities thus calculated that are smaller or equal to the probability of the observed titer. This test value is then interpreted by comparison with a prespecified value such as 0.05.

COMMENT 2: This test is computer intensive. It is normally used only if the observed cell count (in a *contingency table**) is less than 5.

FIXED COSTS: Syn: indirect cost, overhead Costs that are incurred regardless of the level of production or the activity level of an enterprise.

EXAMPLES: Real estate taxes, insurance, and salaried labor are examples of fixed costs.

COMMENT 1: Fixed costs can be divided into cash and noncash costs. *Depreciation** on buildings and equipment is an example of fixed noncash costs.

COMMENT 2: These costs are fixed as long as the size of the enterprise remains stable.

See also *variable costs.*

FOCUS OF DISEASE: See **Nidus**

FOLLOW-UP INVESTIGATION: Syn: follow-up survey Probe of a disease outbreak undertaken to find possible secondary outbreaks.

COMMENT 1: A follow-up investigation occasionally provides the opportunity to identify potentially exposed *populations,* * which may lead to control measures designed to prevent *secondary* or tertiary *outbreaks.* *

See also *traceback* (Figure T2).

FOLLOW-UP SURVEY: See **Follow-Up Investigation**

FOMES: See **Fomite**

FOMITE: Syn: fomes An object or material that is not in itself harmful, but on which pathogens may be conveyed.

EXAMPLES: Bedding, feeding equipment, harness, boots.

See also *vector, indirect transmission, indirect contact.*

FOOD HYGIENE: See Food Safety

FOOD SAFETY: Syn: food hygiene Sector of veterinary public health that focuses on potential hazards that might be present in foods of animal origin.

COMMENT 1: Activities linked to food safety include meat safety procedures and *monitoring** (e.g., *HACCP**), import/export, *animal health,** research and services.

COMMENT 2: The components of a food safety program generally include:

- Prevention of foodborne *diseases** through safety evaluation and surveillance of bacterial, fungal, viral contaminants as well as parasites in foods.
- Safety assessment of food products, components, and manufacturing practices through the evaluation of food additives, nutritional quality, food composition, food processing practices and methods.
- Safety assessment of chemical and environmental contaminants in foods through evaluation and surveillance of agricultural chemical residues, natural and environmental poisons, product processing contaminants, and extraneous materials.

COMMENT 3: In 1996, it was estimated that approximately 1.5 to 5 million people become ill from foodborne diseases every year in the United States. The economic impact of these diseases is estimated at up to 10 billion U.S. dollars annually.

FREE DISTRIBUTION ANALYSIS: See nonparametric analysis

FREQUENCY: Number of occurrences of an event recorded in a population or a sample, during a given time period.

COMMENT 1: Note the difference between absolute frequency (number of events) and *relative frequency** (number of events/population or sample size).

COMMENT 2: When the term "frequency" is used to describe the number of *cases** or *outbreaks** of a *disease,** it may be referring to incident or prevalent events.

COMMENT 3: It is sometimes difficult to determine the number of individuals exposed to a given risk, limiting one's ability to calculate the corresponding *rate.** In order to avoid being limited to comparing numerator information (absolute frequencies), one may elect to calculate an index other than a *proportion.** For example, the number of reported cases of rabies in foxes in a region may be compared to the number of rabies cases in another region by calculating the number of cases per square kilometer for each region. This comparison would be valid if similarities exist between both regions in terms of case reporting scheme and fox *population** density.

FREQUENCY DISTRIBUTION: See **Cumulative Relative Frequency**

FUTURE VALUE: A predicted value based on the current value and the annual growth rate function.

The formula for calculating a future value is: $FV = PV(1 + i)^n$

where FV: future value
PV: present value
i: annual growth rate (decimal fraction)
n: number of years

EXAMPLE: Considering an original investment of $1000.00, the future value of this sum would be $1586.87 after 6 years, given an annual growth rate of 8%.

COMMENT 1: The above function assumes *compound growth.* *

COMMENT 2: This type of estimation is used in *cost–benefit analysis.* *

See also *cumulative relative frequency, cost–benefit, present value.*

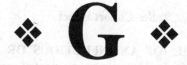

GAMMA ERROR: Syn: type III error Error occurring when concluding that a difference exists, but in the opposite direction to that which is actually correct.

EXAMPLE: To conclude that product "b" gives better results than product "a," whereas the reverse is true.

COMMENT 1: This situation arises because rejection of the *null hypothesis* * can be stated as non null or more specifically as "greater or less than." In all these cases the null hypothesis is rejected, but the consequence of the interpretation of the alternate *hypothesis* * can lead to a gamma error. Thus, the alternate hypothesis must be stated properly and in accordance with the *objectives* * of the *study.* *

COMMENT 2: The gamma risk corresponds to the probability of committing a gamma error.

See also *error* (Figure E3).

GAUSSIAN DISTRIBUTION: See **Normal Distribution**

GEARING: See **Leverage**

GENERAL POPULATION: Syn: **reference population** Exhaustive population for which we want to extrapolate conclusions for an epidemiologic study.

EXAMPLE: All dairy farms in a country (Figure P3, *population**).

COMMENT: The general population can be considered as the *target population** if accessible and not accessible individuals are included.

See also *population, target population* (Figure T1).

GENERATION: Group of individuals born during the same time period (in general, during the same year).

EXAMPLE: All baby foxes born during the spring of 1997 in Fontainebleau forest (France).

COMMENT 1: A generation is a special type of *cohort,** defined by the event "born during the same time period."

COMMENT 2: This word is rarely used in veterinary epidemiology in the context of commercial animal production. For example, although the above definition could apply to all piglets born during the same week in an all-in/all-out farrowing unit, they are usually referred to as a farrowing *group** or batch.

See also *cohort, group.*

GENERATION EFFECT: See **Cohort Effect**

GENERATION TIME (OF AN INFECTIOUS OR CONTAGIOUS DISEASE): The time interval between the moment of contamination of a host by a microorganism and the instant when the host is most contagious or infectious (Figure G1).

EXAMPLE: The generation time for influenza-related *diseases** in different species is normally less than 4 days.

COMMENT 1: This applies to clinical cases as well as to *inapparent infections.**

COMMENT 2: The expression generation time is also commonly used to refer to the time interval between the birth of a parent and the birth of an offspring. For example, bacteria have a relatively short generation time.

See also *latency period, preshedding period, communicable period, period of infectiousness.*

GENETIC EPIDEMIOLOGY: Study of the role and importance of inherited factors (particularly hereditary factors) and their relation with exogenous factors in the occurrence of disease in populations.

EXAMPLE: Segregative analysis used to pinpoint groups of animals (the same family ancestry; the equivalent of family in human genetic epidemiology) with higher *risk** of *disease.**

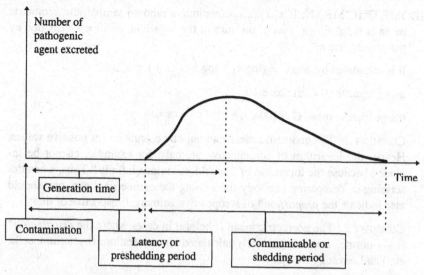

FIGURE G1. Schematic representation of different periods related to contagiosity or infectiousness. This figure does not include recurrent infections.

COMMENT: At the origin of each disease there may be one or more environmental factors (*extrinsic factors**) and/or genetic factors. Depending on the disease, the role of one or the other is more or less important.

GEOGRAPHICAL INFORMATION SYSTEM (GIS): An electronic data system for the collection, analysis, and display of data having a spatial orientation.

COMMENT: Geographical information systems can best be conceived as having three components: an input module, a data management system, and an output module that often contains a cartographic tool.

Input of data can employ several techniques including electronic transfer of standard *databases** such as geological surveys or census data, digitization of existing maps, and capture of remote sensing outputs, which utilize orbiting satellites to picture the earth's surface. Geographical information systems make it possible to overlay multiple layers of data to form a visual and/or statistical picture of geographically referenced data. Symbols of various shapes, sizes, and colors can be used to display patterns and *trends.**

*Data analysis** can consist of simple visual overlays of farms and *disease** status, employ buffers and polygons for pattern recognition, or use spatial statistical packages to assess *risk.**

Output can be in the form of tables, charts, or maps varying in size and detail. Principles of cartography dictate appropriate map construction. A distinction should be drawn between geographical information systems (GISs), which have become sophisticated and powerful in the last decade, and medical geography, which dates back considerably earlier than John Snow's cholera maps of London during the mid-19th century.

GEOMETRIC MEAN: If $x_1, x_2, ..., x_n$ constitute a random sample, the geometric mean is the antilogarithm of the sum of the logarithm of all n x's divided by the sample size n.

It is calculated by: $\log G = (\log x_1 + \log x_2 + ... + \log x_n)/n$

using logarithms to the base 10,

the geometric mean $G = 10^{(\log x_1 + \log x_2 + ... + \log x_n)/n}$

COMMENT 1: The geometric mean can only be calculated for positive values. Hence, the logarithm of seronegative animals, for example, cannot be included because the logarithm of 0 would be "minus infinity." Thus, when describing or comparing antibody titers using the geometric mean, one should also indicate the *proportion** of seropositive animals, irrespective of titers.

COMMENT 2: The geometric mean is helpful in cases where the *distribution** is log-normal. It is thus generally calculated for numerations (bacterium, cells, etc.) and serology results.

COMMENT 3: The geometric mean of a log-normal *variable** corresponds to the *median.**

GOLD STANDARD: Refers to the means by which one can assess whether a disease, or any other event of interest, is truly present or not.

EXAMPLES: Under experimental conditions: The experimental *infection** of animals with a bacterium followed by a microbiological culture to confirm the presence of the infection.

Under field conditions: The post-mortem determination of pneumonic lesions in pigs at the abattoir as a gold standard for the evaluation of thoracic radiography on live pigs just prior to slaughter.

COMMENT 1: The function of gold standards is to act as a quality-control device to assess, for example, the *sensitivity** and the *specificity** of a diagnostic test.

COMMENT 2: While a simple microbiological culture or blood smear may be sufficient to confirm the presence of infection, it is often not enough to confirm its absence. Hence, even with more elaborate and expensive tests, which come with their own inherent *accuracy,** it is often difficult to have access to an appropriate gold standard.

GRADIENT OF INFECTION: Different degrees of response of a host to an infection, ranging from subclinical infection to fatal illness.

COMMENT: Depending on the *disease,** the gradient of infection can be narrow, all infected subjects being affected in a similar way (for example, rabies), or wide, ranging from inapparent *infection** to death (for example, equine infectious anemia).

GROSS MARGIN: Difference between gross income and variable costs.

COMMENT 1: Gross margin analysis is a practical method for assessing enterprise productivity, and is widely used in farm management economics.

COMMENT 2: Also known as "profit before fixed costs."

GROUP: Set of individuals with some common characteristic(s).

COMMENT: Differences between *individuals** of a same group correspond to the *intragroup variation.**

GROWTH RATE: In animal production: Rate of increase in body weight per unit of time.

COMMENT 1: The growth rate is often expressed as an average daily gain. It is a valuable outcome in epidemiologic studies related to animal production, in particular in clinical *trials.**

COMMENT 2: This expression is also frequently used in microbiology (growth of microorganisms) and in economics (see below).

In economics: $\dfrac{\text{Growth during a given time period}}{\text{Value at the beginning of the period}}$

COMMENT 3: The growth rate can be simple (*simple growth**) or compound (*compound growth**).

COMMENT 4: The period often used to calculate growth rates is 1 year (annual growth rate).

COMMENT 5: The growth rate (or *rate** of increase) may be obtained if *present values** (PV) and *future values** (FV) as well as the period are known.

$$i = \sqrt[n]{(FV / PV)} - 1$$

where i is the annual growth rate (decimal fraction), and n is the number of years.

See also *present value, future value, rate.*

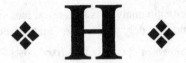

H

H_0: See **NULL HYPOTHESIS**

H_1: See **ALTERNATIVE HYPOTHESIS**

H_A: See **ALTERNATIVE HYPOTHESIS**

HACCP: See **Hazard Analysis and Critical Control Point**

HAPHAZARD SAMPLE: Syn: convenience sample, empirical sample, non-random sample A sample drawn without consideration of representativeness of the source population of sampled units.

EXAMPLE: Selection of the first 10 animals captured in a *herd.**

COMMENT 1: Haphazard samples are drawn principally for matters of convenience, namely, when more-valid and more-structured methods of sampling are not possible. The trade-off for convenience is the potential nonrepresentativeness of the sample (*bias**), which in turn impedes the generalization of the study results.

COMMENT 2: A haphazard or convenience sample differs from *random** and *systematic samples.** Contrary to the former, a method of randomization is used to select all units in random sampling, as well as the first unit in systematic sampling (all other units are obtained by selecting every *n*th unit starting from the first randomly chosen unit).

HAZARD: Any biological, chemical, or physical agent that could have a negative impact on health.

See also *risk analysis.*

HAZARD ANALYSIS and CRITICAL CONTROL POINT (HACCP): The evaluation of all procedures during the production, processing, distribution, and use of raw materials or food products; a hazard detected during this process may be eliminated at specific key junctures referred to as critical control points.

EXAMPLE: A HACCP approach is used in the poultry industry in order to reduce bacterial cross-contamination of carcasses at slaughterhouses. The following six critical control points have been identified: (1) holding area; (2) scalding; (3) defeathering; (4) washing; (5) eviscerating; and (6) chilling.

COMMENT 1: HACCP can be implemented in areas other than *food safety.* *

COMMENT 2: HACCP is based on seven guiding principles:

1. The conducting of hazard analysis. This includes the preparation of a list of steps to identify hazards and the description of preventive measures.
2. The identification of critical control points (CCPs).
3. The establishment of critical limits for preventive measures associated with each CCP.
4. The establishment of *monitoring* * requirements, including procedures for using the results of monitoring to adjust the HACCP process and maintain control.
5. The establishment of corrective actions to be taken when monitoring flags a deviation from a critical limit.
6. The establishment of an effective record-keeping system to document HACCP.
7. The establishment of procedures designed to verify the ongoing validity of the HACCP program being implemented.

HAZARD RATE: See **Instantaneous Incidence**

HEALTH: The World Health Organization describes health as "a state of complete physical, mental, and social well-being and not merely the absence of disease or infirmity."

Health has also been defined as the dynamic balance between a host and its environment.

COMMENT 1: The second definition offers a continuum between the ideal state of well-being and *disease.* * In this regard, optimal health in veterinary medicine is often associated with the optimization of an individual's genetic potential. This view has been criticized in North America for being more a characteristic of performance (productivity) than health per se.

COMMENT 2: In the context of animal production, one may add that the environment should be free of hazards to the producer or the consumer. The concept of financial profitability is also important in the context of farm health.

COMMENT 3: A major role for the *epidemiologist* * is the identification and description of the circumstances and factors leading to an imbalance in the relationship between host and environment.

HEALTH FACTOR: Factor having a beneficial or detrimental health effect, and statistically identified as such based on experimental or observational studies.

EXAMPLES: A balanced diet has been shown to be a beneficial health factor. Overcrowding has been shown to be a detrimental health factor.

HEALTH INDICATOR: Variable depicting a component of the health status of a population.

EXAMPLES: Calving rate; veterinary expenses by cow per year; morbidity rate; attack rate.

COMMENT: An indicator tends to measure or represent a specific *occurrence** or *characteristic** of an individual or group (pen, herd, flock, etc.). An index can be created from several indicators to provide a global assessment of the health status of these individuals or groups.

See also *indicator, index.*

HEALTH MANAGEMENT: Syn: planned animal health and production services The action of implementing a strategy or set of measures designed to sustain or improve health in animal-based operations.

EXAMPLE: Regular follow-up of swine farrowing units by a veterinarian using a *recording** system such as PigCHAMP or PigTale, and implementation of measures designed to reach certain production target values.

COMMENT 1: As indicated in the example above, improving production and the economic efficiency of a farm is an integral part of herd health management in food animal-producing operations. Some authors may refer to production medicine as the medicine focusing on the economic well-being of the farm.

COMMENT 2: In companion animals, health programs are, in principle, similar to the ones in animal production (comment 3), with emphasis on well-being, disease-free status, and, in some cases, performance.

COMMENT 3: Components of a herd health management program include: regular farm visits by a veterinarian, constant *monitoring** of production performance, *biosecurity** procedures to minimize the *risk** of *disease** outbreaks,* attention to animal well-being and environmental concerns, and an awareness of product quality.

COMMENT 4: Health managers require knowledge of veterinary medicine (*etiology,* pathogenesis,* diagnosis,** and treatment of diseases), animal behavior, nutrition, animal management and production, housing, *epidemiology** and economics. The necessity of having a working knowledge of these disciplines is clearly illustrated in Figure H1.

COMMENT 5: The successful implementation of any health management program depends on the participation of the owner or manager of the animal population. Therefore, health managers require strong people skills.

COMMENT 6: Although health management principles apply across species, due to the knowledge required in several disciplines as well as in the animal industry per se, health managers are almost by necessity species oriented.

HEALTH PHENOMENON: A phenomenon linked to the health of an organism or a population.

COMMENT: It is necessary to differentiate "health phenomenon" from *health factor.** A health factor has an impact on the state of *health** (favorable or unfavorable), while a health phenomenon indicates a state of health.

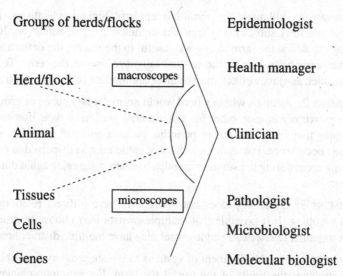

Groups of herds/flocks	Epidemiologist
Herd/flock macroscopes	Health manager
Animal	Clinician
Tissues microscopes	Pathologist
Cells	Microbiologist
Genes	Molecular biologist

FIGURE H1. Position of health professionals depending on the level of biological organization. The dashed lines represent the extent of the vision of clinicians focusing on individual animals. Because the health manager goes beyond individuals and needs to fully appreciate events at the population level, recording systems and data management are required (macroscopes).

HEALTHY CARRIER: Syn: asymptomatic carrier Carrier of a specific infectious agent who does not exhibit any clinical signs associated with the disease throughout the duration of the infection.

EXAMPLES: Birds and rodents harboring arboviruses.

Mary Mallon, nicknamed "Typhoid Mary," who was a carrier of typhoid, was employed as a cook for eight different families in the United States. Although never affected by the disease herself, she was associated with over 200 cases of typhoid before she was identified as a healthy carrier and forced to retire.

See also *carrier* (Figure C1).

HERD: A relatively stable collection of animals, usually a single species, living as a group, more or less closely associated with each other.

EXAMPLES:

1. A group of zebra that graze and travel together.
2. A cattle feedlot that collects animals from multiple sources, then houses and feeds them on one defined location for an extended period of time.
3. A grouping of pigs that are on one farm/location for an extended period of time.
4. A collection of sheep that, while owned by multiple persons in the village, are commonly allowed to intermingle. They may be periodically separated from the village.

COMMENT 1: Although the term has epidemiologic implications, its use should not stray substantially from the common English definition. It is not enough to define the term in any way useful to the reader; the definition must remain essentially true to the normal language use of the term. Technical terms, such as cluster effect, may be more appropriate for certain applications.

COMMENT 2: Animals within a herd would normally be housed or grouped in close proximity to each other for a substantial portion of their lifetime. This grouping may be continuous or periodic. Periodic *groups** should be regular in their occurrence. For example, a herd of cattle may be dispersed to multiple grazing areas during the summer months, but then congregate again during the winter.

COMMENT 3: Ownership does not necessarily have a direct relationship to herd grouping. It is possible that multiple owners may choose to group animals together. Likewise, a single owner may have multiple distinct herds.

COMMENT 4: The development of systems to isolate progeny from their parents stretches the limits of the use of the term. For example, chicken production commonly occurs with birds that are closely grouped for egg production, with hatching occurring in another location, and the chicks being dispersed to separate locations without ever being congregated again. One would normally recognize each group of birds found at these separate locations as a flock (word equivalent to herd when referring to birds or sheep). The advent of segregated early weaning in swine with multisite production is a comparable example. The term "herd" or "flock" may be useful in such settings when a pool of caregiving personnel are allowed access to a grouping of animals on a regular and frequent basis. This grouping may be based on physical proximity, or based on functional proximity, such as along a roadway or waterway. In many cases it may be preferable to avoid the term altogether, in favor of descriptive terms or expressions such as "group" or "production system."

COMMENT 5: Shared risk for disease does not, by itself, constitute the necessary conditions for a group to be called a "herd." For example, farms in close proximity to one another may be at increased risk of disease transmission. This does not constitute a herd effect, however, if the animals are kept at distinct locations.

COMMENT 6: The grouping should remain intact and relatively stable for a substantial portion of either the animals' lifetimes or of a calendar year, whichever is shorter.

COMMENT 7: The use of the expression herd effect should be limited to those effects that depend on stable groupings of animals in relatively close proximity over a sustained time period.

HERD HEALTH MANAGEMENT PROGRAM: See Health Management

HERD HEALTH PROGRAM: See Health Management

HERD IMMUNITY: The ability of a group of animals generally of the same species to resist becoming infected or to minimize the extent of infection and/or disease in terms of severity and incidence.

EXAMPLES: Herd immunity resulting from a vaccination program (e.g., foot-and-mouth disease vaccine in cattle; oral vaccination of foxes against rabies); the feeding of intestinal tissues and content of piglets that died of transmissible gastroenteritis to sows in an attempt to limit the extent of an epidemic; feeding of the same material to gilts and any other incoming reproductive males and females in order to maintain the immune status of the herd and prevent disease.

COMMENT 1: This protection corresponds to a considerable reduction in the probability of any susceptible members of the *herd** of coming in contact with the pathogen because of the reduction, or even the suppression, of the transmission of the *infectious** agent within the herd.

COMMENT 2: The scenario presented in comment 1 often results from the high prevalence of immune individuals within the herd. This prevalence is generally dependent on the *infectiousness** of the agent, the period of communicability, the degree of *population** mixing and herd density. It is possible for a disease to disappear even if the herd or population is not 100% immune (for example, smallpox in humans).

HERD SAMPLE: Sample in which the sampled unit is a herd, irrespective of the size of a herd.

EXAMPLE: In a given county, sampling herds belonging to 10 producers regardless of the composition and size of these 10 *herds.**

COMMENT: The *sample** should be distinguished from a *cluster sample** in which the *sample unit** may be a subpopulation within a herd.

HERD SENSITIVITY: See **Sensitivity**

HEREDITARY DISEASE: Disease transmitted to descendants by the reproductive cell.

EXAMPLE: Hemophilia.

See also *congenital disease, vertical transmission.*

HETEROSCEDASTICITY: This condition reflects the inequality of variance among sampled groups.

COMMENT: It is the converse of the homogeneity of *variance.**

HIERARCHICAL CLASSIFICATION: Method of automatic classification, aiming to group individuals in a certain number of classes in such a way that the classes are both the most homogeneous and the most different from each other.

COMMENT 1: The hierarchical classification starts with the individuals and groups them according to their similarities.

COMMENT 2: Other types of classification proceed the other way around, starting with the whole *group** and then dividing them into different subsets according to their differences.

COMMENT 3: Classification generally follows a *contingency table analysis.** The joint utilization of these two *methods** allows one to judge the real state of nature (*distribution** of individuals in factorial plans) and their relative positions. Using an explanatory approach, the *classification** completes and enhances the results from a preliminary contingency table analysis.

See also *classification, multifactorial analysis, contingency table analysis.*

HIGHLY PATHOGENIC AGENT: Microorganism whose pathogenicity is expressed in the vast majority of contaminated individuals.

EXAMPLES: Rabies virus.
Many H5 and H7 influenza viruses in chickens.

COMMENT: In contrast with *opportunistic agent.**

HILL'S POSTULATES: Fundamental elements of causation proposed by Hill in 1965, which pertain well to epidemiology.

Considering a cause A and an outcome B:

1. Temporality: A precedes B.
2. The strength of the statistical association: A and B are highly correlated.
3. Confirmation by randomized experiments: The conditions of observation exclude biases, including confounding.
4. Specificity and consistency: One must reach the same conclusions when results are obtained for different specimens.
5. Biological gradient (dose-responsiveness): An increased dose of A results in an increase in B in terms of severity.
6. Coherence: The findings are biologically plausible based on the current status of knowledge.

See also *Evans's Postulates.*

HISTOGRAM: Graphic presentation, in the form of rectangles, of the frequency of values taken by a continuous variable grouped in classes.

EXAMPLE: See Figures B3 and B4 (*bimodal distribution**).

COMMENT 1: Class intervals are shown on the x-axis and the relative or absolute frequency on the y-axis. Each rectangle surface has to be proportional to the observed size of the *class.** In the case of classes with equal amplitude, the height of each rectangle is proportional to the class size.

COMMENT 2: To be differentiated from the *bar diagram,** which is used with qualitative *variables** and whose rectangles are always separated.

HISTORICAL DATA: Data collected in the past and available for epidemiologic investigations.

EXAMPLE: Production data collected on a farm over the past 5 years and used as part of a nonconcurrent *cohort study.* *

HORIZONTAL TRANSMISSION: Transmission of a pathogen from an individual hosting the agent to another individual, independent of the parental relationship of those individuals.

COMMENT 1: Horizontal transmission excludes transmission inside the female's body (by *infection* * of the gametes, embryo, or fetus), which is defined as *vertical transmission.* * However, horizontal transmission does include venereal transmission, which corresponds to contamination of an individual by another (in general from one of different sex) during sexual activities.

COMMENT 2: Some pathogens can be transmitted in a vertical or horizontal manner, depending on the circumstances. Thus, the virus of mucosal disease (bovine viral diarrhea) can be transmitted horizontally from an animal that is permanently infected and immunotolerant, and can also be transmitted vertically by a cow that is infected during gestation, to its fetus.

HOSPITAL CONTROL: Control selected from a list of patients from a hospital or clinic.

EXAMPLE: *Case–control study* * on skin cancer in dogs. Controls were selected from a list of dogs that were hospitalized at the same veterinary hospital and during the same period of time as the *cases.* * Only dogs with a previous history of cancer or tumors were not considered for the selection of the *control group.* *

HOST: Organism (usually multicellular) that lodges and maintains in natural conditions a pathogen.

EXAMPLES: Vertebrates and rabies virus; ruminants and *Brucella*; dogs and *Toxocara canis.*

COMMENT 1: In a host, *infectious agents* * multiply or find conditions favorable for their survival. Parasitic agents are maintained, develop, and, in some cases, replicate.

COMMENT 2: The nature of the association between a host and another organism can range from one of *symbiosis* (beneficial for the host) through commensalism (neutral for the host) to parasitism (detrimental to the host).

See also *commensal, symbiont.*

HOST DETERMINANT: See **Characteristic**

HOST FACTOR: See **Characteristic**

HYPERENDEMIC: Characteristic of an endemic disease affecting a large number of individuals.

EXAMPLE: Rabies in the Canadian fox population in 1996.

COMMENT: As opposed to hypoendemic.

See also *endemic, hypoendemic.*

HYPOENDEMIC: Characteristic of an endemic disease affecting a small number of individuals.

EXAMPLE: Human tuberculosis in developed countries.

COMMENT 1: As opposed to hyperendemic.

COMMENT 2: The limit between a hypoendemic disease and a sporadic disease can sometimes be difficult to establish.

See also *endemic, hyperendemic, sporadic disease.*

HYPOTHESIS: A proposition on one or more related events of interest, arrived at from observation or reflection, and that must be formally tested using a scientific approach before it can be accepted or rejected.

EXAMPLES: Flies are a *vector** in the *transmission** of coronaviruses in swine and turkeys.

Squamous cell carcinoma in cats is caused by ultraviolet radiation.

COMMENT 1: The purpose of most hypotheses is to articulate one's understanding of a given situation. Therefore, it is *explanatory* in nature. It may also be essentially descriptive if the hypothesis is limited, for example, to a supposition about the *prevalence** of a *disease.**

COMMENT 2: The hypothesis is a key component of the scientific method. It is the junction between the *induction** and the *deduction** processes. It is said to be conceptual or operational. These two adjectives are meant to emphasize the distinction between the idea (conceptual hypothesis) and the proposition that can be formally tested (operational hypothesis). For example, the hypothesis listed above linking ultraviolet radiation to squamous cell carcinoma is a conceptual hypothesis. The operational hypothesis could be that the incidence of the disease is higher in white cats living outdoors (exposed to sunlight) than in white cats kept indoors. Several operational hypotheses could be derived from one conceptual hypothesis.

See also *null hypothesis, deduction, induction.*

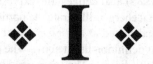

IATROGENIC DISEASE: Disease resulting from the professional activity of health personnel (Greek, *iatros* = physician) (Figure I1).

EXAMPLE: Abscess provoked by an injection.

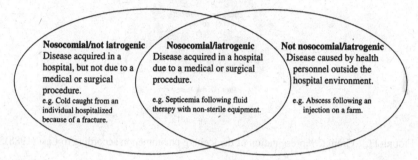

Nosocomial/not iatrogenic
Disease acquired in a hospital, but not due to a medical or surgical procedure.
e.g. Cold caught from an individual hospitalized because of a fracture.

Nosocomial/iatrogenic
Disease acquired in a hospital due to a medical or surgical procedure.
e.g. Septicemia following fluid therapy with non-sterile equipment.

Not nosocomial/iatrogenic
Disease caused by health personnel outside the hospital environment.
e.g. Abscess following an injection on a farm.

FIGURE I1. Schematic representation of the relationship between nosocomial and iatrogenic diseases.

See also *nosocomial*.

ICEBERG PHENOMENON: Analogy with the submerged part of an iceberg to illustrate the portion of a disease that remains clinically inapparent (Figure I2).

COMMENT 1: The submerged portion of the 'iceberg' varies depending on the *disease*.* For example, it can be as little as less than 1% (e.g., rabies) or as much as over 99% (e.g., bovine viral leukosis).

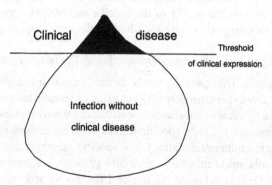

Clinical disease

Threshold of clinical expression

Infection without clinical disease

FIGURE I2. Schematic representation of the iceberg phenomenon.

COMMENT 2: Last (1988) also defines this expression as an analogy with the submerged part of an iceberg to illustrate the portion of a disease that remains unrecorded and/or undetected at any given point in time. This is a different concept from the first definition listed above. The tip of the iceberg represents confirmed *cases** of the disease. The submerged portion comprises cases that have not been accurately diagnosed, whether they are medically attended or not, as well as diagnosed cases that go unreported (Figure I3).

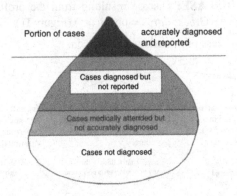

FIGURE I3.   Graphic representation of the iceberg phenomenon according to Last (1988).

ILLNESS: See **Disease**

IMMUNE: Individual possessing a state of immunity to or protection from a pathogen.

COMMENT 1: Generally, subjects immune to a pathogen reflect the total number of vaccinated subjects, the number of subjects that were sick, and those that had a *subclinical infection** but acquired protection/*immunity** after exposure to the pathogen.

COMMENT 2: At the *population** and individual level, one cannot always assume that vaccinated individuals are immune. Indeed, the immune status is dependent on the quality of the vaccine and of the vaccination procedure. A good vaccine poorly delivered often results in inadequate protection.

IMMUNITY: State of resistance/protective ability of an organism to a pathogen.

COMMENT: The immunity can be innate (natural or nonspecific host defenses) or acquired spontaneously (via induction of specific host defenses) after an infection (clinical or subclinical) or artificially through human intervention (e.g., vaccination). It can be specific (directed toward a given agent) or nonspecific (general immunostimulation). The specific immunity can be active (vaccination, subclinical infection) or passive (through maternal antibodies or serum transfer). It is achieved via humoral (antibody) and cellular (T-lymphocyte) pathways.

IMMUNIZATION: Process that confers immunity.

COMMENT: Immunization can be active (via vaccination) or passive (via maternal antibodies or transfer of serum). Active immunization involves exposing an individual to a pathogen, rendered innocuous in some way, that results in establishing a state of protection or *immunity* * by activating the immune system.

IMMUNOASSAY: A laboratory procedure used in the identification of an infectious agent or to quantify a substance by using a specific antibody.

EXAMPLES: Enzyme-linked immunosorbent assay (ELISA); gel agglutination; immunofluorescent techniques; precipitation; radioimmunoassay, etc.

COMMENT: Technical advances in immunoassays over the past two decades have greatly contributed to the development of *sero-epidemiology.* *

IMPORTED CASE: Case of disease contracted in a country other than the one where it is observed.

EXAMPLE: Dog with clinical signs of rabies in Paris, France, on its return from a trip to Morocco where it contracted the *disease.* *

COMMENT: As opposed to *indigenous case.* * The concept of importation refers to the movement of goods (or in this case, disease) from one country to another. In large countries such as the United States, Russia, China, Canada, or Brazil, some authors may use the expression "imported case" when referring to cases transported from an infected to a disease-free region within the same country. For example, some states of the United States are considered free of pseudorabies (Aujeszky's disease). Any case occurring in these states would be considered imported. Alternatively, one could say that the disease has been "introduced" or "reintroduced" into this region.

INAPPARENT DISEASE: Condition that is never observed clinically.

EXAMPLE: Subclinical mastitis.

INAPPARENT INFECTION: Syn: silent infection Infection that does not produce detectable clinical signs or performance losses.

COMMENT 1: Many infections remain inapparent (see *iceberg phenomenon**). Although some authors equate inapparent to *subclinical,* * the above definition proposes to limit the expression "inapparent infection" to infections where no applied evidence (signs, altered performance parameters) exists.

COMMENT 2: Some inapparent infections may not even be detectable via direct or indirect tests. In most cases, this is probably the result of current technical limitations.

See also *subclinical infection, latent infection.*

INCIDENCE: The number of new health events (infection, disease, etc.) experienced by a given population over a specified period of time.

EXAMPLE: In 1996, the annual incidence of brucellosis-infected herds in France was approximately 300.

COMMENT 1: It is necessary to differentiate incidence (new cases) from *prevalence** (all existing cases) (Figure P9, prevalence). Both expressions may be used in reference to a specific period of time (a week, a month, a year, etc.).

COMMENT 2: Incidence is sometimes inappropriately used interchangeably with *incidence rate** and incidence proportion. Incidence is in units (e.g., cows, pens, herds); incidence rate is the number of new cases or *outbreaks** per unit of time and is in units of 1/time; incidence proportion is the proportion of a *population at risk** that becomes affected in a given period of time and is unitless.

COMMENT 3: Incidence may also be used when referring to *subclinical** cases identified via a *screening** procedure.

See also *incidence rate*.

INCIDENCE DENSITY: See **Instantaneous Incidence**

INCIDENCE DENSITY RATE: See **Incidence Rate**

INCIDENCE DENSITY RATIO: See **Relative Rate**

INCIDENCE RATE: Syn: **incidence density rate**

$$\frac{\text{Number of new events (infection, disease, etc.) occurring}}{\text{Number of individual (or herd)} - \text{time at risk}} \text{ during a given period}$$

The denominator represents the sum of the time at risk of all individuals (or groups/herds/flocks, depending on the unit of interest) during the observation period.

EXAMPLE: The incidence rate of cattle *herds** *infected** with brucellosis in France for the year 1996 was 0.04 per 100 herd-years.

COMMENT 1: This *rate** does not only apply to clinically expressed *diseases.**

COMMENT 2: In practice, the denominator is often obtained by calculating the average *population at risk** during the period of interest:

(number of individuals/herds at risk at the beginning of the observation + number at the end of the observation) × 0.5.

COMMENT 3: When a *study** is conducted over a long period of time (a year or more, for example), an *individual** may be affected by the same disease more than once. In some cases, the investigators may elect to limit the period of observation in such a way as to avoid this situation, or they may consider that an individual is no longer at risk of becoming diseased once it has been diagnosed with it. For example, a cow may be afflicted with mastitis more than once in a given year. The yearly incidence rate of cows with mastitis could be calculated by dividing the number of cows that had mastitis at least once during the year (one case) over the total number of cows at risk in the population during that year. Of course, this would only give an estimate of the true incidence rate. For more *accuracy*,* one would have to calculate the *animal-time** at *risk** (see *rate**).

This situation also offers the opportunity to calculate the incidence rate of occurrences of mastitis. The yearly incidence rate of mastitis would then be calculated by dividing the number of mastitis cases (a cow affected with mastitis twice during the observation period counting for two) observed during the year over the number of cows present in the population at risk. This *proportion** is not a true rate.

See also *incidence, rate.*

INCIDENCE RATE RATIO: See **Relative Rate**

INCIDENTAL RESERVOIR: Animate or inanimate object serving as reservoir for a given pathogen because of fortuitous circumstances, and generally without prevailing in this role.

> EXAMPLE: Clothing *contaminated** with smallpox virus and stocked by the army for 15 years before being marketed as surplus.

See also *reservoir.*

INCIDENT CASE: Syn: new case New case of a disease occurring during a given period.

> COMMENT: As compared to *prevalent case.* *

> EXAMPLE: Of 120 healthy cats included in a prospective study at the beginning of 1994, 23 developed a housesoiling behavior problem during that year.

See also *incidence, prevalence.*

INCLUSION CRITERIA: See **Eligibility Criteria**

INCOME: Cash inflows that are considered taxable.

> COMMENT: While *revenue** refers to all cash inflows, income refers only to those items that are considered taxable.

INCOME STATEMENT: A financial report of revenues, expenses, and net income (or loss) for a specific period of time.

> COMMENT: An income statement may be prepared on a *cash basis** or *accrual basis** method of *accounting.* *

See also *revenue, expenses.*

INCUBATION PERIOD: See **Disease Cycle**

INCUBATORY CARRIER: Carrier shedding the pathogen before the appearance of the first clinical signs.

> EXAMPLE: A dog shedding the virus at the end of the incubation period for rabies.

INDEPENDENT VARIABLE: Syn: explanatory variable, predictor Variable measured and hypothesized to explain one or more outcomes of interest (dependent variables) in the context of a given study.

EXAMPLES: Variation in the fox population density explains some of the variation in the incidence of rabies.

Ambient temperature variation (independent variable) is associated with an increase in preweaning diarrhea in pigs (*dependent variable**).

COMMENT: The *association** between an independent variable and a dependent variable does not necessarily imply *causality.**

See also *dependent variable.*

INDEX: Plural: indices A quantitative representation of the health status of a population, usually by constructing a composite of one or more scores.

Simple index: A ratio of two measurements taken from either one population at different times or two *populations** at identical times, used to show a proportionate change.

EXAMPLE: $I = G1/G0 \times 100$ where $G1$ = the quantity at time 1 and $G0$ = the quantity at time 0.

Complex index: A composite weighted measure of several elementary indices that together provide a more complete synopsis of *health** status or of any other situation.

EXAMPLES: Index of cleanliness in dairy cows developed by I.N.R.A. (Institut National de Recherche Agronomique; a French institution performing agriculture-related research). This index is based on a "score of cleanliness" given for each of a series of defined areas on the surface of the body of a cow.

Crude index: Index calculated on a population without adjustment to take into account any of the characteristics of this population or of its environment.

EXAMPLE: Crude morbidity rate.

COMMENT: A crude index can be modified by *standardization** or *adjustment** to take into account characteristics such as age and race.

See also *indicator.*

INDEX CASE: First case reported that calls attention to the existence of an outbreak.

COMMENT: The index case is not necessarily the *primary case,** which corresponds to the actual first case that has occurred (and that may not have been reported first). This applies to new and well-known conditions. When confronted with what is believed to be a new *disease,** it is not unusual to discover, once diagnostic tests become available, that evidence exists that the disease, or at least its *agent,** was present for some time prior to the first reported case. The evidence could be serologic, histopathologic, genetic, clinical, etc. Porcine pleuropneumonia and acquired immunodeficiency syndrome (AIDS) are two examples where serologic testing of serum banks supports the assertion that the *infectious** agents associated with these diseases (and potentially cases) were present years before these conditions became recognized.

See also *primary case.*

INDEX OF CONCORDANCE: Proportion of agreement between a diagnostic test and a gold standard.

Diagnostic method	Number of diseased individuals	Number of nondiseased individuals
Positive response	a	b
Negative response	c	d

Index of concordance = (a + d) / (a + b + c + d)

COMMENT 1: The ideal index of concordance would represent the *proportion** of *individuals** (or *herds,** flocks, etc.) correctly identified as diseased and nondiseased (or *infected** and noninfected) by a diagnostic test. However, in reality, the true status of individuals or herds may not be known. This is why, in practice, this index is used to quantify the degree of agreement between an established test or *gold standard** and another diagnostic test.

EXAMPLE: The index of concordance for a tube agglutination test, developed in 1983 to determine the infection status of pigs to *Actinobacillus pleuropneumoniae,* was 0.77 or 77%, based on a comparison with the complement fixation test, which was the *gold standard** at that time.

COMMENT 2: The index of concordance can be calculated under various circumstances. For example, it can be used to compare the clinical diagnoses of two clinicians who have examined the same individuals (e.g., two people examining the same group of cows for clinical mastitis). It may also be used to compare results obtained using the same test on the same individuals but at two different times (e.g., the index of concordance for *A. pleuropneumoniae* serological results obtained using a tube agglutination test at 3 days and at 8 weeks of age on the same pigs was 52%).

COMMENT 3: Some authors use the expressions "test *efficiency"** or "degree of agreement" as equivalent to index of concordance.

COMMENT 4: Do not confuse this index with the *kappa statistic,** which measures the degree of agreement beyond chance.

See also *kappa statistic.*

INDICATOR: Descriptive measure, quantitative or not, depicting a specific aspect of a system.

EXAMPLES: *Incidence** and *prevalence rates.**

COMMENT: To be differentiated from complex indices, which are always quantitative and aimed at describing the entirety of a system. Indeed, while an indicator is a measure of a specific event or characteristic of a system (i.e., herd, organization), an *index** is designed to achieve a global perspective, which could be accomplished by pulling several indicators together.

See also *index*.

INDICATOR VARIABLE: A variable used in regression analysis to indicate which of two possible levels of a variable an individual belongs to.

COMMENT: This is a quantitative variable that identifies (or indicates) the *classes** of a qualitative variable. More than one indicator variable can be used together, when a *variable** has more than two categories, to indicate what category an *individual** belongs to. In general, when a variable has k levels, the number of indicator variables required is k – 1.

EXAMPLE 1: An indicator variable can take on 0 or 1 to indicate the presence or absence of a covariate.

EXAMPLE 2: For a covariate that has three distinct levels, two indicator variables are necessary and sufficient to describe an individual's *classification*.* In a *study** on dermatofibrosarcoma in dogs, each animal included in the study was classified using the *qualitative variable** "breed type" (hounds, gun dogs, terriers, non-sporting dogs, working dogs, draft animals, and toy breeds). For analytical purposes, an indicator variable, also referred to as a dummy variable, was created for each class. Hence, the indicator variable, "hounds," had a value of 1 if the dog was included in this class and a value of 0 if it was not.

INDICES: See **Index**

INDIGENOUS CASE: Syn: native case Case of disease contracted by a subject in the country where it lives.

EXAMPLE: Cases of rabies in foxes in Canada.
Cases of porcine pleuropneumonia type I in Canada.

COMMENT: As opposed to *imported case.**

INDIRECT ASSOCIATION: Association of a factor X with an event of interest Y by way of one or several intermediate or intervening factors Z_1, Z_2, etc.

$X \to Z \to Y$.

EXAMPLES: Increase in the standard of living (X) → increase in the number of vehicles (Z) → increase in the number of road accidents (Y).

Age → Teat sphincter function → Mastitis in cows.

INDIRECT CONTACT: Relationship between two subjects via fomites or through an intermediate subject.

EXAMPLES: Fomites: farm equipment (trough, drinkers, milking equipment, etc.). Transmission of *Brucella abortus* between cows from an infected dairy herd and cows from a brucellosis-free herd by means of an infected dog or a dog carrying virulent material.

See also *direct contact, contagion.*

INDIRECT COST: See Fixed Cost

INDIRECT TRANSMISSION: Passage of a pathogen from one individual to another by the intermediary involvement or action of another individual, object, or substance.

COMMENT 1: In the strictest sense, the term *vector** should be reserved for biological *agents,** such as biting insects, but it is often used in a broader sense to apply to any intervening *individual,** object, or substance involved in the transmission of disease agents. Inanimate objects and substances are sometimes referred to as *fomites.**

COMMENT 2: The indirect transmission of a disease can be:

• by *contact** between a new *host** and a *vector** (in the broad sense) that has previously been contaminated by contact with the individual hosting the pathogen. Such vectors would include other, nonsusceptible individuals; objects, such as grooming equipment and buildings; water; air; foods; etc. (for example, aerial transmission of the virus of foot-and-mouth disease over a distance of kilometers or transmission of ringworm by contact with spore-contaminated stalls and equipment).
• by arthropods (vector in the strict sense) (for example, transmission of arboviridae by mosquitoes).

COMMENT 3: A vector may be active (for example, arthropod transmission of an infectious agent) or passive (contamination of food, water, equipment).

COMMENT 4: An insect vector involved in indirect transmission can be a *mechanical vector,** when it simply transmits the disease agent mechanically (for example, tabanid transmission of equine infectious anemia by mouthpart contamination during feeding), or a *biological vector,** when the disease agent multiplies (e.g., arthropods and arbovirosis) or undergoes a stage of its life cycle within the vector (for example, malaria).

COMMENT 5: As opposed to *direct transmission.**

See also *contagious disease* (Figure C9).

INDIVIDUAL: A unit member of a population.

Statistical sense: Elementary statistical unit.

EXAMPLES: Animal, herd, observation.

COMMENT 1: In an epidemiologic context, the terms "unit" and *case** are also used as synonyms.

COMMENT 2: In *health management,** individual is often used as record-keeping jargon in reference to data specific to one animal (i.e., individual record).

See also *sampling unit,** *epidemiologic unit.**

INDUCTION: Syn: inductive inference The act or process of deriving general principles or laws from particular observations.

EXAMPLE: The fact that a statistically significant *association** exists between a factor and an event of interest may lead to the induction of the *hypothesis** that this is a *risk factor** for this event.

COMMENT 1: Descriptive epidemiologic *studies** and *statistical inferences** use inductive reasoning.

COMMENT 2: In veterinary medicine, induction is a term often used to refer to the act or process of causing something to occur, such as anesthesia or parturition. It may also be used in the expression "induction period," which refers to the period needed for a particular *cause** to produce *disease** [see *disease cycle** (incubation period) and *latency**].

INDUCTIVE INFERENCE: See Induction

INFECTION: Invasion by microorganisms capable of reproducing identical entities in receptive individuals.

EXAMPLE: A pregnant cow exposed to *Brucella abortus* and becoming the site of multiplication of this bacterium.

COMMENT 1: Infection is not synonymous with clinical *disease** because an infection can remain inapparent. The essential characteristic of an infection is the multiplication of the agent in the *host.**

COMMENT 2: The word infection is mainly used for *pathogenic** microorganisms. However, the above definition does not exclude *commensals.** Indeed, although infections often trigger a response or a reaction from the host (local cellular injury due to competitive metabolism, toxins, intracellular replication, antigen–antibody response), this is not essential.

COMMENT 3: Infections are often characterized based on the location in the host (enteric, pulmonary, apical, local, general, etc.), the mode of transmission (airborne, dustborne, waterborne, vector-borne, etc.), the origin (*nosocomial,** pyogenic, *endogenous,** *exogenous,** etc.), the duration (acute, chronic), the relation with other agents (mixed, secondary, cross), or the presence (*clinical**) or absence (*subclinical,** *latent**) of signs.

COMMENT 4: Infection applies only to living matter and is to be distinguished from *contamination,** which does not imply multiplication and which is not limited to living organisms. Indeed, "contaminated" or "soiled" are attributes that can also be used in reference to inanimate material or objects.

COMMENT 5: Unicellular microorganisms (bacteria, fungus, protozoa, etc.), viruses, and prions are the *agents** involved in infections.

COMMENT 6: Infection is to be differentiated from *infestation*,* which is a term used in relation to *parasites*.*

INFECTION IMMUNITY: See **Premunition**

INFECTIOSITY: See **Infectiousness**

INFECTIOUS: Syn: infective Caused by or capable of being transmitted by infection.

> EXAMPLES: Infectious *agent;** infectious rhinotracheitis (a highly *infectious disease** of cattle).

> See also *infection, infectious disease.*

INFECTIOUS DISEASE: Disease caused by infection.

> EXAMPLES: All viral, bacterial, and fungal *diseases.**

> COMMENT 1: Infectious disease should be differentiated from parasitic disease, which is caused by an *infestation.**

> COMMENT 2: Infectious diseases are not necessarily *contagious** (for example, tetanus). Some can only be transmitted by a *vector** (transmissible disease) (for example, equine viral encephalomyelitis).

> See also *infection, contagious disease* (Figure C8).

INFECTIOUS DISEASE CYCLE: See **Chain of Infection**

INFECTIOUS DOSE 50 (ID50): Number of organisms required to produce an infection in 50% of a named species, under specified conditions.

> EXAMPLE: The ID50 of *Bacillus anthracis* for sheep is 600 spores.

> COMMENT: The ID50 is lower the greater the *virulence** of the pathogen and when the *resistance** of the recipient is low.

INFECTIOUSNESS: Syn: infectiosity A relative quantification of the ease with which a disease organism is transmitted from one host to another.

> EXAMPLES: Diseases transmitted by aerosols are generally more infective than those transmitted by arthropod vectors.

> The equine encephalitides are highly infective whereas bovine viral leukosis is not.

> COMMENT 1: Infectiousness applies to a *disease** or to a source of microorganisms.

> COMMENT 2: Infectiousness is to be distinguished from contagiousness, which concerns only contact transmission, whether direct or indirect, and excludes *vector** transmission. Thus, equine viral encephalomyelitis is essentially noncontagious.

COMMENT 3: Infectiousness should also be distinguished from *infectivity.* Infectivity corresponds to the phase of entry into the *host** (or capacity to start an *infection** with a certain number of microorganisms), whereas infectiousness refers to the departure phase from the host (or the amount of microorganisms produced by the host and available for the transmission).

COMMENT 4: Infectivity is inversely proportional to the number of units of a microorganism necessary to produce an infection. Infectiousness is proportional to the number of units of a microorganism produced by the host and available for the transmission to other organisms.

INFECTIVE: See Infectious

INFECTIVITY: The characteristic of a microorganism that allows it to infect and subsequently survive and multiply within a susceptible host.

EXAMPLE: Ebola Reston is highly infective for some species of monkeys.

COMMENT 1: The degree of infectivity can be expressed by the number of microorganisms necessary to provoke an *infection** in a particular *host.** For example, a strain of rabies virus of vulpine origin has a higher infectivity for foxes than for dogs or cats. The opposite is true for a strain of canine origin.

COMMENT 2: Infectivity and *virulence** should be differentiated.

COMMENT 3: The specific infectivity of a microorganism is directly associated with the *receptivity** of the host.

INFERENCE: The act or process of reaching a conclusion from observations or premises that are considered valid.

EXAMPLES: A field *study** was designed to establish the role of an *infectious** *agent** A in cattle abortions. One should not make inferences on the role of agent A in abortions unless a series of observations (obtained by *sampling** the cattle *population**) and statements regarding this study are considered valid. For example, the following statements or findings could be expected:

The relationship between agent A and abortions:
1. When antibodies against agent A (Ab A) were detected, abortions consistently occurred.
2. Abortions due to causes other than A were identified, including cases when cattle were also found positive to A (Ab A present).
3. The infection (agent A) preceded the abortion.

The validity of the protocol:
4. The investigative procedures did not produce significant artifacts, such as many *false positives,** which could have occurred with a serological test with low *specificity.**
5. The study design and its execution were consistent with the *objectives** of the study (analytical approach: *case–control** or, more likely, *cohort study**).

6. The sampling methodology allowed the comparison of representative *samples.* *
7. *Extrapolation** of the results was limited to populations similar to the study samples.

Although not exhaustive, this series of statements would have to be made and found valid before one could infer that agent A plays a role in the occurrence of abortions in cattle. This is why all scientific studies, in particular field work, have to be thoroughly discussed before results may be extrapolated.

COMMENT: *Induction** and *deduction** are inferences (Figure I4).

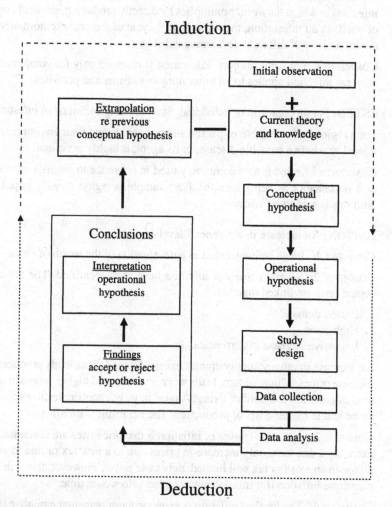

Induction

Deduction

FIGURE I4. Conceptualization of the scientific method as a cycle showing the role of inference (deduction and induction).

See also *induction, deduction.*

INFESTATION: Parasitic aggression or subsistence on the surface of the host's body of ectoparasites (insects, mites, ticks, etc.) and invasion of the tissues or organs by endoparasites.

EXAMPLES: *Sarcoptes scabiei* in swine resulting in pruritis and reduced growth rate.*

Fasciola hepatica found in the liver parenchyma and bile ducts of sheep, cattle, and several other domesticated species, as well as humans.

COMMENT 1: The word infestation is used for *parasites** in the same way that the word *infection** is used for bacteria, viruses, fungi, etc. In contrast with an infection in which the *agent** multiplies by directly producing identical copies of itself, in an infestation, the reproductive cycle of the parasite normally includes a series of different developmental stages.

COMMENT 2: For some authors, infestation is reserved only for ectoparasites, whereas infection applies to all other microorganisms and parasites.

INFESTED: For an organism or individual: State of being victim of an infestation.

For a region or farm: State of people and/or animals and their environment in a locality where a parasitic disease, or its agent, is highly prevalent.

COMMENT: Infested is also commonly used in reference to animals perceived as a nuisance or as being harmful. For example, a region densely populated with rats is said to be infested.

INFLATION: An increase in the general level of prices.

COMMENT 1: It can be considered as a devaluation of the worth of money.

COMMENT 2: Several causes of inflation have been identified. The most accepted ones are linked together:

1. Excess demand
2. High costs
3. Excessive increase in currencies.

An increase in money supply creates excess demand. This leads producers to increase prices, which, in turn, leads workers to demand higher wages in order to maintain their standard of living. A raise in wages contributes to excess demand and to higher costs of production. The net result is inflation.

COMMENT 3: A critical feature of inflation is that price rises are sustained. For example, a one-time only increase in prices due to a new tax or due to an increase in an existing tax will immediately raise prices. However, this will only constitute inflation if it translates into higher prices over time.

COMMENT 4: The level of inflation is expressed as a percentage relative to the previous level of prices. This is why inflation can exceed 100%. It is referred to as the inflation rate.

INFORMATION BIAS: See **Bias**

IN-PERSON INTERVIEW: See **Questionnaire, Unstructured Interview, Structured Interview**

INSTANTANEOUS INCIDENCE: Syn: incidence density, instantaneous risk, hazard rate. Theoretical measure of the probability of occurrence of a disease at time t, when Δt tends toward zero:

$$\frac{\text{(Probability that an unaffected individual at } t \text{ develops the disease between } t \text{ and } t + \Delta t)}{\Delta t}$$

COMMENT 1: The instantaneous incidence is used in many *mathematical models** in *epidemiology.**

COMMENT 2: Because it is impossible to calculate the instantaneous incidence for the infinitude of times that exist, *incidence rates** are calculated over periods of time under the assumption that, during the measurable time period, the instantaneous incidence rate is constant. For example, an incidence rate for time 1 to time 2 can be calculated as the number of incident events between time 1 and time 2 divided by the sum of the individual times at risk between time 1 and time 2. This incidence rate corresponds to the average instantaneous incidence rate between time 1 and time 2.

INSTANTANEOUS RISK: See **Instantaneous Incidence**

INTERACTION: In biology: The interdependence of two or more determinants to produce an effect.

In statistics: A quantitative effect involving two or more variables that can be expressed in a model.

EXAMPLES: Biology: The combination of high dust concentration in a chicken house and *Aspergillus* resulting in an increase in respiratory problems in a broiler operation.

Statistics: The need for a product term in a linear regression model.

COMMENT: Two factors are said to interact if the difference in mean responses for two levels of one factor is not constant across levels of the other factor.

INTERCURRENT: Occurring during the course of an existing disease.

COMMENT 1: It is the attribute of a *disease** or an *infection** occurring while another condition (infectious or not) is already present in the individual or group of interest.

COMMENT 2: An intercurrent infection is said to be a *secondary infection** when the initial disease is also infectious. For example, pasteurellosis following a viral respiratory disease or infection in cattle. In contrast, osteomyelitis occurring following an open fracture would be considered intercurrent, but would not be known as a secondary infection.

COMMENT 3: The temporal *distribution** of two diseases or infections is not always easy to determine. In the cattle example presented in comment 2, it is assumed that *Pasteurella* infected the animals after the viral infection. In fact, the opposite could be true.

COMMENT 4: The words *relapse** or *recurrence** would apply instead of intercurrent when the same disease or infection reoccurs in the same individual or group.

See also *secondary infection, relapse, recurrence.*

INTEREST: Charge made for the use of borrowed money, which is levied as a percentage of the debt over a determined period of time.

COMMENT 1: As described above, interest is a charge for the borrower, but it is a source of *income** for the lender.

COMMENT 2: Interest is also used in economics as a general term referring to a right or share in something (a company, grazing land, a valuable animal used for reproduction, etc.).

See also *capital, simple interest, compound interest.*

INTEREST RATE: Price paid for the use of borrowed funds over an agreed time period.

COMMENT 1: Interest payments represent *income** to the lender, and an *expense** to the borrower.

COMMENT 2: Interest may be charged on a simple or compound basis.

COMMENT 3: In order to make a profit from a cash investment, the interest rate has to be higher than the *inflation rate.** The actual interest earned (*benefit**), if any, corresponds to the interest rate minus the inflation rate.

See also *compound interest, simple interest.*

INTERGROUP VARIATION: Syn: between-group variance A measure of dispersion among the central values of a variable for several groups of individuals.

COMMENT: The *variances** can be estimated from the components of a variance method.

See also *analysis of variance.*

INTERINDIVIDUAL VARIATION: A measure of the total dispersion between the values of the same variable measured on many individuals.

COMMENT 1: See comment 1 of the definition of *intragroup variation.**

COMMENT 2: The total *variance** is a measure of the interindividual variation.

See also *analysis of variance.*

INTERMEDIATE HOST: A term in parasitology to indicate a host in which a parasite undergoes development with or without replication but in the absence of sexual replication.

EXAMPLES: Snails and the giant liver flukes; ruminants for hydatid echinococcosis; terrestrial snails for protostrongylid nematodes.

See also *definitive host*.

INTERNAL RATE OF RETURN (IRR): The rate of return on an asset investment.

COMMENT 1: Used as a method for ranking investment proposals.

COMMENT 2: The internal rate of return is calculated by finding the *discount rate** that equates the present value of future cash flows to the *cost** of the *investment** (i.e., a net present value of zero).

See also *discount rate, net present value, present value*.

INTERNALITIES: Costs and benefits that accrue directly to a project or business.

EXAMPLE: A dairy mastitis control program may include antibiotic therapy (*costs**), increased milk production, and lower *culling rates** (*benefits**). Such items, being internal to the farm's budget, are considered to be internalities. However, the potential impact of antibiotic residues on consumers (considered an undesirable effect) would be considered part of *externalities.** To protect consumers and to internalize such externalities, the government may pass legislation limiting the use of antibiotics and contaminated milk.

See also *externalities*.

INTERNALITY: See Internalities

INTERQUARTILE INTERVAL: See Interquartile Range

INTERQUARTILE RANGE: Syn: interquartile interval A measure of the dispersion of a distribution based on the difference between the values of the third and first quartiles.

See also *quantile* (Figure Q1).

INTERVENTION STUDY: Epidemiologic study designed to determine the relationship between an intervention (therapy, prophylactic measure, policy or regulation, management decision, etc.) and the health status of individuals or populations.

EXAMPLES: Evaluation of two different mastitis control programs under field conditions.

Comparison between two treatments aimed at controlling sarcoptic mange in swine. The outcomes of interest could be skin lesions, clinical signs at the *individual** or *group** (pen) level, growth performance, etc., depending on the *study** design.

Evaluation of *mortality** and *morbidity rates,** and production performances in groups of piglets depending on two different cross-fostering strategies.

COMMENT: Intervention studies are *experiments** or *trials.** Most trials are clinical trials performed in research facilities or directly in the field. Some interventions are not targeted at individual animals or farms but at regions. For example, it could be a control program for bovine viral leukosis implemented in a county. This would be similar to a community trial. In veterinary medicine, one would refer to a regional control program. Its assessment would be an evaluation of the program designed to determine its degree of implementation and success in comparison with other regions.

Interventions can also be assessed as part of *observational studies.** However, the interpretation of results is usually not as straightforward because, by design, the observer has no control over the allocation of individuals to the different treatment groups. Several other factors (age of individuals, severity of clinical signs, variability in application of treatments, etc.) may also contribute to the introduction of significant *biases** in the study. An alternative approach is to nest an intervention study within the observational study. In this case, animals or groups of animals selected for a clinical trial performed under field conditions would also be monitored as part of the observational study.

See also *trial, efficacy, effectiveness, efficiency.*

INTERVIEW: See Questionnaire, Unstructured Interview, Structured Interview

INTRAGROUP VARIATION: A measure of dispersion between the values of the same variable measured from individuals belonging to a specific group.

COMMENT 1: The intragroup variation is equal to the *interindividual variation** of all individuals within the group and is equal to, or less than, the total interindividual variation.

COMMENT 2: The *variances** can be estimated by the components of a variance method.

See also *analysis of variance.*

INTRAINDIVIDUAL VARIATION: A measure of the dispersion of the values taken by a single variable for a single individual as a function of time.

EXAMPLES: Body growth, individual seasonal variations, diurnal variation of the rectal temperature or the level of glycemia.

INTRINSIC FACTOR: Syn: endogenous factor Characteristic of an individual that could modulate its performance or receptivity to diseases.

EXAMPLES: Species, breed, sex, age, and some genetic factors.

COMMENT: As opposed to *extrinsic factor.**

INVASIVENESS: 1. A measure of the ability of a microorganism or neoplasm to propagate through cells, tissue, organs, etc.

EXAMPLE: *Leptospira typhimurium* is a highly invasive organism.

COMMENT 1: Some bacteria have a great invasiveness for some species in which they readily provoke septicemia (for example, *Bacillus anthracis* for herbivores) and a more limited invasiveness for other species (for example, cutaneous anthrax in humans). Other bacteria have a weak invasiveness and produce only localized diseases (for example, *Moraxella bovis*).

COMMENT 2: No strict parallels can be drawn between virulence and invasiveness. Some microorganisms can be highly invasive yet do not produce any clinical signs (for example, arboviruses in birds and rodents) or only mild symptoms (for example, blue tongue virus in adult cattle) (Figure I5).

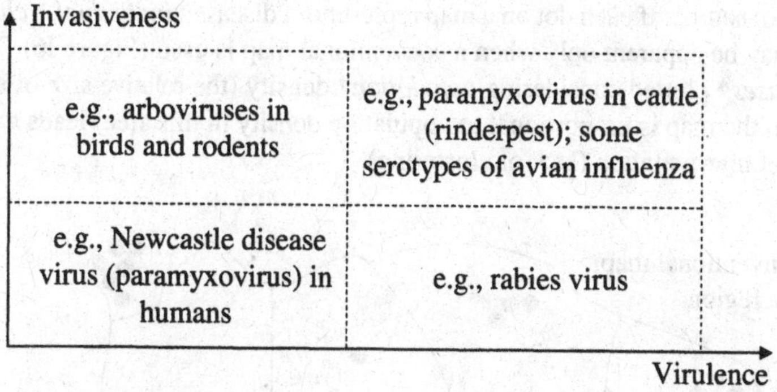

Invasiveness		
e.g., arboviruses in birds and rodents	e.g., paramyxovirus in cattle (rinderpest); some serotypes of avian influenza	
e.g., Newcastle disease virus (paramyxovirus) in humans	e.g., rabies virus	

Virulence

FIGURE I5.   Schematic representation of the independence between invasiveness and virulence.

2. The degree to which a medical procedure or examination penetrates a body cavity or orifice.

EXAMPLE: Bowel resection is invasive, whereas, usually, an ophthalmic examination is not.

INVESTMENT: Real capital formation (e.g., maintenance or production of equipment, livestock, building construction on a farm, etc.) with the purpose of producing goods and/or services for future sale or consumption.

In common usage, the laying out of money in the purchase of assets.

COMMENT 1: The first definition written above focuses mainly on the purchase of capital goods, which is also known as capital investment. In contrast, the purchase of *assets,** such as securities, bank deposits, etc., with the primary goal of creating income or capital gain, is known as financial investment.

COMMENT 2: One may refer to gross investment (investment inclusive of *depreciation**) or to net investment (investment minus depreciation).

COMMENT 3: The decision to invest by an individual or a firm is based on many criteria:

Motivation to invest;

Return on investment (criteria set for the *net present value,** the *internal rate of return,** and the *pay back period** allow one to analyze the future return on investment);

Financial position of the individual/firm;

Ability of the individual or firm to exploit investment opportunities;

Availability of internal or external financial resources;

Ability to integrate new investments into the organization.

COMMENT 4: Livestock is considered a particular investment because it cannot be depreciated, and generally is quite liquid (can be quickly converted into cash at little loss).

ISODEMIC MAPPING: Cartographic device to examine geographic clustering of cases after adjusting for population density (population-by-area cartogram).

COMMENT: If each dot on a map represents a diseased *individual,* * *clustering* * may be apparent only when a conventional map is used (Figure I6). The same *cases* * plotted considering *population* * density (the relative size of each area on the map is proportional to population density in this area) leads to a different interpretation (lack of clustering).

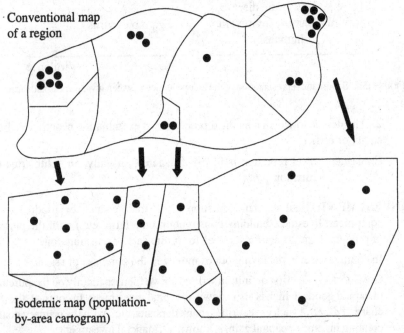

FIGURE I6. Geographical distribution of cases on a conventional map and on an isodemic map.

ISOLATION: Separation of infected subjects (diseased, contaminated, or even just suspected of being infected) during the period of communicability, in such conditions as to avoid all possible direct or indirect transmissions of the infectious agent to susceptible subjects.

COMMENT 1: This is a *primary prevention* * approach.

COMMENT 2: The word isolation is also used in food animal production when animals believed to be *disease** free (replacement animals) are put in *quarantine** in order to deliberately expose them to specific *agents** prior to their introduction in the *herd.**

COMMENT 3: Modern commercial animal operations are expected to have isolation facilities separated from any other animals by at least 2 to 4 km and with proper *biosecurity,** including waste management, pest control, and strict access regulations.

See also *quarantine*.

ITEM: In questionnaire design, one of the options available in a multiple-choice question.

EXAMPLE: Question with five items:

How many cattle were bought during the last 36 months?

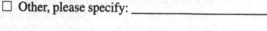

☐ 0
☐ 1 to 5
☐ 6 to 10
☐ 11 to 20
☐ > 20

COMMENT: To be valid, *multiple-choice* (or *closed*) *questions** must include all necessary items corresponding to possible answers. Hence, the following items are often added:

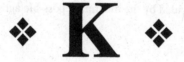

☐ Don't know
☐ Do not apply
☐ Other, please specify: _____

❖ K ❖

KAPLAN–MEIER METHOD: Nonparametric method of estimation of the survival function that is part of the life table family of methods.

COMMENT 1: Survival is the *probability** that an *individual** from a *population** or a *cohort** is still alive following an initial moment (time 0, which can be defined by an event). This probability can be estimated once the exact time of death events is known.

COMMENT 2: This *method** is based on the idea that to still be alive at instant *t*, it is necessary to be alive until just before *t* and not to die during that instant t. *Rates** of survival are estimated on successive time intervals during the study period T.

COMMENT 3: The intervals ($t1$, $t2$, ...) separate two deaths (or a certain number of successive deaths). Intervals are not chosen a priori and are not necessarily of equal length, as opposed to the *actuarial method.**

COMMENT 4: This method is particularly useful for small *samples** with censored observations.

COMMENT 5: Being *nonparametric,** it does not require any assumptions about the form of the function that is being estimated.

See also *survival function, actuarial method.*

KAPPA COEFFICIENT: See Kappa Statistic

KAPPA STATISTIC: Syn: kappa coefficient Index measuring the extent of agreement between two matched categorical variables.

EXAMPLES: Comparison of skin test readings for tuberculosis performed independently by two veterinarians on the same subjects.

As part of a *validation** effort, some questions were used to evaluate the internal consistency of responses within a *questionnaire** on *biosecurity.** Answers to the following two questions: "For a production cycle, are all animals received onto the farm at the same time?" and "For a production cycle, are all animals shipped from the farm at the same time?" were compared to: "Do you practice all-in/all-out production on your farm?" A positive response to the first two questions was considered equivalent to a positive response to the last one. The agreement within the *survey** was moderate to good (kappa = 0.57 ± 0.22).

COMMENT 1: In the calculation of the kappa coefficient (k), the difference between the observed proportion agreement and the chance proportion agreement ($p_o - p_c$) is divided by the maximum possible agreement beyond chance ($1 - p_c$).

Test B		Test A +	–	Total		Standard test +	–	Total
+		a	b	f_1	For example: New test +	42	58	100
–		c	d	f_2	–	38	862	900
	Total	n_1	n_2	N	Total	80	920	1000

*Apparent prevalence:** Standard test = 80/1000 = 8%
New test = 100/1000 = 10%

Observed proportion agreement $(p_o) = \dfrac{a+d}{N}$ $\qquad \dfrac{42+862}{1000} = 0.904$

Chance proportion agreement $(p_c) = \dfrac{a'+d'}{N}$ $\qquad \dfrac{8+828}{1000} = 0.836$

where $a' = \dfrac{n_1 f_1}{N}$ is the expected number (by chance) of occasions with both tests being positive.

$d' = \dfrac{n_2 f_2}{N}$ is the expected number (by chance) of occasions with both tests being negative.

also, $b' = \dfrac{n_2 f_1}{N}$ and $c' = \dfrac{n_1 f_2}{N}$

hence, kappa (k) $= \dfrac{p_o - p_c}{1 - p_c} = \dfrac{2(ad - bc)}{n_1 f_2 + n_2 f_1} = 1 - \dfrac{b + c}{b' + c'} \qquad \dfrac{0.904 - 0.836}{1 - 0.836} = 0.41$

Note that this calculation of kappa involves the following assumptions:

- The patients or the material to be evaluated are collected independently.
- Neither rater is aware of the results of the other rater's assessment.
- The rating categories are mutually exclusive and exhaustive.

COMMENT 2: The kappa statistic is very useful when comparing two tests, particularly a well-accepted one and a new one, such as in the example above. It is the most practical and the simplest tool to measure agreement between categorical results performed by two techniques or by two observers.

COMMENT 3: The agreement can be tested (*null hypothesis:** kappa = 0) using the standard error of kappa and Student's t *distribution.** No agreement beyond chance gives a kappa of 0, and a kappa of 1 indicates perfect agreement. All possible values can be interpreted as follows:

Excellent	if kappa is included	between 0.81 and 1,
good		between 0.61 and 0.8,
moderate		between 0.41 and 0.6,
weak		between 0.21 and 0.4,
very weak		between 0.01 and 0.2,
poor		if ≤ 0.

COMMENT 4: Some disagreement between two raters or two tests may be considered more serious than others. For example, when evaluating the distance between two farms, two observers were given the following options: < 0.5 km, 0.5 to 1 km, 1 < x < 3 km, $\geq$ 3 km. A disagreement between < 0.5 and $\geq$ 3 is more critical than between < 0.5 and 0.5 to 1. Therefore, to account for the magnitude of the discrepancy, one could assign weights to reflect the seriousness of the disagreements between raters or tests. This produces a weighted kappa. The reader is referred to Shoukri and Edge (1996) for further information on this issue and on the kappa statistic in general.

KOCH'S POSTULATES: A series of four postulates proposed by Robert Koch, a German bacteriologist (1843–1910), regarding the ideal conditions required to demonstrate causality for an infectious agent.

1. The *agent** must be shown to be present in every case of the *disease** by isolation in pure culture.
2. The agent must not be found in cases of other disease.
3. Once isolated, the agent must be capable of reproducing the disease in experimental animals.

4. The agent must be recovered from the experimental disease produced.

COMMENT: This series of postulates is not suitable for diseases with *multifactorial etiology*.* New series of postulates have been proposed by Evans (*Evans's postulates**) and Hill (*Hill's postulates**).

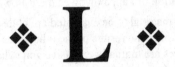

LABORATORY SENSITIVITY OF A TEST: See **Detection Limit**

LAPLACE–GAUSS DISTRIBUTION: See **Normal Distribution**

LATENCY: **In a strict sense:** State in which a pathogen is present in the host in a quiescent state.

In a broad sense: State (and period) during which the pathogen cannot be demonstrated in the infected host or is shed intermittently.

EXAMPLES: In a strict sense, *infections** with certain viruses (e.g., a member of the herpesvirus group, some retroviruses). The pathogen cannot be recovered by conventional means, and may simply be integrated in the form of genetic information in the nucleus of some cells of the host. One example is infection with *Varicella-zoster*, the virus of chicken pox. The virus may persist as a latent infection for decades before resuming a pathogenic role.

In a broad sense, the term of latency is sometimes used to denote the long interval for virus infections with a long incubation period (for example, scrapie, a so-called slow virus infection).

LATENCY PERIOD: **Syn: preshedding period** Interval between the time of contamination of an individual by a pathogen and the time when it becomes a source of this agent.

EXAMPLE: The latency period for rabies in foxes is around 20 to 30 days (period between *contamination** and appearance of the virus in the saliva).

COMMENT: To be differentiated from period of contagion and from incubation period.

See also *generation time* (Figure G1).

LATENT CARRIER: In France: carrier with a particularly long incubation period (latent infection).

In North America: This expression is seldom used.

EXAMPLE: A cow infected with bovine viral leukosis.

COMMENT: An organism that hosts the nonexpressed genome of a pathogen (e.g., herpes virus) is a particular case of latent carrier.

See also *latent infection*.

LATENT INFECTION OR DISEASE: Infection or disease that remains subclinical for a period of time far in excess of the expected incubation period for the disease of interest.

EXAMPLE: Adult swine infected with pseudorabies (Aujeszky's) virus for several months before presenting any clinical signs, when the usual incubation period is only a few days.

COMMENT: Animals with a latent infection are also said to be in a *carrier* * state or to have a chronic *infection.* * These animals may hamper the *control* * of the *disease* * if they are not identified.

See also *latency, disease cycle*.

LEASE: A long-term rental agreement.

LEAST SQUARES METHOD: See **Method of Least Squares**

LETHALITY: The capacity of an agent or disease to cause death.

COMMENT 1: This risk is expressed by the *case fatality rate.* * Although this *rate* * is occasionally used as synonymous with lethality, this usage is not recommended.

COMMENT 2: Do not confuse with *mortality.* *

LEVEL OF SIGNIFICANCE: A probability considered to be too unlikely to be attributable to chance when the null hypothesis is assumed to be true.

COMMENT 1: The level of significance is often symbolized by the p value.

EXAMPLE: $p < 0.05$ implies that, if a particular sample-derived test procedure was repeatedly performed, the magnitude of the test statistic (and the set of those with a greater magnitude in the sense of a probability tail distribution) would occur in less than 5% of the replicates when the *null hypothesis* * is correct.

COMMENT 2: The lower this probability is, the more significant is the test statistic (e.g., a test statistic with $p = 0.0001$ is less likely under the null hypothesis, and hence more significant, than a test statistic with $p = 0.05$).

COMMENT 3: The p value should not be confused with α (alpha). The latter is a probability fixed a priori by the statistician and used for decision making (i.e., to reject or not reject the null hypothesis); it is not a probability associated with any test statistic, unlike the level of significance that is dependent on data. If the p value is less than the α level, then a test statistic is considered statistically significant. The choice of alpha should depend on the relative costs of making *alpha* and *beta errors.* *

See also *alpha error.*

LEVERAGE: Syn: gearing The use of debt to increase the expected return on equity.

COMMENT: Financial leverage is measured as the ratio of long-term debt to long-term debt plus equity.

See also *expected return.*

LIFE EXPECTANCY: Syn: expectation of life Average number of days, weeks, months, or years of probable life of a subject, taken at a given age, in function of known age-specific mortality rates.

EXAMPLE: In France, the life expectancy of a fox is 1 year.

COMMENT 1: Life expectancy can be calculated from birth or starting at a given age. It varies according to the species, sex, time, region, etc. Life expectancy at birth may be referred to as lifespan.

COMMENT 2: In commercial animal production, life expectancy is largely dependent on market conditions.

COMMENT 3: Life expectancy may be shorter at birth than later on, after a known critical period.

LIFE TABLE: Syn: cohort life table Representation of risk as a function of time.

COMMENT: It is used in particular to represent the *risk** of dying as a function of age. It can be generalized to apply to any type of risk. There are two risks used to obtain these tables: the risk of surviving up to a certain period and the risk of dying during that period. The table consists of the risk of mortality and the cumulative risk of survival for a *cohort** of individuals followed over sequential periods of time.

EXAMPLE: Used in domestic animals to study *mortality** (Table L1) and *culling** patterns.

TABLE L1. **Life table of mortality in pigs during the first 4 days postpartum in a large cohort**

Age at death (days)	Number of pigs			Percent dead	Cumulative survival
	At risk	Censored[a]	Dead		
1	551,154	1074	18,743	3.40	0.966
2	531,337	634	12,226	2.30	0.944
3	518,477	467	10,019	1.93	0.926
4	507,991	361	6,339	1.25	0.914

[a]Censored: lost to follow-up (removed or weaned)

LIFETIME PREVALENCE: Total number of individuals, for a given population or cohort, that had a given disease during their life.

EXAMPLE: Percentage of cows that experienced mastitis throughout their productive life.

See also *prevalence.*

LIKELIHOOD: Given a random sample, the likelihood is the joint density of the variable(s) of interest evaluated at the observed values obtained from the sample.

EXAMPLE: If one randomly picks five animals from a large *population** with a *proportion** p of *disease** (M) and $(1 - p)$ of nondisease (M-) and one has observed: (M, M-, M, M, M). The likelihood of this *sample,** noted L, is equal to:

$$L = p \times (1 - p) \times p \times p \times p = p^4 (1 - p).$$

COMMENT 1: In the case of a *quantitative variable,** the likelihood is calculated using its distribution law (for example, normal, log-normal, or any other possible law).

COMMENT 2: The likelihood thus calculated is a function of the distribution of the studied *random variable.** In the case of a *normal distribution,** one obtains an expression depending on the *mean** and the *standard deviation.**

COMMENT 3: The *maximum likelihood method** is a method of estimation that selects values of *parameters** in such a way as to give maximal likelihood based on the observed *data.**

See also *estimate, maximum likelihood method.*

LIKELIHOOD RATIO (TEST OF MODEL): Ratio of two likelihoods used as a test to compare a restricted to a complete model for the observed data.

COMMENT: The likelihood ratio test or *statistic** can be compared to the *chi-square distribution** with *degrees of freedom** equal to the number of *parameters** in the larger *model** minus the number of parameters in the smaller model.

LIKERT SCALE: Measurement technique used to rank people's judgments of objects, events, animals or other people.

COMMENT 1: Statements are presented to respondents who are asked to indicate their degree of agreement or disagreement with them.

EXAMPLE: Indicate your degree of agreement or disagreement with each of the following statements about GATT (General Agreement on Tariffs and Trade) and swine production by circling one of the following letters:

SA = Strongly agree
A = Agree
U = Undecided

D = Disagree
SD = Strongly disagree

1. GATT will have a beneficial impact on swine production in the USA by increasing exports   SA   A   U   D   SD
2. Because of GATT, I am planning on increasing the size of my herd   SA   A   U   D   SD

COMMENT 2: A Likert-type scale includes only statements that are clearly favorable or clearly unfavorable. Neutral or borderline statements are eliminated during the design process by a panel of experts on the topic considered in the *questionnaire**.

COMMENT 3: The statements are arranged in *random** order in the questionnaire. Favorable statements are scored from 5 to 1 (Strongly agree = 5, Agree = 4, Undecided = 3, Disagree = 2, Strongly disagree = 1); unfavorable statements are scored in the reverse direction from 1 to 5. Finally, scores for all items are summed.

COMMENT 4: The simplicity of the Likert scoring system makes this procedure very attractive to researchers. It is used, for example, in studies on human–animal bonds and in clinical trials assessing pet owners' perception of the effect of a drug on their animal's behavior.

COMMENT 5: *Validity** is often assessed by administering the scale to individuals known to hold strong opinions on both sides of an issue. *Reliability** is tested using the test–retest method (the scale is given to the same person on two occasions and the results are compared), the split-half method (involves splitting the scale into two halves, which are then compared), or the equivalent forms (when two different scales on the same topic are compared).

COMMENT 6: There is an ongoing debate about the validity of attitude scale in predicting behavior. People's opinions on a topic like GATT and its impact on animal production may be multidimensional and a single favorability score may not reflect specific concerns.

LIQUIDITY: The ability to provide cash when needed.

COMMENT: Typical liquidity measures are:

Current ratio = Total current assets/Total current liabilities
Working capital = Total current assets – Total current liabilities

See also *current asset, current liability*.

LOGISTIC REGRESSION: Statistical method used to model the relationship between the probability of occurrence of a dichotomized event (disease/nondisease for example) and a number of qualitative or quantitative independent or explanatory variables, and whose purpose is to describe, explain, or predict.

COMMENT 1: It is called logistic regression because it uses the logistic transformation of the *probability** of occurrence of the event under study. Given that (p): probability of occurrence of the event: logit (p) = log [$p/(1-p)$] = log [*odds** (p)]

COMMENT 2: It is the method most frequently used in *analytical epidemiology* (*cohort* and *case–control studies*).

COMMENT 3: If one applies logistic regression to one factor only (x: coded 0 when absent and 1 when present), it should read: logit $(p) = a + bx$, where b is the logarithm of the *odds ratio* measuring the relationship between, for example, a *disease* and a *risk factor.*

If one applies logistic regression to two factors (x_1 and x_2 coded 0 when absent and 1 when present) it should read: logit $(p) = a + b_1x_1 + b_2x_2$, where b_1 and b_2 measure the corresponding relationships between the disease and factors x_1 and x_2. The relationship between the disease and x_1 is adjusted for the presence of x_2 and the relationship between the disease and x_2 is adjusted for the presence of x_1. This is only true in the absence of interaction between the two factors.

COMMENT 4: In the context of a case–control study, the intercept a should not be interpreted.

EXAMPLE: When studying the relationship between *neonatal mortality* of lambs and their birthweight (x_1) and barn temperature (x_2): with logit $(p) = a + b_1$ (birth weight), one finds that b_1 is statistically significant; with logit $(p) = a + b_2$ (barn temperature), one concludes that b_2 is significant; however, considering logit $(p) = a + b_1x_1 + b_2x_2$, only b_1 comes up significant. The explanation is that the distribution of the two factors is linked inducing a synergy between the presence of thin lambs and low barn temperatures. Thus, the relationship observed between mortality and barn temperature, in this study, is due to the other factor—birth weight (see *confounding*).

See also *adjustment, association, logit, odds ratio.*

LOGIT: Syn: log-odds Natural logarithm of the odds of an event.

Let p be the *probability* of occurrence of an event, then its logit is log $[p/(1 - p)]$.

COMMENT: This is used in logit *models,* *logistic regression,* and log-linear models.

See also *odds, logistic regression.*

LOGNORMAL DISTRIBUTION: A random variable X follows a lognormal distribution if the variable Y, defined as the Neperian logarithm of X, follows a normal distribution.

COMMENT: Many biological *variables* have a lognormal distribution.

EXAMPLES: Count variables, such as milk somatic cell count, often show a lognormal distribution; the frequency distribution of serological titers is also generally lognormal.

See also *normal distribution.*

LOG-ODDS: See Logit

LOG-RANK TEST: A nonparametric test that compares survival functions between two groups.

EXAMPLE: To compare two treatments based on the survival of the animals in each group.

See also *survival function.*

LONGITUDINAL STUDY: An observational study in which regular observations are made in a population that is being followed for a relatively long period of time.

EXAMPLE 1: A serological *study** involving testing 50 dairy herds for the bovine viral leukosis virus every month for 3 years.

EXAMPLE 2: A 3-year study of 50 dairy herds in which *observations** about multiple clinical diseases, *subclinical diseases,** production, and reproductive performances are recorded.

COMMENT 1: A longitudinal study is a particular category of *prospective study.** A prospective study includes at least two periods of observation (at the beginning and at the end). A longitudinal study includes more than two periods of observation (often a lot more).

COMMENT 2: Many longitudinal studies allow for the examination of relationships between multiple *factors** of interest and multiple outcomes of interest (see also example 2).

COMMENT 3: Longitudinal studies are nearly always carried out prospectively but in selected instances, when very good historical data are available, longitudinal studies may be carried out retrospectively.

See also *cross-sectional study.*

LOSSES: Negative profits.

COMMENT 1: Negative profits may result from decline in output, or increased production costs, or a combination of both.

COMMENT 2: One should be careful to distinguish between direct and indirect losses.

Direct losses can be expressed in term of "products," e.g., *mortality,** *abortion*, decline in feed conversion efficiency, decline in days to market, etc.

Indirect losses, such as prohibition of access to export markets, cannot be expressed in terms of products, and are thus more difficult to quantify.

See also *profits.*

LOST TO FOLLOW-UP: Subject leaving a prospective study.

COMMENT: Several events may result in lost to follow-up: death or migration, which may lead to withdrawal bias; lack of adherence to therapy, which may produce a compliance bias.

See also *bias.*

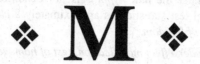

M

MAIN HOST: See **Definitive Host**

MAIN VECTOR: Syn: **principal vector** A vector that, under natural conditions, is largely responsible for the transmission of a pathogen compared to others vectors.

EXAMPLES: Broad sense: goat cheese and human brucellosis due to *B. melitensis*. Strict sense: *Ixodes ricinus*, and *Ixodes persulcatus* for tickborne encephalitis, in Western Europe and Eastern Europe, respectively.

COMMENT: For a given *disease,** the same species of arthropod may be the main vector in one geographical region, a *secondary vector** or accidental vector in another, and even incapable of achieving *transmission** elsewhere.

MANIFESTATION RATE: The proportion of the total number of diseased individuals or *outbreaks** that is actually identified, calculated as:

$$\frac{\text{Number of diseased individuals or outbreaks identified}}{\text{The true number of diseased individuals or outbreaks}}$$

COMMENT: This *proportion** is clearly an approximation because it is usually not possible to determine accurately the true number of diseased individuals or *outbreaks.**

EXAMPLE: It is assumed that, for every case of salmonellosis recorded in humans in the United States, at least nine are not reported. Therefore, the manifestation rate would be around 1/10 or 10%.

MANIFESTATIONAL VARIABLE: See **Dependent Variable**

MANTEL–HAENSZEL CHI-SQUARE TEST: See **Mantel–Haenszel Test**

MANTEL–HAENSZEL TEST: Syn: **Mantel–Haenszel chi-square test** A chi-square test of independence between two dichotomous variables (i.e., risk factor and disease), after adjusting for one or more confounding factors by the use of stratification.

COMMENT 1: It is only applicable in the absence of interaction between the two *variables** and the *confounder** (i.e., the confounding factors must not be effect modifiers).

COMMENT 2: Under the *null hypothesis** of conditional independence, the Mantel–Haenszel test statistic has approximately a *chi-square distribution** with one *degree of freedom.**

See also *confounder, effect modification, test of homogeneity.*

MARGINAL COST: The additional cost of producing one more unit of output.

EXAMPLE: The production of 60 quintals of wheat per hectare cost 480 dollars/ha. In similar conditions, the production of 61 quintals of wheat per hectare costs 488 dollars/ha. The marginal cost for the production of a quintal of wheat is then 8 dollars.

MARGINAL REVENUE: The additional gross revenue produced by selling one additional unit of output.

MARGINAL TAX RATE: The tax rate applicable to the last unit of income.

MARKET PRICE: The price of a raw material, product, service, etc., in an open market.

COMMENT 1: The economic concept of price includes exchanging commodities either for money or for each other.

COMMENT 2: In a free-market economy, prices are theoretically determined based on supply and demand. However, mainly with agricultural products, governments may have price support policies that prevent prices from falling below an agreed level.

COMMENT 3: In a formal market (stock exchange, commodity market, etc.), there is usually a margin between the buying and selling price. In this case, there are two market prices.

MARKET VALUE: The most likely cash price that an asset would bring if sold fairly in an open and competitive market.

COMMENT 1: It is a method of *asset** valuation.

COMMENT 2: An alternative to *book value.**

COMMENT 3: When land is involved, one may want to differentiate between the market value in its present use and that in some alternative use. For example, agricultural land would be valued differently in a company's accounts if it were to be listed as building land.

See also *asset, book value.*

MASS SCREENING: Syn: mass testing Systematic examination applied to the vast majority of individuals in a population.

EXAMPLE: Mass screening for bovine brucellosis in France, the United Kingdom, the United States, Canada, etc.

COMMENT 1: As opposed to *selective screening.**

COMMENT 2: Quality (*sensitivity,* * *specificity**), *cost,** and *practicality** are important considerations when selecting a test for mass screening. For example, allergic tests are less practical than serological tests.

COMMENT 3: Although mass screening often refers to regional or national screening efforts sponsored by a government, this approach may also be implemented by large integrated companies in their quest to control or *eradicate a disease.** For example, in the mid-1980s, a number of swine companies in Canada systematically tested all reproductive animals (including replacement animals) as part of a strategy aimed at controlling porcine pleuropneumonia.

See also *screening.*

MASS TESTING: See **Mass Screening**

MATCHING: Method of subject selection that provides for equal distributions of certain factors (usually confounders) between comparison groups.

COMMENT: Matching is most often performed in *case–control studies,** where controlling for levels of factors uncommon in an unmatched *sample** of potential *controls** would otherwise be impractical.

EXAMPLE: In a case–control study of environmental determinants of cancer in dogs, it may be necessary to match controls to *cases** on potential *confounders** including sex, age, breed, and location of residence.

MATHEMATICAL EXPECTATION: Syn: **expected value of a variable** Theoretical mean of a distribution.

For a random variable x, the mathematical expectation $E(x)$ is the sum of values of the random variable x weighted by their probability of occurrence. Hence, given values $x_1...x_k$ with probabilities of occurrence $p_1...p_k$ (with $p_1 + p_2 +... p_k = 1$), the mathematical expectation $E(x)$ is:

$$p_1x_1 + p_2x_2 +... p_kx_k$$

EXAMPLES: The mean of a normally distributed *random variable.** The *proportion** of a dichotomous variable with a *binomial distribution.**

MATHEMATICAL MODEL: An abstract representation of reality using mathematical language (sets, functions, equations, or systems of equations) to describe or predict the behavior of the phenomenon or process under study.

COMMENT 1: There are two types of mathematical models: *deterministic models** and *probabilistic models** (or stochastic).

COMMENT 2: In *epidemiology,** *models** are normally constructed to describe or predict patterns of *disease** occurrence as well as the likely variations in these patterns given the application of various control strategies.

See also *deterministic model, probabilistic model.*

MAXIMUM LIKELIHOOD METHOD: Statistical method of estimation of one or several parameters based on maximizing the likelihood function (obtained from a sample), which is a general estimation procedure that yields sufficient asymptotically minimum unbiased estimators whenever they exist.

COMMENT 1: This *method* * considers every possible value of a given parameter, and, for each value, computes the *likelihood* * that this particular observation would have occurred. Hence, the *estimate* * is the one for which the likelihood of the actual observation is the greatest.

COMMENT 2: Maximum likelihood or least squares can be used in a regression situation, although maximum likelihood is often more complicated. The parameter estimates from these two methods do not have to be identical. However, when the observations are independently, identically, and normally distributed, they will yield identical results.

COMMENT 3: This method was proposed in the 1920s by R.A. Fisher, one of the foremost English statisticians.

See also *estimate, method of least squares, likelihood.*

MEAN: See **Sample Mean**

MEASUREMENT: Assessment of an object or a phenomenon with the purpose of comparing it to a reference.

COMMENT: There are many kinds of measurements: quantitative, nominal or categorical, and qualitative or ordinal:

- For quantitative measurements, the comparison is made using a standard unit and the measurement produces a result expressed in an amount of units (e.g., weight of animals expressed in kilograms).
- For categorical measurements, each measurement establishes the membership of an observation in a predetermined category. Hence, this type of measurement produces a disjointed set of elements (e.g., species, breeding lines).
- Qualitative measurements are more subjective and categories are ordered without reference to a standard unit (e.g., body condition ranked from 1 to 5; 1 (poor), 3 (good), 5 (overweight).

MEASUREMENT BIAS: See **Bias**

MEASUREMENT ERROR: A false or mistaken assessment of a parameter.

COMMENT: There are two main characteristics associated with measurement errors: lack of *validity* * and lack of *repeatability.* *

See also *error.*

MECHANICAL CARRIER: Syn: **passive carrier** Individual contaminated with an infectious agent that does not multiply or replicate in the host.

EXAMPLE: Chickens may act as mechanical carriers for *Mycoplasma* before becoming infected.

COMMENT 1: In North America, this expression may be used in everyday conversations. However, because *carriers** are considered, by definition, to be infected or infested individuals, the preferred term is "contaminated animal or individual." The equivalent term for an object would be *fomite.**

COMMENT 2: In most cases, the pathogen eventually infects or infests the individual or dies out because of conditions that are unsuitable for its survival. Therefore, the mechanical carrier stage is often short.

COMMENT 3: Infected or infested carriers are labeled *active carriers** by authors who do not consider that infection or infestation is a prerequisite for the status of carrier. This term is offered in contrast to mechanical or passive carrier.

See also *carrier*.

MECHANICAL VECTOR: Syn: Passive vector A vector that acts as a mode of transportation for the pathogen being transmitted, without development or multiplication of the agent within the vector.

EXAMPLES: Broad sense: human beings are passive vectors of the foot-and-mouth disease virus, which can lodge in the nasal pits for 1 to 2 days. Strict sense: the stable fly, *Stomoxis calcitrans*, can carry the equine infectious anemia virus for a maximum of 30 minutes.

COMMENT 1: The efficiency of this type of *vector** depends essentially on the resistance of the pathogen, and the activity of, and distances traveled by, the vector.

COMMENT 2: This is in contrast to *biological vector.**

MEDIAN: Syn: second quartile A measure of central tendency of the population defined as the value of the random variable that would divide individuals if they were classified into increasing (or decreasing) order in two equal frequency groups (i.e., each group contains 50% of the total population).

COMMENT 1: In a symmetrical *distribution** (for example, *normal distribution**), the median and the mean are the same.

COMMENT 2: In an asymmetrical distribution, the median could be preferred to the mean, because it is less dependent on extreme values.

See also *mode* (Figure M1), *quantile* (Figure Q1).

MEDICAL PROPHYLAXIS: Prophylaxis by medical means (use of biologics and pharmaceuticals).

EXAMPLES: Vaccination, antisera (e.g., tetanus antitoxin) and prophylactic use of antibiotics, parasiticides and coccidiostats.

COMMENT 1: Medical prophylaxis is usually applied in association with sanitary measures.

COMMENT 2: For a number of *diseases,** in particular, those of viral origin, this approach is not effective.

MESO-ENDEMIC: That has the characteristics of an endemic of medium prevalence.

EXAMPLE: Human tuberculosis in some developing countries.

METHOD: Set of orderly and planned steps used to reach a goal.

COMMENT 1: Method and *procedure** are often used interchangeably. However, method refers mainly to the thinking process involved in mapping out the approach needed to reach a goal, while procedure refers more to its technical aspect.

COMMENT 2: In a research context, methods are described in one section of a *protocol** or a publication (Materials and Methods), and typically include a description of the data collection (sampling, inclusion and exclusion criteria, etc.), manipulation, and analysis.

COMMENT 3: Along with the materials, the methods should be complete and accurate enough to provide the reader with all necessary information to replicate the study.

See also *protocol, methodology.*

METHOD OF LEAST SQUARES: **Syn: least squares method** A curve-fitting technique that is used to estimate the parameter's value of a model by minimizing the sum of the squared difference between the values predicted by the model and the corresponding values obtained from a set of observations.

EXAMPLES:

- To estimate the *mean** of a *sample** of size *n*, the criterion to minimize is:

$$f(m) = \sum_{i=1}^{n} (x_i - m)^2$$

the solution is: $m = \dfrac{\Sigma x_i}{n}$; the *arithmetic mean.**

- To estimate *parameters** for a *regression** line: $y = ax + b$, the criterion to minimize is:

$$\sum_{i=1}^{n} [y_i - (ax_i + b)]^2$$

$[y_i - (ax_i + b)]$ measures the deviation between the observed value and the value calculated from model $y = ax + b$. The estimates of a and b by the least squares method provides the smallest sum of the square of deviation from the *model.**

COMMENT 1: As opposed to *likelihood,** the least squares method does not involve the distribution laws (or *probability**) of the *random variables** under study.*

COMMENT 2: This method was suggested in the early 19th century by the French mathematician Adrien Legendre.

See also *estimation, maximum likelihood method, regression.*

METHODOLOGY: Scientific study of methods.

COMMENT 1: Methodology consists of all principles allowing the development of a method (for example, sampling) whose practical application can be used in various studies. The report of these epidemiologic studies will present a section describing the method(s) used (not the methodology).

COMMENT 2: Do not confuse with the *methods** themselves.

See also *method, protocol, procedure.*

MINIMUM DETECTABLE LEVEL: See **Detection Limit**

MODAL DISTRIBUTION: Syn: unimodal distribution Distribution presenting only one mode or one region of high frequency of observations.

See also *mode* (Figure M1).

MODE: Given a discrete variable distribution, it is the most frequent value of a random variable.

COMMENT 1: When the *variable** is continuous, one can only define the mode class that corresponds to the maximal *frequency** (Figure M2).

COMMENT 2: Given a unimodal symmetrical *distribution** (for example, *normal distribution**), the mode, mean, and *median** are the same (Figure M1). This is not the case when the distribution is asymmetrical (Figure M1).

COMMENT 3: A distribution may have one or more modes (*modal, bimodal,* or multimodal *distribution**).

See also *median, sample mean.*

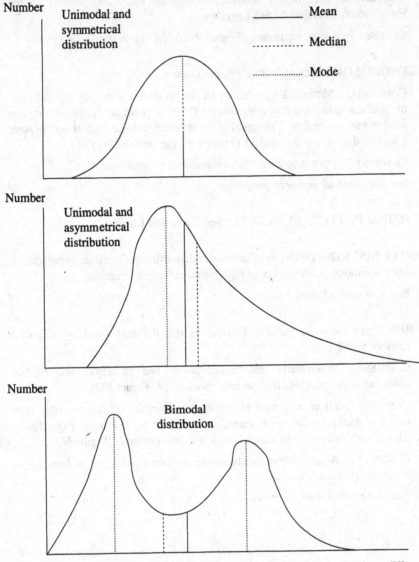

FIGURE M1. Schematic representation of the mean, median, and mode given different distributions.

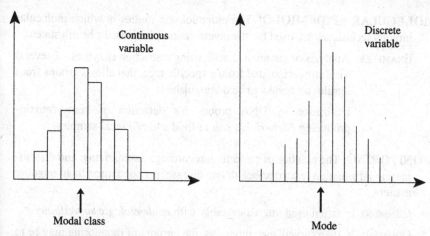

FIGURE M2.   Schematic representation of the modal class (continuous variable) and of the mode (discrete variable).

MODEL: Definition 1: Statistical and mathematical models are summarizations or representations used to recognize patterns in data that are not obviously apparent.

EXAMPLE 1: Linear or log-linear models (See also *mathematical model**).

Definition 2: Biologic models employ animals (or their components) as a sub-stitute for humans in research.

EXAMPLE 2: Use of mice to model human diseases.

Definition 3: An aggregation of individuals (not necessarily a random sam-ple) under study that is used for extrapolating results to a population.

EXAMPLE 3: Use of canine rabies vaccination in a model community can be used to judge the efficacy of mass canine vaccination in a rabies *endemic** county.

COMMENT: One can classify models according to their formalism (mathemat-ical, nonmathematical), but also according to their purpose. One then speaks of descriptive, explanatory, or predictive models.

MODEL ERROR: Error occurring when using an inappropriate model to test one or more hypotheses.

COMMENT 1: The resulting lack of fit will produce wrong estimates of the *alpha* and *beta errors,** which will often lead to improper conclusions. This is an *error** due to the inappropriateness of the test rather than due to *sampling.**

COMMENT 2: Such an error is sometimes referred to as a type 3 (not to be con-fused with *gamma error**) or type 4 statistical error, due to a lack of under-standing of the problem at hand.

MOLECULAR EPIDEMIOLOGY: Epidemiologic studies in which molecular biology techniques are used for the investigation of disease or health states.

EXAMPLES: Analysis of the nucleic acid, using restriction enzymes, of several viral strains isolated from a specific area, that allows groups from similar outbreaks to be distinguished.

Utilization of DNA probes for detection of verocytotoxin-producing *Escherichia coli* in food and calf fecal samples.

MONITORING: The practice of collecting, recording, summarizing, and disseminating information related to health and disease in a population in an ongoing manner.

COMMENT 1: Often used interchangeably with *epidemiologic surveillance.**

COMMENT 2: Like surveillance programs, the purpose of monitoring may be to enumerate and describe the frequency of *disease** occurrences, to record changes in productivity, to evaluate disease-control programs, or to assess the temporal and spatial patterns of disease or the occurrence of new diseases. However, some authors claim that monitoring differs from surveillance in two aspects:

1. The number of diseases or events being observed. Monitoring would be the preferred expression when data are gathered for only one disease or one main outcome; surveillance being the terminology used when data are gathered for many different diseases or outcomes.
2. The population under study. Monitoring would be used when only one species is considered, whereas surveillance would be the favored expression when two or more species are investigated.

An exception to such a classification scheme is the use of the word monitoring in the title of the American national animal surveillance program known as *National Animal Health Monitoring System*. In this particular case, it was decided to avoid using the word surveillance because of its negative connotation (i.e., being watched by the government).

COMMENT 3: In large animal *populations,** several computer recording systems are available to support monitoring activities (e.g., PigCHAMP, Pig-Tales, Swine Graphics, DairyCHAMP, DAISY, etc.).

See also *epidemiologic surveillance*.

MONOFACTORIAL DISEASE: See **Monofactorial Etiology**

MONOFACTORIAL ETIOLOGY: Other spelling: **monofactorial aetiology** Syn: **unifactorial etiology, unifactorial disease, monofactorial disease** Expression used in reference to the concept of a single cause being responsible for a particular pathological condition.

EXAMPLES: Trauma producing a bruise.

A sudden intake of an excessive amount of nitrogenous nutrients is sufficient to provoke alkalosis in dairy cows.

The virus responsible for rabies.

MONOVARIATE: Syn: univariate Refers to a single variable from a sample of individuals taken from a population.

COMMENT 1: As opposed to *multivariate.* *

EXAMPLE: A monovariate *evaluation* * such as determining the average weight of *individuals* * in a *sample* * of a *population* *.

COMMENT 2: A simple linear regression ($y = ax + b$) or the comparison of average weights between males and females in the same population is considered a monovariate analysis by some *epidemiologists* * because only one independent variable is present. Others prefer the expression "bivariate analysis" because the dependent variable also needs to be measured.

MORBIDITY: 1) State of being diseased. 2) Frequency of diseased individuals.

COMMENT 1: Two definitions are provided because morbidity can be used either to express the fact that a morbid condition is present or in reference to the *incidence* * or *prevalence* * of clinical *cases* * observed in general or in *association* * with a particular condition within a *population* * (e.g., 8% of dogs in a kennel were affected with flea allergy dermatitis).

COMMENT 2: The second definition is the only one used in practice in *epidemiology.* * It corresponds to the number of disease cases observed in a population during a given period of time or at one point in time. It is often referred to as percentage of morbidity or *morbidity rate.* *

MORBIDITY RATE:

$$\frac{\text{Number of diseased individuals}}{\text{Population at risk}}$$ at a given time or during a given time period

EXAMPLE: The morbidity rate in a herd of calves was 40% between March and June (i.e., of 100 calves, 40 were sick).

COMMENT 1: This definition takes into consideration the common usage of this expression, where "time" is not necessarily an integral part of the denominator. In this context, the morbidity rate can be calculated using all *cases* * (*prevalence* *) and not only new cases (*incidence* *). However, to be more accurate, the morbidity rate for a given time period should include the number of individual-time in the denominator (see *animal-time* *). This calculation is very much higher than a *point prevalence,* * if one is investigating an acute condition.

COMMENT 2: Because the *disease* * of interest may be limited to, or more prevalent at, a certain age or stage of production, it is preferable to specify the *population at risk* * when reporting the morbidity rate. The unit of interest may also need to be defined. For example, in a farrowing operation, the morbidity rate due to transmissible gastroenteritis may be 90% of piglets among affected litters, but with only one-third of the litters being affected (litter morbidity rate of 33%).

See also *population at risk, rate.*

MORTALITY: Frequency of deaths.

COMMENT 1: It corresponds to the number of deaths in a *population** during a given time period. It is often expressed as the *mortality rate.**

COMMENT 2: Not to be confused with *lethality.**

COMMENT 3: Mortality is often used in composite expressions, such as overall or total mortality (mortality due to all causes of death in a population), differential mortality (difference in mortality between two or more groups), endogenous mortality (mortality due to an internal cause), and exogenous mortality (mortality due to a cause external to the subject).

MORTALITY DENSITY: See **Mortality Rate**

MORTALITY RATE: Syn: **mortality density** Number of deaths divided by the number of individual-time at risk in a defined group or population.

EXAMPLE: 1.3 per 10,000 dog-years was the mortality rate for skin cancer in a particular region.

COMMENT 1: In practice, percent mortality is often referred to as the mortality rate. For example, if 10 out of 100 calves present in a *herd** during the summer months died, one may say that the mortality rate was 10% during that period. As for any other *rates,** it is important to consider in the denominator only the animals at *risk** during the time period of interest.

COMMENT 2: Mortality rate should be distinguished from *case fatality rate.**

COMMENT 3: Death rate is considered synonymous with mortality rate. However, in veterinary medicine, "mortality rate" is more commonly used than "death rate." Also note that, for some authors, death rate is used only when referring to the total mortality rate for all *diseases** in a *population.**

MOVING AVERAGE: Syn: **rolling average** Technique used to remove some of the random variation in temporal patterns of disease occurrence or of any other variable plotted against time.

Example of calculation:

Month in 1993	% of litters with fostering events	4-month moving average
January	60	
February	35	58.25
March	70	53.75
April	68	57.5
May	42	
June	50	

$(60 + 35 + 70 + 68)/4 = 58.25 =$ moving average for March 1 (center point for the months of January to April, inclusively (Figure M3).

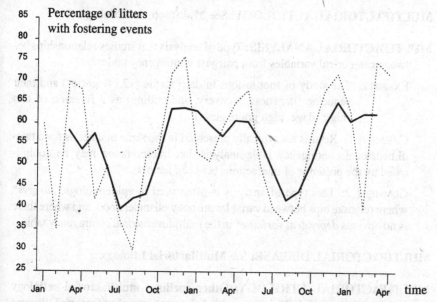

85 — Percentage of litters
80 — with fostering events
75
70
65
60
55
50
45
40
35
30
25

Jan   Apr   Jul   Oct   Jan   Apr   Jul   Oct   Jan   Apr   time

FIGURE M3.   Scatter plot of the percentage of pig litters from farm A with fostering events. Monthly information, January 1993 to April 1995. Dotted line, monthly data; solid line, 4-month moving average.

COMMENT 1: This allows a better visual identification of any underlying patterns.

COMMENT 2: Moving averages of 3 to 5 months are useful for investigating seasonal patterns; 15- to 25-month moving averages are recommended for cyclical patterns; and 34- to 40-month moving averages are used for long-term (secular) trends.

MULTIANNUAL VARIATION OF INCIDENCE: Biologically meaningful difference in the annual incidence of a disease over several years.

EXAMPLE: Multiannual cycle (probably 4 years) of fox rabies in Western Europe.

COMMENT: Many diseases have periodic cycles of 3 to 10 years in addition to their seasonal fluctuations of *incidence.**

MULTICENTER TRIAL: Syn: cooperative trial A trial in which several observers located in different sites participate, according to a common protocol, and by uniting their data to produce a collective report.

EXAMPLE: A rabies vaccine *trial** in dogs conducted at the four French veterinary schools.

COMMENT: *Observational studies** (*case–control,** *cohort,** *cross-sectional**) may also be performed in different locations, such as veterinary clinics and especially in large referral centers where rare *diseases** are more likely to be observed.

MULTIFACTORIAL AETIOLOGY: See **Multifactorial Etiology**

MULTIFACTORIAL ANALYSIS: Type of analysis that studies relationships between categorical variables from pairwise contingency tables.

EXAMPLE: The study of foot lesions in dairy cattle (12 categories) and their sequelae (lameness, recovery, and culling) as a function of diet (high silage, high grain, grass).

COMMENT 1: Results are typically presented in the same manner as for a two-dimensional contingency table analysis, but interpretation may be complicated by the presence of interactions between factors.

COMMENT 2: This type of analysis is often used in epidemiologic *surveys** where relationships between variables are not well understood, and where there is no obvious *dependent variable** in the multidimensional contingency table.

MULTIFACTORIAL DISEASE: See **Multifactorial Etiology**

MULTIFACTORIAL ETIOLOGY: Other spelling: **multifactorial aetiology** Syn: **multifactorial disease, multiple causation, plurifactorial disease (seldom used)** Expression used in reference to the concept of more than one cause being responsible for a given pathological condition.

COMMENT: Each *causal factor** participates in the *pathological** process, but only their combined action is responsible for the observed condition. The vast majority of *diseases** are considered to be multifactorial.

EXAMPLE: Mastitis may be caused by the *association** between microbes, poor milking and drying management, and a faulty milking machine.

MULTIPHASIC SCREENING: See **Multiple Screening**

MULTIPLE CAUSATION: See **Multifactorial Etiology**

MULTIPLE CHOICE QUESTION: See **Closed Question**

MULTIPLE CORRELATION COEFFICIENT: Coefficient measuring the maximum degree of linear relationship between one variable and a linear combination of a set of other variables.

COMMENT: To be differentiated from the *canonical correlation coefficient.**

MULTIPLE SCREENING: Syn: **multiphasic screening** Simultaneous examination of a population for more than one disease.

EXAMPLE: Blood or milk samples are concurrently collected in France for the screening for brucellosis and bovine viral leukosis.

See also *screening.*

MULTISTAGE SAMPLE: See **Multistage Sampling**

MULTISTAGE SAMPLING: Sampling that occurs in two or more distinct stages that are characterized by their hierarchical ordering.

EXAMPLE 1: Two-stage sampling: Within one county, *herds** (the primary units) are initially randomly selected (first stage), and animals (the secondary units) are then randomly selected within herds (second stage).

EXAMPLE 2: Three-stage sampling: As above, but certain counties are randomly selected within a state.

COMMENT: The *sample** obtained with this sampling strategy is referred to as a multistage sample.

MULTIVARIATE: A statistical analysis involving three or more variables.

COMMENT: Sometimes used in a more restricted sense to refer to more than one *dependent variable.**

MULTIVARIATE ANALYSIS: Analysis that allows the study of several variables simultaneously.

EXAMPLES: Factorial analysis, principal component analysis, clustering, discriminant analysis, manova, logistic regression.

COMMENT: Some methods are descriptive while others are inferential in nature (Tables M1 and M2).

TABLE M1. **Principal descriptive multivariate analytical methods**

One group of variables	
Continuous	Principal component analysis
	Hierarchical classification
Qualitative	Contingency table analysis
	Multifactorial analysis
	Hierarchical classification
Two groups of variables	Correlation analysis

TABLE M2. **Principal inferential multivariate analytical methods**

Method	Independent variables	Dependent variable
Multiple linear regression	n quantitative	1 quantitative
Logistic regression	n qualitative or quantitative	1 qualitative
Analysis of variance	n qualitative	1 quantitative
Discriminant analysis	n qualitative or quantitative	1 qualitative

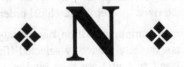

❖ N ❖

NATIVE CASE: See **Indigenous Case**

NATURAL ENVIRONMENT OF A DISEASE: See **Nidus**

NATURAL FOCUS OF A DISEASE: See **Nidus**

NATURAL HISTORY OF A DISEASE: Successive steps in the evolution (appearance or recognition, development or progression, disappearance) of a disease in a population, when there is no intervention.

COMMENT: Knowledge of the natural history of a disease is important to establish efficacious individual or collective intervention programs. However, in commercial animal production, intervention programs are usually already in place and *efficacy** is determined by comparing existing program(s) to alternative ones.

NATURAL NIDALITY: See **Nidality**

NEGATIVE PREDICTIVE VALUE (PV–): Probability that an individual found negative to a test is truly free of the disease or outcome of interest for which the test was performed.

COMMENT 1: In the contingency table included with the definition of *positive predictive value,** the negative predictive value is equal to $d/c + d$.

COMMENT 2: The negative predictive value depends on the two intrinsic *characteristics** of the test (*sensitivity,** *specificity**), and also on the *prevalence** of truly affected individuals. The relationships of PV– to sensitivity (SENS), specificity (SPEC), and prevalence (P) are expressed in the following equation:

$$PV– = SPEC \times (1 – P)/[SPEC \times (1 – P) + (1 – SENS) \times P]$$

Hence, when prevalence decreases, the PV– increases and when it increases, the PV– decreases (see Figure P7).

EXAMPLE: In the example presented for the positive predictive value, the negative predictive value for a prevalence of 20% is 96.2% (7600/7700) and for a prevalence of 1% is 99.95% (9405/9410).

COMMENT 3: A frequent error is to refer to a lack of sensitivity when negative test results are confirmed a posteriori to be false, using the equation $c/(c + d)$. This, in fact, is simply the complement of the negative predictive value $(1 – PV–)$, which has nothing to do with sensitivity: $a/(a + c)$.

COMMENT 4: The factors affecting the predictive value of a negative test used at the herd or flock level (assessment of groups of individuals) are somewhat similar to those at the individual level. However, the elements in the equation are group level information:

$$HPV- = \frac{(1-HTP) \times HSPEC}{(1-HTP) \times HSPEC + HTP \times (1-HSENS)}$$

Where HPV– is the herd negative predictive value, HTP is the true prevalence of affected herds, HSENS is the herd sensitivity of the test, and HSPEC is the herd specificity. Therefore, factors affecting HSENS and HSPEC must also be taken into account. Hence, assuming the test in the example above is used at the population level (individual sensitivity and specificity of 0.95), and that 10 individuals are tested in herds with 30% of the animals diseased, the HSENS and HSPEC would be 98% and 60%, respectively, if one reactor is considered sufficient to indicate the presence of disease. Given an HTP of 40%, the HPV– would be 0.978 or 97.8%, but for an HTP of 5%, the HPV– would be 0.998 or 99.8%.

See also *sensitivity, specificity, positive predictive value.*

NEONATAL DISEASE: Disease occurring within a few days following birth.

COMMENT 1: The period at risk varies depending on the species. For example, in humans, it is 28 days; in cattle, 7 to 21 days; in swine, 3 to 7 days; and in poultry, 1 to 10 days. These numbers tend to vary depending on the author reporting the information.

COMMENT 2: To be differentiated from *congenital disease,** which begins in utero and is observed at birth.

NEONATAL MORTALITY: Mortality among liveborns occurring within a few days following birth (postpartum deaths).

EXAMPLES: Mortality occurring during the first 24 hours after hatching in chickens. Mortality among piglets during the first 3 days of life.

COMMENT 1: The number of days the animals are considered at *risk** varies with the species and, at times, with herd management. For example, in pigs, it is often limited to 3 days because this corresponds to the most critical period in terms of survival. With the advent of medicated early weaning, some may consider the first 10 days to 2 weeks of life. Normally, mortality occurring between birth and weaning would be referred to as preweaning mortality, which may also include *stillbirths.**

COMMENT 2: Not to be confused with stillbirth.

COMMENT 3: In many animal production units, neonatal mortality is one of the principal determinants of herd productivity and profitability. The following are three major categories of neonatal mortality:

Low viability: Animals unable to survive under standard husbandry conditions because they are born weak and/or undersized.

Trauma: Lethal internal and/or external injuries, often inflicted by the dam.

Scours: Death from infections of the alimentary tract.

See also *neonatal mortality rate.*

NEONATAL MORTALITY RATE:

$$\frac{\text{Number of deaths occurring in a population within a few days following birth}}{\text{Total number of individuals born alive in this population}} \quad \text{over a given period of time}$$

COMMENT 1: This *rate** is usually expressed as a percentage. The period after birth is mainly defined according to each species.

COMMENT 2: To be differentiated from *perinatal mortality rate.**

See also *rate, neonatal disease.*

NESTED CASE–CONTROL STUDY: Case–control study performed in the context of a concurrent longitudinal study.

EXAMPLE: While conducting a *prospective study,** researchers may observe a rare outcome (e.g., a rare form of cancer). Because of the limited number of cases, researchers may elect to investigate further by selecting a *control group** among the individuals monitored prospectively. They can then go retrospectively (looking for additional *risk factors** not included in the prospective study), focusing on a limited number of *cases** and controls.

See also *case–control study.*

NET INCOME: The profit (or loss) of a business that appears on the income statement.

COMMENT: *Profits** in the form of net income may be distributed as dividends or contribute to owners' equity as retained earnings.

See also *income statement, profit.*

NET PRESENT VALUE (NPV): The present value of future returns minus the present value of the cost of the investment.

$$NPV = \sum_{t=1}^{t=n} \frac{A_t - C_t}{(1+r)^t}$$

Where A = total returns over a 1-year period
C = total costs over a 1-year period
n = number of years
t = 1 year
r = discount rate expressed as a decimal fraction

$$\sum_{t=1}^{t=n} : \text{sum of all } \frac{A_t - C_t}{(1+r)^t} \text{ for each value of } t, \text{ from } t = 1 \text{ to } t = n$$

COMMENT 1: Used as a method for ranking *investment** proposals.

COMMENT 2: An NPV > 0 indicates that a project may be profitable.

COMMENT 3: Calculating NPV often involves highly subjective assessments (i.e., future *interest rates**). Hence, simpler calculations, such as *payback period,** are used.

See also *present value, payback period, internal rate of return.*

NET WORTH: Assets minus liabilities.

COMMENT 1: Also known as owners' equity.

COMMENT 2: Calculated from a *balance sheet.**

COMMENT 3: On a cost value balance sheet, the net worth figure reflects retained earnings and *contributed capital.**

COMMENT 4: On a market value balance sheet, the net worth provides an *estimate** of what would be left if the business was liquidated.

See also *balance sheet, contributed capital.*

NEW CASE: See Incident Case

NIDALITY: Syn: natural nidality Process by which a pathogen can persist in well-defined nidi associated with specific climatic, geographic, and ecological conditions.

EXAMPLE: Nidality of plague in Iran.

COMMENT 1: For some pathogens, certain regions offer climatic and ecological conditions favorable to one or more species acting as *reservoir** or *vector.** *Disease** occurrence may then be dependent on the availability of these reservoirs or vectors (which may result in long interepidemic periods). For example, Rocky Mountain spotted fever, a rickettsial disease of rodents transmitted by ticks, is limited to specific areas of North America.

COMMENT 2: Nidality is not an English word. It was introduced by the Russian Pavlovsky in the late 1950s. The theory born from the concept of nidality is regarded as the first precondition of landscape *epidemiology,** also known as medical *ecology.** Although the concept of nidality is valid, this word has rarely been used in the English medical literature over the past 15 years.

See also *nidus.*

NIDUS (OF A DISEASE) (Plural: nidi): Syn: focus of a disease, natural focus of a disease, natural environment of a disease, nosogenic territory Geographical location where the environment offers favorable conditions leading to the occurrence, maintenance, and propagation of a disease.

EXAMPLE: Nidi of plague in Iran.

COMMENT 1: The nidus of a disease represents any area where the *disease**
can be found, as well as any area where the disease may not be apparent, but
where the essential environmental conditions exist for this disease to occur.

COMMENT 2: Nidus is also commonly used in medicine to refer to the focus of
a morbid process in an individual (e.g., a urolith; bacterial growth in a particular tissue or organ, known as a nidus of *infection**).

See also *nidality, nosoarea.*

NONCOMMUNICABLE DISEASE: Syn: nontransmissible disease Disease
whose cause(s) cannot pass or be carried from one animal to another directly
or indirectly.

EXAMPLES: Milk fever, fractures, tetanus.

COMMENT: Conditions other than almost all *infectious diseases** and those
resulting from *infestations** or genetic transmission are considered noncommunicable.

NONCURRENT ASSETS: Assets that are used to operate the business.

EXAMPLE: Buildings, equipment, machinery, automobiles, breeding livestock,
and land are examples of noncurrent assets.

NONPARAMETRIC ANALYSIS: Syn: free distribution analysis Method of
statistical analysis that does not require specification of an underlying sampling process that generates a statistical distribution.

EXAMPLES: Mann–Whitney test, chi-square test, Kruskal–Wallis test.

NONPARAMETRIC TEST: Statistical test that does not assume a specific form
for the distribution function of the variable.

COMMENT 1: As opposed to *parametric test.**

COMMENT 2: In general, each parametric test corresponds to a nonparametric
test; the latter being, most often, less powerful.

COMMENT 3: These tests are often used when the *sample size** is small or the
density function of the *variable** has an unusual shape.

NONRANDOM SAMPLE: See **Haphazard Sample**

NONRESPONDENT: Syn: nonresponder Individual included in a survey who
does not participate.

COMMENT 1: The vast majority of nonrespondents are individuals who elect
not to participate (also labeled nonparticipants). The reasons associated with
this refusal can be quite diverse. Common reasons are concerns over confiden-
tiality, lack of interest in the *study** or the problem being investigated, perceived lack of value of the study, and assumption that an adequate feedback (results of study) will not be provided. Some individuals labeled nonrespondent
may, in fact, be people who were never contacted (i.e., *questionnaire** sent to

the wrong address and not returned). Although the researcher may request return of the questionnaire from people who elect not to participate (questionnaire returned but not filled out), people do not always follow instructions.

COMMENT 2: Nonrespondents may differ from respondents, which could introduce a *bias** in the study. For example, in a study on farrowing-to-conception interval in swine, nonrespondents may be less likely to use a computerized recording system than respondents. Therefore, it is advisable to identify some characteristics of nonrespondents in order to compare them to respondents.

NONRESPONDER: See Nonrespondent

NONRESPONSE: Missing answer to a questionnaire, either partial (one or more questions unanswered) or total (no reply to the entire questionnaire).

> EXAMPLES: In a mail *questionnaire,** a short *question** following a long one at the bottom of a page was missed by 7% of respondents.
>
> In a *survey** of swine producers in Minnesota, several respondents declined to answer financial questions related to their operation.

COMMENT 1: Nonresponses may introduce a *bias** if their occurrence is dependent on one or several *characteristics** of respondents and *nonrespondents.**

COMMENT 2: Good questionnaire design tends to minimize nonresponse. Good follow-up will reduce the percentage of questionnaires not returned (hence, increases the *response rate**).

NONTRANSMISSIBLE DISEASE: See Noncommunicable Disease

NORMAL DISTRIBUTION: Syn: Laplace–Gauss distribution, Gaussian distribution. Probability distribution of a continuous variable, represented by a modal and symmetrical curve (Figure N1).

The density function for the normal distribution of the *variable** x is:

$$f(x) = \frac{1}{\sqrt{2\pi}\sigma} e^{-(x-\mu)^2/2\sigma^2}, -\infty < x < \infty$$

where π and e are the constants 3.14159 and 2.71828 (these are approximations), respectively; the two *parameters** of the distribution are μ, the mean, and σ, the *standard deviation.**

COMMENT 1: The properties of a normal distribution are:

- It is a continuous distribution, symmetrical, with the two extremities spreading to infinity;
- The arithmetic mean, the mode, and the median are identical;
- 95.44% of the values of the variable are included in the interval between the mean ± two standard deviations;
- Its shape is completely determined by the mean and the standard deviation. Different values of μ shift the curve along the x-axis and different values of σ determine the degree of flatness or peakedness of the graph of the distribution.

COMMENT 2: When the mean is equal to zero and the standard deviation equals 1, it is known as the unit normal or standard normal distribution.

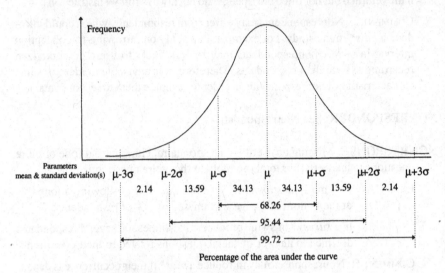

FIGURE N1. Example of a normal distribution.

NOSOAREA: Region where a particular disease is present.

COMMENT: This expression is seldom used in English.

See also *nidus*.

NOSOCOMIAL: Pertaining to or originating in a hospital or clinic.

EXAMPLES: Multiresistant staphylococcus infection contracted during hospitalization.

Salmonellosis in a horse acquired following surgery in a veterinary hospital.

COMMENT: Term used in association with *disease** or *infection.** It should be differentiated from *iatrogenic.**

See also *iatrogenic*.

NOSOGENIC TERRITORY: See Nidus

NOTIFIABLE DISEASE: Syn: reportable disease Disease required to be reported to federal, state, or local health officials when diagnosed, and whose detection may trigger a set of disease-control measures as defined by government authorities.

EXAMPLES: Foot-and-mouth disease, rinderpest, African swine fever, rabies, brucellosis, hog cholera, and tuberculosis are examples of notifiable diseases in countries of the European community and in North America.

COMMENT 1: Most countries have two lists of notifiable diseases, one for human and one for animal *diseases*.*

COMMENT 2: A disease may be notifiable even if absent from an area, if its introduction could be damaging to the *health** of animals or to the economy of the country, in particular via trade restrictions. It may also be notifiable if it is a zoonotic disease or if a control program is in place within a defined area.

COMMENT 3: Notifiable diseases are often, but not always, *contagious*.* For example, anthrax is *infectious*,* but noncontagious; equine encephalomyelitis, bluetongue, and African horse sickness are arboviral diseases, and consequently, although they are transmissible, they are not contagious.

NOTIFICATION RATE:

$$\frac{\text{Number of declared cases or outbreaks}}{\text{Number of identified cases or outbreaks}} \text{ during a given time period}$$

COMMENT 1: This expression is rarely used in veterinary *epidemiology*.* It is largely limited to government functions related to *notifiable diseases*.* The notification rate of such diseases is quite variable; it is sometimes very low (around 2%) for both human and animal *diseases*.* Several factors may explain the underreporting of animal diseases. The most frequent factors are the perception that the disease is not a serious one, the lack of appropriate information, distrust of governmental authorities, and the shortage (or limited amount) of compensation funds or of any other incentives.

COMMENT 2: Note that the denominator is limited to identified *cases** or *outbreaks*,* which only approximate, at best, the actual number of such events.

See also *rate*.

NULL HYPOTHESIS (H₀): The original or current hypothesis one wishes to test statistically by using observed data to either refute or not refute the hypothesis.

EXAMPLE: In a clinical trial in which one wants to show the *efficacy** of a treatment (A) as compared to a placebo (B), the null hypothesis of identical treatments is:

$$H_0: A = B \text{ (same effect)}$$

The *alternative hypothesis** is:

$$H_1: A > B \text{ the effect of A is superior to B.}$$

COMMENT 1: The null hypothesis is often labeled H_0. The alternative hypothesis (labeled H_1) in the example above postulates that there is a significant difference between *groups** which chance alone cannot explain, or at least within a given *error** level. The null hypothesis does not have to be one of no difference.

COMMENT 2: The possible conclusions of a statistical test are:

- To fail to reject the null hypothesis (we have not been able to show significant differences based on the observations and with the specified power).

or

- To reject the null hypothesis (with some risk of error) in favor of the alternative hypothesis.

NYCTEROHEMERAL: See **Nyctohemeral**

NYCTOHEMERAL: Syn: Nycterohemeral Pertaining to the day-and-night cycle.

COMMENT: To be differentiated from *circadian**, which refers to a 24-hour cycle.

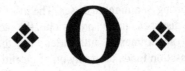

OBJECTIVE: Expected result of an action.

COMMENT 1: Objectives should not be stated in terms of activities (for example, to perform a serology test), but only in terms of results (the *herd* infection* rate** must be decreased by 5%).

COMMENT 2: In business, the acronym SMART is often used to describe the qualities of good objectives. SMART objectives are:

Specific: Focusing on a particular topic or issue; yet, the objective should be strategically coherent with the main goal(s).

Measurable: Can be quantified or assessed.

Achievable: Realistic. Allows a range of variation in the expected outcome; this criterion takes into account fluctuations due to measurement errors. Outside this range, the result might be considered as a failure or a success. Adequate funding is another important consideration.

Result oriented: The achievement of different objectives is verified by comparing observed results with the planned objectives.

Time limited: There is a clear and acceptable time frame considered to reach the objective.

EXAMPLE 1: An objective could be to bring a herd infection rate down to 5% in 3 years.

COMMENT 3: The term *objective* should be reserved for precise statements conforming to the above criteria. The word goal should be used in reference to broader end points, such as the eradication of a disease. SMART objectives are objectives designed to reach goals. For example, improving the entry-to-service interval in a swine operation is one objective leading to the producer's goal: increased profitability.

EXAMPLE 2: A *descriptive* epidemiologic *study** is conducted to "determine the importance of a disease." Objectives are to measure herd infection rate, infection rate within infected herds, and to evaluate the corresponding costs of infection. This action is driven in such a way as to be able to assess the appropriateness of a possible intervention decision.

COMMENT 4: In epidemiology, objectives can be categorized as:

• Descriptive: Aiming at determining the frequency and distribution of a *health factor** or condition.
• Explanatory: Aiming at detecting or characterizing the relationship between *risk factors** and a *health** or *disease** condition.
• Operational: Aiming at modifying the health status of a *population.**

OBSERVATION: See **Entry**

OBSERVATIONAL STUDY: Epidemiologic investigation characterized by the absence of manipulation of the study factor by the investigator.

EXAMPLES: Descriptive study; case–control study; cohort study (Figure O1).

COMMENT 1: Observational studies may be *descriptive** or *analytical.** The feature that distinguishes *experimental studies** from observational studies is the assignment of subjects to treatments or *groups.** For both *experiments** and clinical *trials,** the assignment of subjects to treatment groups is done by the investigator. In observational studies, subjects are usually grouped based on their attributes and the investigator cannot control the timing of exposure of these subjects to the factor(s) of interest, nor can he or she choose the conditions under which such exposure occurs (time, intensity, etc.).

COMMENT 2: One major limitation of observational studies results from the limited control the investigator has over the study situation, making these types of studies more susceptible to distortion. Given the potential sources of *error** and *bias,** the analysis stage of these studies is particularly critical.

See also *analytical study, descriptive study, trial, experiment.*

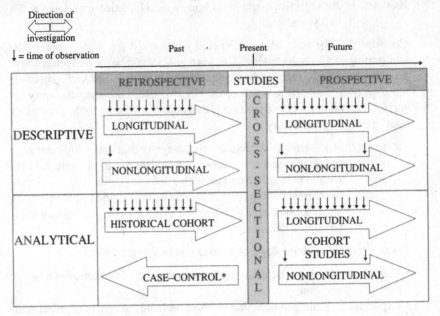

FIGURE O1.   Different types of observational studies.

* The observation periods or times for case–control studies varies. One period of observation corresponds to the identification and selection of cases and controls. The time or period observed (retrospectively) for the assessment of risk factors may be a specific point or period in the past, or, in practice, it may be the current exposure status of cases and controls at the time of their selection.

OCCUPATIONAL HEALTH: Aspect of environmental health concerned with people's working environment.

EXAMPLES: Salmonella *infection** in abattoir workers and chronic bronchitis in postal workers exposed to varying levels of air pollution are considered occupational *diseases.**

COMMENT: An important part of this domain involves the description and analysis of the relationship between chronic diseases and toxic components present at, or around, the work area. It is a domain of intervention in *public health.**

OCCURRENCE: An incident or event.

EXAMPLE: The international registry of animal *diseases** compiles occurrences.

COMMENT: When an occurrence or event is recorded, it is an *entry** in a *recording** system.

See also *entry, recording.*

ODDS: Ratio of the probability of occurrence of an event to that of nonoccurrence.

Given an event E with probability p (with $0 \leq p \leq 1$); the probability of nonoccurrence is $(1 - p)$. Hence, the odds in favor of E are $p/(1 - p)$.

EXAMPLE: The prevalence rate of a disease D in a given population is 20%. Therefore, the odds in favor of this disease are: $0.2/(1 - 0.2) = 0.25$.

COMMENT: The capital Greek letter omega (Ω) is usually used to designate the odds in favor of an event. Using the known symbols for a two-by-two table:

		Disease		
		D+	D–	Total
Test	+	a	b	a+b
	–	c	d	c+d
	Total	n_1	n_2	N

Odds in favor of D+ = $\Omega = n_1/n_2$, and odds in favor of D– = $n_2/n_1 = 1/\Omega$.
See also *odds ratio*.

ODDS RATIO (O.R.): Syn: cross-product ratio Ratio of two odds.

COMMENT 1: Consider a two-by-two table where π_{ij} is the joint probability for the cell in row I and column J. Then, the odds ratio is: $(\pi_{11}/\pi_{12})/(\pi_{21}/\pi_{22}) = (\pi_{11}\pi_{22}/\pi_{12}\pi_{21})$.

COMMENT 2: In practice, odds ratios are calculated using sample cell frequencies from a two-by-two table. If n_{ij} is the number of observations in row I and column J, then the sample version of the odds ratio is: $(n_{11}n_{22}/n_{12}n_{21})$.

EXAMPLE: Based on the table presented with the definition of *odds*,* the odds ratio for the *disease*,* depending on the result of the diagnostic test, would be (a/b)/(c/d) or ad/bc.

COMMENT 3: The odds ratio is equal to the *ratio** of two likelihoods: $\Omega =$ L1/L2. It is a measure of the quality of a diagnostic test and it is independent from the *population** size N and from the disease *prevalence.**

COMMENT 4: In *epidemiologic studies,** the odds ratio measures the intensity or the degree of *association** between a *risk factor** and an outcome. The degree of association increases as the odds ratio increases.

COMMENT 5: The odds ratio is a measure of the intensity of the relationship between a risk factor and an outcome that is not dependent on the type of *study.** Indeed, the odds ratio can be estimated in *case–control studies,** cohort studies,** and *cross-sectional studies.** On the other hand, the *relative risk** can only be estimated in cohort studies or cross-sectional studies.

COMMENT 6: In cases where the outcome (e.g., disease) is rare, the value of the odds ratio is close to the value of the relative risk (Table O1). Hence, when this occurs in a case–control study, the odds ratio is considered a good *estimate** of the relative risk.

COMMENT 7: When *controls** from a case–control study are representative of the population free of the outcome of interest, and when this population is considered stable at the time of the selection of *cases,** then the calculated odds ratio is equal to the relative risk.

TABLE O1. Odds ratio values depending on disease prevalence and relative risk.

Disease prevalence	Relative risk	
	RR=2	RR=10
10^{-3}	2.00	10.05
10^{-2}	2.02	10.50
10^{-1}	2.22	20.00

OFFENSIVE PROPHYLAXIS: Translation of a French expression referring to prophylaxis applied in an environment where the disease or infection of interest already exists.

Terminology not used in English. Equivalent: Prevention program in a diseased area.

COMMENT: It is an application of *secondary* or *tertiary prevention.**

See also *defensive prophylaxis.*

ONE-SIDED TEST: Syn: unilateral test Statistical test in which the null hypothesis is rejected when values of the test statistic are more extreme than the critical value of the test.

EXAMPLE: We want to compare the *rate** of *infection** of *herds** before and after the start of a disease *prevention** program. A priori, the second rate of infection should be smaller than the first, suggesting the use of a one-sided test.

COMMENT: The use of a one-sided test instead of a *two-sided test** leads to a gain in *power,** in the sense that the number of subjects needed to attain a given power is smaller for a one-sided test than for a two-sided test.

See also *statistical test, two-sided test.*

ONE-STAGE SAMPLING: Sampling that arises in one stage, leading to a simple sample.

EXAMPLE: Random selection of bulk milk samples arriving at a laboratory on a given day.

OPEN-ENDED QUESTION: Question that allows the respondent to answer freely in his or her own words.

EXAMPLE 1: How many cows do you have in your herd?

EXAMPLE 2: In the context of a questionnaire sent to dog owners, the following question was asked:

What behavior(s) are you concerned about?

COMMENT 1: As opposed to *closed question.* * Open-ended questions are valuable when a continuous variable response is expected. It allows unanticipated responses and relieves the tedium of too many closed questions (example 2).

COMMENT 2: Coding is often difficult and can be a source of error. Underreporting of an event is more likely as people often forget unless prompted.

COMMENT 3: This type of question is not recommended when the level of education of respondents is considered low.

See also *closed question.*

OPEN TRIAL: Syn: before and after trial Trial including only one group in which the comparison focuses on the state of individuals before and after the intervention.

COMMENT 1: This method differs from other trials by the absence of a *control* * group (Figure T3, *trial* *).

COMMENT 2: In some instances, researchers compare results of this trial with prior results obtained from another population (historical control), though it is often difficult to guarantee the *comparability* * of these two *populations.* *

COMMENT 3: Care must be taken in interpretation of these studies because of a phenomenon called *"regression* * to the mean." When repeated *measures* * are taken on the same group at two different times, extreme values tend to get closer to the mean. This could lead to erroneous conclusions regarding the variability of the measure or the factor studied.

OPERATING CHARACTERISTIC RATIO (OCR): Quotient of the frequencies of the results of a test in diseased and nondiseased individuals.

$$OCR = \frac{\text{Probability of the result of a test for individuals affected by a given disease}}{\text{Probability of the same test result for nonaffected individuals}}$$

When a test can provide either a positive or a negative result, two OCRs are possible: one positive (OCR+) and one negative (OCR–).

OCR+ = Se/(1 – Sp) = (1 – beta)/alpha

OCR– = (1 – Se)/Sp = beta /(1 – alpha)

Where Sp = specificity
Se = sensitivity
alpha = false positive risk
beta = false negative risk

COMMENT: The positive OCR can vary from 0 when the sensitivity is null, to infinity when the specificity tends to 1. The negative OCR is null when the sensitivity is 1; it is equal to beta when the test is completely specific. An

OCR+ of 3 means that the positive result of the test is three times more frequent in diseased that in nondiseased individuals.

See also *receiver operating characteristic curve.*

OPERATING COST: Expression considered synonymous to total production cost; although in North America, it is often used as synonymous with variable cost only.

See also *total production cost, variable cost.*

OPERATIONAL EPIDEMIOLOGY: Use of epidemiologic methods to study specific health problems that include a decision-making process seeking the optimal result for the control of these problems.

EXAMPLE: *Study** concluding in the choice of a *disease** control strategy in a given region.

COMMENT 1: The type of intervention chosen refers to three alternative *prevention** strategies: primary, secondary, and tertiary.

COMMENT 2: Epidemiologic research conducted at this level has also been referred to as pragmatic or action oriented. It is the *epidemiology** of intervention as opposed to the epidemiology of knowledge. These two levels of epidemiology involve fundamentally different interests, research strategies, and *hypotheses.** Consequently, researchers operating at different levels may respond to the same body of empirical evidence in very different ways.

See also *primary prevention, secondary prevention, tertiary prevention.*

OPPORTUNISTIC AGENT: A microorganism that does not ordinarily cause disease but becomes pathogenic under certain circumstances.

EXAMPLE: *Pathogenic** action of some bacteria, such as *Bordetella bronchiseptica* after viral pulmonary infection.

COMMENT 1: Most frequent circumstances favoring an opportunistic agent:

• An impaired immune system resulting from other *disease** or drug treatment.
• Weakening of anatomical barriers (nonspecific immunity) due to environmental challenges (cuts, dust, major temperature variations, etc.).

COMMENT 2: *Agents,** such as *Pasteurella multocida,* may be opportunistic only in a selected number of animal species and under specific circumstances.

OPPORTUNISTIC VECTOR: A vector responsible for transmitting a pathogen in an accidental manner.

EXAMPLES: Broad sense: cat and tularemia.
Strict interpretation: fly and blackleg (*Clostridium chauvoei*).

OPPORTUNITY COST: Value of the best alternative that must be forgone when an action is taken.

EXAMPLES: A farmer has the option of selling a ton of home-grown corn or feeding it to his livestock. The opportunity cost of feeding the corn to his livestock is the expected *market price*,* net of the transport and marketing *costs** required to complete the sale.

A self-employed small animal veterinarian makes a *profit** of $45,000 a year but pays himself/herself no wage; this person needs to consider alternative uses of his/her time. For example, this veterinarian could be making $65,000 a year working for a pet food company as a member of its technical service division. This is the opportunity cost of this person's time. Of course, other factors, such as the intangible benefits of self-employment, would play a significant role in this case.

COMMENT: This is considered the true cost of an action or decision (e.g., production of a product). It includes the *benefits** lost by not employing a resource in the most profitable alternative way.

See also *cost*.

OR: See **Odds Ratio**

ORDINAL VARIABLE: Variable classified into ordered qualitative categories.

COMMENT: A numerical value may be associated with each category (see example). These categories have a distinct order, but no numerical distance exists between them. Hence, for the example below, category 4 represents a higher frequency than 2, but it does not mean that 4 is twice as frequent as 2.

EXAMPLE: Presence of coughing in a swine unit:
1. never
2. sometimes
3. often
4. very often

See also *attribute*.

OUTBREAK: The confirmed presence of disease, clinically expressed or not, in at least one individual in a defined location and during a specified period of time.

COMMENT 1: An outbreak is closely circumscribed to an *epidemiologic unit*.* Although an outbreak may be limited to one *case,** the term often implies that several *individuals** are affected. In fact, in some animal production operations, such as poultry, an outbreak may encompass several thousand cases. Like *epidemic,** outbreak conveys a certain sense of unexpectedness or, at least, a sense that a certain threshold has been reached. For example, a few pigs out of 2000 housed in a grow–finish operation have atrophic rhinitis. One would report that a few cases of this disease are present in this herd (assuming it is *endemic** in the area). However, if 200 cases were observed, it would certainly be referred to as an outbreak.

Some authors use outbreak and epidemic interchangeably. This practice is quite current in lay publications and in everyday conversations.

COMMENT 2: The grouping of several individual cases under one single outbreak is sometimes arbitrary. For example, cases of kennel cough occurring over a short period of time in dogs that can be *traced back** to the same canine boarding house can logically be considered as part of the same outbreak (same source of *contamination**). However, it would be more difficult to reach the same conclusion if cases were more spread out in time and location, and if no exposure factor linked them in any meaningful way.

COMMENT 3: It is sometimes difficult to pinpoint the exact boundaries of an outbreak in space and time. The World Organization for Animal Health (OIE) defines an outbreak as the "occurrence of *disease** in an agricultural establishment, breeding establishment or premises, including all buildings as well as adjoining premises, where animals are present." Although this definition is limited to food animals, it could well be adapted to other domesticated animals. For nomadic herds, the OIE proposes to count as one outbreak all cases of disease occurring within a 50 km^2 area. The geographical distribution of an outbreak may also be defined based on ownership. For example, an outbreak of atrophic rhinitis in pigs could include animals housed in several buildings (belonging to the same owner) spread out in different locations.

In terms of time, recurrence of disease within a *herd** can be considered as a new outbreak if the time between the first and the second occurrence of disease exceeds the maximum incubation period. However, this guideline is not very useful for infections with long *latency periods.** In this situation, one may have to establish arbitrarily disease-specific criteria (e.g., salmonellosis in Great Britain).

See also *epidemic, epidemiologic unit.*

OUTCOME: See **Dependent Variable**

OVERHEAD: See **Fixed Cost**

OVERMATCHING: Matching comparison groups, usually in a case–control study, on the level of one or more factors that is unnecessary, counterproductive, or statistically/economically inefficient.

EXAMPLE 1: Matching on a factor that is not associated with exposure and, hence, is not a *confounder.**

EXAMPLE 2: Matching on a factor that is not an independent determinant of the *health** outcome and, hence, is not a confounder.

EXAMPLE 3: Matching on a factor that is associated with exposure but is not a confounder and, hence, introduces confounding.

COMMENT: Definitions of overmatching that claim that it leads to the creation of *case** and *control groups** that are too similar to be compared for valid results are incorrect. They fail to take into account the fact that unbiased effect measure *estimates** can be obtained after *adjustment,** which is required in all matched case–control analyses.

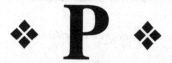

❖ P ❖

PANDEMIC: Disease that propagates over long distances, through several continents, and that affects a considerable portion of the human population (pandemic disease).

EXAMPLE: The flu (influenza).

COMMENT: In North America, pandemic is also used in reference to animal diseases (see *panzootic**).

PANEL: Representative sample of a population normally questioned on a regular basis over a certain period of time (in sociological and marketing studies).

EXAMPLES: Panels used by consumer groups in their assessment of new products or new regulations.

In France, a panel of veterinarians is used to survey the profession on a regular basis on issues related to their professional activities.

COMMENT: Panels are frequently used in research and development of food products and, occasionally, with regards to issues of *food safety.**

PANZOOTIC: Disease that propagates over long distances, through several continents, and that affects an important part of an animal population (panzootic disease).

EXAMPLE: Newcastle disease in chickens.

COMMENT: *Pandemic** may also be used for animal *diseases.**

PARAMETER: A constant that characterizes a mathematical model; when this model is used to represent an animal population, it becomes a characteristic of that population.

EXAMPLES: In the equation a + bx, a and b are parameters and x symbolizes a measured *variable.**

The mean μ and *variance** σ^2 are parameters of the *gaussian (normal) distribution** (Greek letters usually denote parameters). For example, given that milk production is normally distributed, it is characterized by these two parameters.

COMMENT: In practice, for example, one does not know the mean and variance or *standard deviation** of a given *population** when it is very large. These values are then estimated from a representative *sample** of the population. They are called *estimators** and are labeled *m*, *s²*, and *s*, respectively.

Estimators are not considered constant because their values depend on *sampling variation.* *

See also *estimator, estimate, normal distribution.*

PARAMETRIC ANALYSIS: Method of statistical analysis that assumes a sampling process generating a specific statistical distribution.

EXAMPLE: Parametric *analysis of variance** assumes that error terms in the linear *model** follow a standard normal distribution.

PARAMETRIC TEST: Statistical test that postulates a specific distribution function.

EXAMPLES: *Student's* t *test** and the *analysis of variance** that assume normality.

PARASITE: General meaning: Foreign organism that lives at the expense of a host.

In pathology: Foreign uni- or multicellular organism living at the expense of a host and whose life cycle comprises several stages completed with the same host or, sometimes, using several hosts.

EXAMPLES: Unicellular parasite (*Babesia equi*, agent of horse babesiosis); multicellular parasite (*Fasciola hepatica*).

COMMENT: The term parasite is normally associated with a net negative impact on the *host** (see host). The degree of association between an organism and its host will determine whether it is called a parasite, a *commensal,* * or a *symbiont.* *

PARATENIC HOST: See **Transport Host**

PARTIAL CORRELATION COEFFICIENT: A measure of the degree of linear relationship between two variables after adjusting for one or more other variables.

EXAMPLE: Adjusted correlation between weight and height controlling for age.

COMMENT 1: It is a corrected simple *correlation.* *

COMMENT 2: This coefficient is different from the coefficients obtained by *multiple regression.* *

PASSIVE CARRIER: See **Mechanical Carrier**

PASSIVE RESERVOIR: Reservoir ensuring the preservation of a pathogen without multiplication.

EXAMPLES: A barn *contaminated** with *Mycobacterium tuberculosis.*
A field contaminated with *Bacillus anthracis.*

COMMENT 1: The *effectiveness** of a passive reservoir is directly dependent on the survival capabilities of the pathogen.

COMMENT 2: "Passive" and "reservoir" are contradictory terms in the context of the definition of *reservoir,* * as given in this dictionary. However, the association of both words expresses best the concept defined above.

PASSIVE VECTOR: See Mechanical Vector

PATHOGEN: See Agent of Disease

PATHOGENESIS: The way a disease develops in an organism, organ, or tissue.

PATHOGENIC: That which produces disease.

See also *pathogenicity.*

PATHOGENICITY: The host-specific ability of an agent to cause disease or otherwise induce pathological change in a susceptible host.

COMMENT 1: Although pathogenicity is almost exclusively associated with infectious agents in the English literature, this word may also apply to noninfectious agents, as long as they are capable of inducing pathological change (e.g., asbestos is capable of causing malignant mesothelioma and is therefore a pathogen).

COMMENT 2: Pathogenicity is host specific; that is, an agent pathogenic to one genus or species of organism is not necessarily pathogenic to other organisms.

COMMENT 3: *Epidemiologists** quantify pathogenicity using different *rates** or *proportions:* *

• Degree of pathogenicity = Number sick/Number contaminated
• Degree of severity = Number of severe cases/Number sick
• *Case fatality rate.* *

COMMENT 4: Pathogenicity is commonly used as a synonym for *virulence.* * Although the two terms are often used interchangeably, they are not the same. However, there is no consensus in the medical community on the exact meaning of pathogenicity and virulence, or on how they should be measured.

See also *virulence.*

PATHOGNOMONIC: That which indicates an abnormality or abnormalities by which a specific disease or condition may be recognized.

EXAMPLE: Well-circumscribed dark and solid pneumonic areas with fibrinous pleurisy are considered pathognomonic lesions of the peracute form of porcine pleuropneumonia.

COMMENT: Very few diseases produce pathognonomic lesions or signs. However, when these are present, they greatly contribute to the *validity** of the *diagnosis.* *

PATHOLOGICAL: Syn: abnormal Pertaining to changes or abnormalities that a disease or condition produces in organs, tissues, or fluids.

COMMENT 1: The limit between normal and pathological can be difficult to define.

COMMENT 2: The changes can correspond to a clinical disease but also to a *subclinical** disease: asymptomatic *infection,* * *infestation,* * diminution of production, etc.

PATHOLOGICAL PHENOMENON: Abnormal occurrence affecting one or more individuals.

COMMENT 1: Pathological phenomenon refers to a clinical or subclinical condition.

COMMENT 2: In North America, *pathology** is widely used (albeit incorrectly) in oral presentations as synonymous with pathological phenomenon.

See also *pathological, pathology.*

PATHOLOGY: Science that studies the causes and nature of disease; more specifically, the structural and functional changes that occur in organs, tissues, or fluids.

COMMENT: Pathology is wrongly, but commonly, used in daily conversations as synonymous to any anatomical or functional manifestations of *disease.* *

See also *pathological phenomenon.*

PATIENT: Individual presenting clinical signs or lesions caused by a pathogen.

EXAMPLES: A cat hospitalized with epistaxis.
A sow affected with the "thin sow syndrome."

COMMENT 1: The patient is said to be sick, ill, or diseased.

COMMENT 2: The diseased subject can be a human, an animal, a plant, or even a microorganism.

COMMENT 3: The term inpatient may be used to refer to humans or animals who are hospitalized; whereas outpatient refers to individuals receiving treatment without being admitted.

COMMENT 4: The distinction between diseased and healthy is usually based on the presence (or absence) of identifiable clinical signs and/or lesions. However, this classification is more difficult if the patient demonstrates only a slight decrease in production (e.g., decrease in milk production for a cow affected by *subclinical** mastitis).

PAYBACK PERIOD: The length of time it will take for an investment to generate sufficient profit to pay for itself.

EXAMPLE: If a new machine costing $10,000 increases receipts (or decreases *expenses**) by $1000 per year (before *depreciation**), its payback period is 10 years.

COMMENT 1: Because depreciation is a method of offsetting initial cost, it must be omitted in calculation of the payback period.

COMMENT 2: Generally, the shorter the payback period, the more attractive the *investment*. *

COMMENT 3: This criteria is mainly used for the choice of investments in the context where financial resources are limited, or when cash flow is critical.

COMMENT 4: Its disadvantages are numerous:

- Several projects with the same payback period can have very different patterns of net revenue over the period.
- It ignores the length of the life of the investment. Any revenue flows occurring after the end of the payback period are not considered in the calculation.
- It does not show whether or not another investment, using the same resources, would have been more profitable.

PERINATAL MORTALITY RATE:

$$\frac{\text{Number of deaths occurring in a population within a few days around birth}}{\text{Total number of individuals born into this population}} \text{ over a given period of time}$$

COMMENT 1: The period around birth varies depending on the species and the person reporting the rate. The postpartum period included in this expression may be as short as 1 day.

COMMENT 2: This rate includes late abortions, stillborns, and early deaths of liveborns. However, because of the peripartum period under consideration, most perinatal mortality rates are constituted of stillborns and liveborns only. In practice, this is also the information most likely available to veterinarians.

COMMENT 3: Not to be confused with *neonatal mortality rate*, * which is limited to livebirths.

See also *rate, stillbirth, neonatal mortality rate.*

PERIOD OF COMMUNICABILITY: See **Communicable Period**

PERIOD OF INFECTIOUSNESS: Period during which an infected individual may be the source of an infection.

This expression is seldom used in North America.

COMMENT: The infection may be directly (by contact) or indirectly (via arthropods) transmitted. The period of infectiousness differs from the *communicable period* * (*contagious disease* *), which does not include *transmission of a disease* * by arthropods.

See also *generation time* (Figure G1).

PERIOD PREVALENCE: See **Prevalence**

PERIOD PREVALENCE RATE: See **Prevalence Rate**

PERSONAL INTERVIEW: See **Questionnaire**

PERSON-YEAR: Unit of measurement corresponding to a person being exposed to a particular risk during 1 year.

COMMENT: Analogous to *animal-time.**

PHENOMENON: In general, anything that expresses itself to an individual's consciousness, whether through senses or otherwise.

Also said of anything that can be the object of an experience or an observation.

PIE CHART: Graphical representation of the frequency of values taken by a qualitative variable, in the form of segments of a circle, each segment having a surface proportional to its relative frequency.

EXAMPLE: See Figure P1.

COMMENT: The value of the angle formed by each segment is calculated by multiplying 360 degrees by the relative frequency (percentage) of the corresponding value of the variable.

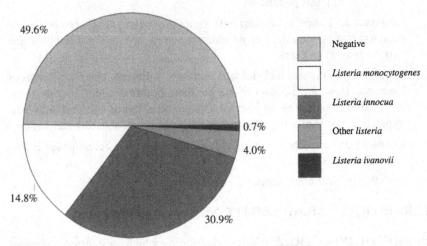

FIGURE P1. Example of a pie chart: Contamination of processed meat with *listeria.*

PILOT INVESTIGATION: See **Pilot Study**

PILOT STUDY: Syn: **pilot investigation** Preliminary small-scale study, performed to test all aspects of a protocol in order to proceed with a larger scale investigation.

COMMENT 1: It allows for the design of a definitive *protocol** and the acquisition of preliminary results.

COMMENT 2: A pilot study is generally conducted before any major investigation, such as a nationwide study on the *prevalence** of a particular *disease.** However, formal pilot studies are rarely performed prior to routine *epidemio-*

logic studies, * such as a *case–control study* * of calf diarrhea in a particular region.

COMMENT 3: A first estimate of a parameter (for example, prevalence of *Streptococcus agalactiae* mastitis in Ontario dairy farms) can be derived from a pilot study and used to calculate the sample size requirement of a larger scale study aiming at estimating this parameter at a given precision for a given *population.* *

PLANNED ANIMAL HEALTH AND PRODUCTION SERVICES: See **Health Management**

PLURIFACTORIAL DISEASE: See **Multifactorial Etiology**

POINT PREVALENCE: Syn: **instantaneous prevalence, spot prevalence** Prevalence at a given point in time.

See also *prevalence.*

POINT PREVALENCE RATE: See **Prevalence Rate**

POINT SOURCE EPIDEMIC: Syn: **common source epidemic** Epidemic in which all cases originate from a single common cause (Figure P2).

EXAMPLE: An epidemic of mulberry heart disease in pigs fed a diet highly deficient in selenium. All *cases* * could be traced back to one feedmill.

COMMENT: When exposure occurs over a very short period of time, the resultant cases develop within the expected *range* * of one incubation period.

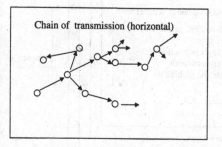
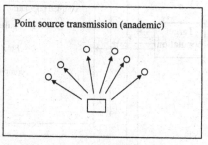

Figure P2. Schematic representation of the transmission of a pathogen during a point source epidemic (anademic) compared with the individual-to-individual (horizontal) transmission observed under most circumstances (i.e., independently of the *disease* * *incidence* * pattern, e.g., *epidemic,* * *endemic,* * *sporadic* *).

See also *epidemic.*

POPULATION: General meaning: Totality of the individuals of the same kind that share or have in common certain attributes.

Statistical meaning: All the units that enter a study (Figure P3).

EXAMPLES: Living beings, objects, events.

COMMENT 1: In a definition of the word *epidemiology,** population is used in a restrictive sense to indicate only human population, limiting the definition to the study of human *health phenomena.** A less restrictive use of epidemiology includes the statistical meaning and considers health phenomena in more diverse populations: humans, animals, plants, and microbes.

COMMENT 2: Because the *study** *objective** of epidemiology is constituted by populations, it is not surprising that some epidemiologists distinguish several categories of populations. Several of these definitions are presented in this dictionary. The associated terminology, especially among different countries, is not always well defined in the scientific literature, which compounds the problem. This is why each type of population defined herein will be illustrated by a specific example relating to the following fictitious case: one wants to conduct an *epidemiologic study** on the *association** between dairy cows with mastitis and the impact of the disease on production performances. Hence, dairy farms must be sampled as part of this study.

See also *population at risk, study population, general population, eligible population, population exposed, sampled population, target population, source population.*

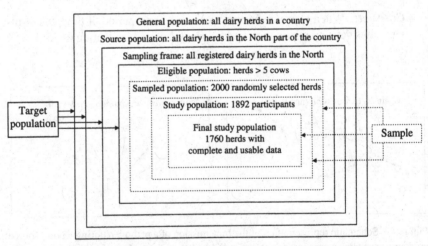

FIGURE P3. Different populations considered in epidemiologic studies, illustrated with a specific example.

POPULATION AT RISK: Part of a general population that is susceptible to develop an event of interest under specific circumstances or study conditions.

COMMENT 1: The notion of population at risk is independent from the exposure to the *risk factor**. The population at risk corresponds to a susceptible population for a given *risk** (see Figure P4).

COMMENT 2: When the population at risk is exposed to the risk factor or *disease** determinant, this population is said to be at a higher risk of developing the event or pathological phenomenon (see Figure P4).

COMMENT 3: There are several levels of risk for the population at risk. Thus, the level of risk for foot-and-mouth disease is not equal for all cattle and will vary according to whether the animals are vaccinated against the disease, and according to whether they are found in an *outbreak** of this disease, or situated 150 meters, 5 kilometers, or 60 kilometers from the outbreak (see Figure P5).

POPULATION ATTRIBUTABLE FRACTION: See **Population Attributable Risk Fraction**

POPULATION ATTRIBUTABLE RISK: A measure of how a risk factor contributes to the overall incidence of disease in a population.

Population attributable risk =

(Incidence in exposed population – incidence in nonexposed population) $\times$ proportion of population exposed.

POPULATION ATTRIBUTABLE RISK FRACTION: Syn: population attributable fraction, population attributable risk proportion (often multiplied by 100), population etiologic fraction Proportion of the disease in a population associated with a specific risk factor.

Population attributable risk fraction =

$$\frac{\text{(Incidence in exposed population – incidence in nonexposed population)} \times \text{proportion of population exposed}}{\text{Incidence in the population}}$$

or

$$\frac{\text{(Incidence in population – incidence in nonexposed population)}}{\text{Incidence in population}}$$

or

$$\frac{\text{(Prevalence of exposure in the population)} \times (RR - 1)}{1 + \text{(Prevalence of exposure in the population)} \times (RR - 1)}$$

RR = *Relative risk**

COMMENT 1: This calculation provides an *estimate** of the reduction in *disease* incidence** in a *population** that will potentially occur if exposure to the *risk factor** is eliminated and if no confounding was present when the association between exposure and disease was assessed.

COMMENT 2: For rare exposures, the population attributable risk fraction is small, even when the *risk factor** is strongly related to the disease of interest (Table P1).

TABLE P1. Population attributable risk fraction, expressed as a percentage, depending on the prevalence of exposure to the risk factor (also expressed as a percentage) and on the relative risk

Prevalence of exposure	Relative risk				
	0.5	1	2	5	10
0.5	0.25	0	0.50	1.96	4.31
10	4.76	0	9.09	28.57	47.37
50	20.00	0	33.33	66.67	81.82
95	32.20	0	48.72	79.17	89.53

POPULATION ATTRIBUTABLE RISK PROPORTION: See **Population Attributable Risk Fraction**

POPULATION ETIOLOGIC FRACTION: See **Population Attributable Risk Fraction**

POPULATION EXPOSED (TO A RISK FACTOR): Syn: exposed population
Population that has been effectively subjected to a given risk factor or causal agent, independently of the fact that it may or may not be susceptible to the disease associated with the exposure.

EXAMPLE: For a *study** on bovine tuberculosis in a *herd**, the population exposed includes noninfected and infected animals with tuberculosis, because all have been exposed to the *risk.**

COMMENT: The *population at risk** includes all individuals or herds susceptible to the condition of interest, independently of the fact that they may or may not have been exposed to a given *risk factor** (Figures P4 and P5).

See also *population at risk*.

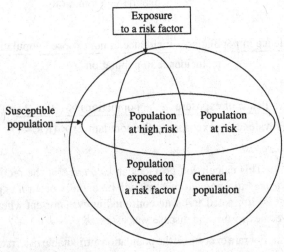

FIGURE P4. Populations based on risk.

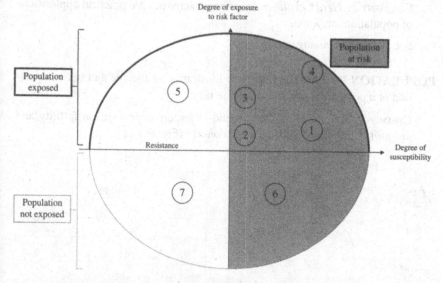

FIGURE P5. Relationship between risk and exposure for foot-and-mouth disease. The circled numbers correspond to the comments below.

- Population at risk
  1. Cattle not vaccinated in a country where foot-and-mouth disease is sporadic.
  2. Cattle vaccinated in the same country as in (1).
  3. Cattle vaccinated but located close to a farm experiencing an outbreak.
  4. Ruminants and pigs not vaccinated and located on a farm experiencing an outbreak (high-risk population).
- Population exposed but not susceptible
  5. Carnivores located on a farm going through an outbreak.
- Population at risk but not exposed
  6. Cattle in a country free of the disease.
- Population not at risk and not exposed
  7. Carnivores in a country free of the disease.

POPULATION MEDICINE: The medical discipline pertaining to animal populations.

COMMENT 1: It consists of the clinical evaluation of the health status of populations based on field observations, laboratory tests, and on-farm data collection pertaining to the population itself and to its management and environment. It also involves directed actions (applied prevention, control strategies and therapeutic treatments) for the optimization of *health*.* Optimization of health, in practice, is determined in part by the economic viability of the operation (e.g., company) overseeing the population.

COMMENT 2: *Herd* health management** activities are practical applications of population medicine.

See also *health management.*

POPULATION PYRAMID: Graphical illustration of the age and sex composition of a population at a given point in time.

COMMENT: The shape of the pyramid is largely dependent on fertility and *mortality** associated with each age *cohort** (Figure P6).

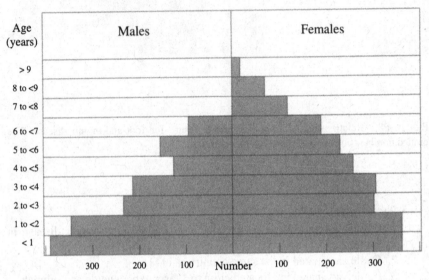

FIGURE P6.   Example of a population pyramid.

POSITIVE PREDICTIVE VALUE (PV+): Probability that an individual found positive to a test is truly affected by the disease or outcome of interest for which the test was performed.

COMMENT 1: Considering the following contingency table, the predictive value of a positive test is equal to $a/(a + b)$:

Test results	Number of subjects		
	Truly affected	Not affected	Total
Positive	a	b	a + b
Negative	c	d	c + d
Total	a + c	b + d	N = a + b + c + d

COMMENT 2: The positive predictive value depends on the two intrinsic *characteristics** of the test (*sensitivity,* * *specificity**), and also on the *prevalence** of truly affected individuals. The relationships of PV+ to sensitivity (SENS), specificity (SPEC) and prevalence (P) are expressed in the following equation: PV+ = SENS × P/[SENS × P + (1 − SPEC) × (1 − P)]. Hence, when prevalence decreases, the PV+ decreases; and when it increases, the PV+ increases.

EXAMPLE: Given a test with a sensitivity and a specificity equal to 0.95; the following table gives the *distribution* of results under two different scenarios: one when the prevalence is 20%, the other when the prevalence is only 1%.

(20%)	Infected	Healthy	Total	(1%)	Infected	Healthy	Total
+a	1900	400	2300	+b	95	495	590
−	100	7600	7700	−	5	9405	9410
Total	2000	8000	10,000		100	9900	10,000

aIn the first case, the positive predictive value is 82.6% (1900/2300).
bIn the second, it is equal to 16% (95/590).

COMMENT 3: A frequent error is to refer to a lack of specificity when positive test results are confirmed a posteriori to be false, using the equation b/(a + b). This, in fact, is simply the complement of the positive predictive value (1 − PV+), which has nothing to do with specificity: d/(b + d).

COMMENT 4: The factors affecting the predicting value of a positive test used at the herd or flock level (assessment of groups of individuals) are somewhat similar to those at the individual level. However, the elements in the equation are group level information:

$$HPV+ = \frac{HTP \times HSENS}{HTP \times HSENS + (1 - HTP) \times (1 - HSPEC)}$$

Where HPV+ is the herd positive predictive value; HTP is the true prevalence of affected herds; HSENS is the herd sensitivity of the test and HSPEC is the herd specificity. Therefore, factors affecting HSENS and HSPEC must also be taken into account.

Hence, assuming the test in the example above is used at the population level (individual sensitivity and specificity of 0.95), and that 10 individuals are tested in herds with 30% of the animals diseased, the HSENS and HSPEC would be 98% and 60%, respectively, if one reactor is considered sufficient to indicate the presence of disease. Given an HTP of 40%, the HPV+ would be 0.62 or 62%, but for an HTP of 5%, the HPV+ would only be 0.11 or 11%.

See also *sensitivity, specificity, negative predictive value.*

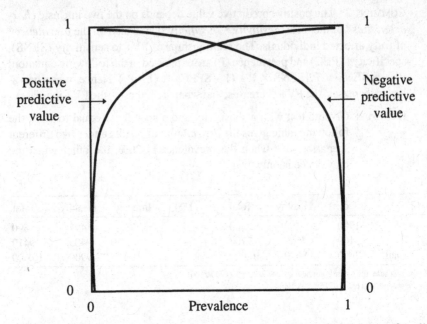

FIGURE P7. Example of the variation in positive and negative predictive values (0 to 1) depending on prevalence of disease (0 to 1).

POSSIBLE VECTOR: A possible vector of a pathogen is one whose potential as a vector has only been studied under laboratory conditions.

COMMENT: This type of vector could take over the role of the *principal vector** if the latter were eliminated. Therefore, possible vectors have to be considered in disease control programs.

POTENTIAL RESERVOIR: Any animate (humans, animals, insects, etc.) or inanimate object (plant, soil, feces, etc.) or any combination of these that is not currently a reservoir but whose biological and ecological characteristics are such that it could become a reservoir for a specific pathogen in a given region and at a given time.

EXAMPLE: Various species of rodents and birds are known *reservoirs** for the West Nile virus, a flavivirus causing West Nile meningoencephalitis in horses. Various rodents and birds inhabiting the Camargue region on the south coast of France, presently free of this virus, are therefore potential reservoirs for this *agent.**

POWER: Probability that a statistical test will reject the null hypothesis when in fact it is false.

COMMENT 1: Power is equal to 1 minus the probability of a *beta error** (type II).

COMMENT 2: In general, when comparing *groups,** the power of a test will increase as the number of *individuals** increases and the *sampling variance** decreases. Since power is dependent on certain elements of the *study** or investigation, it is appropriate to refer to the power of the study (or power of the investigation, power of the experiment, etc.).

COMMENT 3: In a comparison between groups, a very powerful test will consider significant a small difference between groups. In contrast, a test with little power will only consider significant important differences.

COMMENT 4: In a case where the *sample size** is very large, very small differences (usually not biologically meaningful) will become statistically significant, which defeats the purpose of statistical *hypothesis** testing. This is the case when investigations are based on large *data banks.**

PRACTICALITY (OF A TEST): Facility of implementation of a test.

COMMENT: The practicality of a test depends on several factors: the time needed to obtain results, the initial *investments** required, the maintenance and *operational costs,** the degree of technical difficulty and the availability of the necessary equipment and products to perform the test, and the potential *risk** for the operator and the environment.

EXAMPLES: The buffered antigen test (used for brucellosis) is practical. It is very quick, economical, does not require sophisticated technical skills, the material needed to perform the test is readily available, and it is without risk for the operator. Conversely, although they may be excellent tests, radioimmunoassays are not considered very practical: they are slow, expensive, require high technical skills and sophisticated equipment, and they present risks for the operators (radioactivity).

PRAGMATIC APPROACH: Method of approaching and attempting to solve a health problem that need not depend on an exhaustive scientific inquiry of the problem.

EXAMPLE 1: Estimation of the *incidence rate** of bovine leukosis virus infection in dairy cattle using a convenience sample of owners involved in a voluntary breeding program (and are hence not necessarily a representative sample of the owners of all dairy cattle at risk of *infection**).

EXAMPLE 2: Regional health officers elect to clean up a polluted water supply without doing *epidemiologic studies** to examine what health effects the water has, if any, on a population of animals or people.

COMMENT: Such realistic approaches are often taken because of the lack of a viable alternative, and represent a compromise between conducting studies with rigorous scientific standards and doing little or nothing to address a health problem because the desired level of scientific standards cannot practically be met.

PRECIPITATING FACTOR: Factor accelerating the development of a morbid condition.

Expression rarely used in North America.

EXAMPLE: Gestation is a precipitating factor for paratuberculosis.

COMMENT: Some authors consider precipitating factor as equivalent to *triggering factor.** In practice, it is often difficult to differentiate between the concept of acceleration and the concept of inducement of the *disease** process.

PRECISION OF AN ESTIMATE: Measure of dispersion or variance associated with the use of a random sample to obtain the estimated population statistics.

> EXAMPLE: For a *population** which is normally distributed, the precision of the estimate of the *mean** is given by the *sample variance** divided by the *sample size.**

COMMENT 1: The larger the *dispersion,** the worse the precision. Therefore, precision is inversely proportional to the variance of the measure.

COMMENT 2: This measure is related to sample size (see example). However, there is no relationship between the precision of the estimate and the population size as long as the sample size is negligible compared to the population. For example, measurements obtained from a sample of 30 individuals will have the same precision whether the population comprises 10,000, 100,000, or 1,000,000 individuals.

COMMENT 3: This is a characteristic of the measuring process and not of the individuals being measured. However, it is possible that the individuals may not be independent of the measuring process.

COMMENT 4: Do not confuse precision with *accuracy** or lack of *bias.** If one seeks to estimate the average weight of a group of animals whose real value is 721.5 kg, the estimation can be (Figure P8):

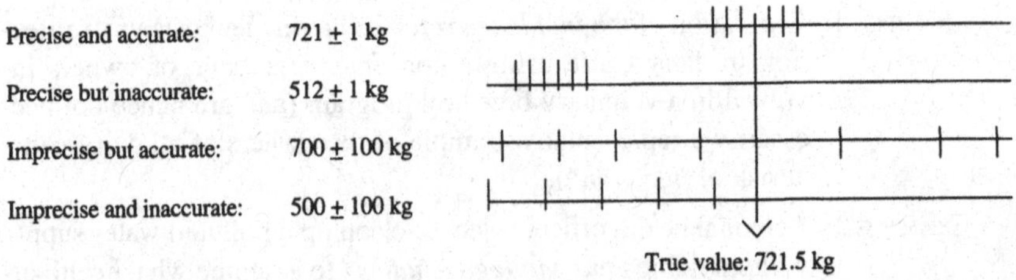

Precise and accurate:	721 ± 1 kg
Precise but inaccurate:	512 ± 1 kg
Imprecise but accurate:	700 ± 100 kg
Imprecise and inaccurate:	500 ± 100 kg

True value: 721.5 kg

FIGURE P8. Graphic representation of the degree of precision and accuracy of an estimate.

PRECISION OF A TEST: Measure of closeness of agreement between values obtained from repeated measurements performed on samples or individuals under specific conditions, usually by the same test.

> COMMENT 1: A precise test gives repeatable results but does not ensure *accuracy** (see Table A1, accuracy).

COMMENT 2: This notion includes the concept of *repeatability** (e.g., repeated measurements taken by the same operator) and sometimes the concept of the level of refinement of the measure (e.g., number of significant digits).

PREDICTOR: See Independent Variable

PREDISPOSING FACTOR: Syn: enabling factor Factor conditioning or priming an individual (i.e., its physiologic, anatomic, or immune characteristics) in such a way that the probability of occurrence of an event is increased.

EXAMPLES: Cold and humid conditions are known as factors predisposing to respiratory diseases. Overcrowding is a predisposing factor for many infectious diseases due to the stress associated with close confinement and due to the higher *contact rate** between individuals (i.e., porcine pleuropneumonia, erysipelas, colibacillosis). High stocking density may also have an impact on nondisease issues such as growth performances.

COMMENT 1: A predisposing factor may or may not be essential to the occurrence of an event.

COMMENT 2: Predisposing factor, *triggering factor** and *precipitating factor** are all expressions that may be used interchangeably by some authors. Of the three, the first two are more commonly used.

PREGNANCY RATE: $\dfrac{\text{Number of pregnant females}}{\text{Number of females bred}}$ over a given period of time

COMMENT 1: The probability of becoming pregnant is usually determined for a specific period after breeding.

COMMENT 2: Pregnancy rates are often expressed and reported as percentages. See also *rate, fecundity rate.*

PREMUNITION: Syn: infection immunity State of resistance in a host harboring a pathogen, to infection by the same or a closely related pathogen that lasts as long as the agent remains in the body.

COMMENT 1: As this definition implies, resistance is dependent on the continued presence of the *agent** and disappears after its elimination. Premunition is mainly used for parasitic *diseases**.

COMMENT 2: Premunition may be complete or partial.

PRESENT VALUE: The value today of a future payment, or series of payments, discounted at the appropriate discount rate.

COMMENT 1: The formula below allows calculation of a present value (PV) from a future value (FV):

$$PV = \sum \frac{FV}{(1+i)^n}$$

Where PV = present value
FV = future value
i = discount rate
n = number of years

COMMENT 2: The calculation of present value is used in *cost–benefit analyses.**

See also *discount rate, discounting.*

PRESENT VALUE OF BENEFITS: See Present Value of Future Returns

PRESENT VALUE OF COSTS: Sum of the present cost values calculated for each year.

COMMENT: The formula is analogous to the one used for the calculation of the present value of future returns once benefits are replaced by costs.

See also *net present value, cost–benefit analysis, discounting.*

PRESENT VALUE OF FUTURE RETURNS: Syn: present value of benefits
Sum of the present values of the benefits calculated for each year.

COMMENT 1: It can be expressed by the following formula:

$$PVB = \sum_{t=1}^{t=n} \frac{A_t}{(1+i)^t}$$

With A = sum of benefits over a year.
n = number of years considered.
t = 1 year.
i = discount rate expressed as a decimal fraction.

$\sum_{t=1}^{t=n}$ = sum of all $\frac{A_t}{(1+i)^t}$ for each value of t, from $t = 1$ to $t = n$.

COMMENT 2: This PVB is used in *cost–benefit analysis.**

PRESHEDDING PERIOD: See Latency Period

PRETESTING (OF A QUESTIONNAIRE): Multistep procedure performed to evaluate the design of a questionnaire and the degree of comprehension of each question by individuals representative of the target population.

EXAMPLE: Several strategies are possible. The following is one approach:

- After a first solid draft is written, the *questionnaire** is reviewed by colleagues (*epidemiologists** and/or individuals involved in the field of interest; i.e., practitioners, animal scientists, etc.).
- The revised version is presented to three to ten individuals who are comparable to the *target population.** The questionnaire is presented to each individual in this group in a format as close as possible to what should be the final version of the questionnaire.

This is particularly critical for mailed questionnaires. Participants are first asked to fill out the questionnaire as if they were included in the study. Written comments should then be obtained from each participant. The ideal scenario is to schedule a meeting of all participants in order to gather their comments and foster a discussion among them about each question.

- The questionnaire is modified according to the participants' recommendations and step 2 is repeated. If needed, this could be done a third time.

COMMENT 1: Participants in the pretest should not be included in the *study*.* However, it is recommended, as a gesture of appreciation, to provide the participants with a summary of the study results (the study conducted using the questionnaire reviewed by these participants).

COMMENT 2: In addition to elicit information to determine whether each question was understood by the participants, a series of key questions should also be asked about the format of the questionnaire: Is there enough space after each question to write down the answer? Are some questions likely to be inadvertently overlooked? How much time did it take to fill out the questionnaire? If skip patterns are used, are they adequate? Are all questions necessary? Have any essential questions been omitted?

PREVALENCE: Total number of cases or outbreaks of a disease or of an infection in a specific population, at a designated time or during a particular time period.

COMMENT 1: A *case** normally refers to a single *individual,** but an *outbreak** can be defined at one of a number of different possible levels. For example, a barn or house; a *herd** or flock (which may include ≥ 1 barn or house); a farm (≥ 1 herd or flock); a company; a region. As for any outbreaks, not all individuals within a group would be expected to have the *disease** or *infection** of interest.

COMMENT 2: Prevalence includes all cases (new cases and those already present at the beginning of the time period), while *incidence** only refers to new cases occurring during the period of time of interest. Hence, prevalence comprises incidence.

COMMENT 3: Prevalence can be calculated for a given period of time (*annual prevalence**, monthly prevalence, weekly prevalence, prevalence over one production cycle, etc.) or for a specific point in time. The former is known as period prevalence and the latter as *point prevalence** (Figure P9).

COMMENT 4: Prevalence, like incidence, is an absolute number. When this number is divided by the number of relevant units (individuals, barns, herds, etc.) of the *population** present at or during a designated time, it is known as the *prevalence rate.** In practice, many authors use prevalence as equivalent to prevalence rate.

COMMENT 5: Prevalence is sometimes used for conditions other than diseases or infections. For example, based on given criteria to assess body condition, one could say that the prevalence of overweight sows in a 1000-sow farm is 200.

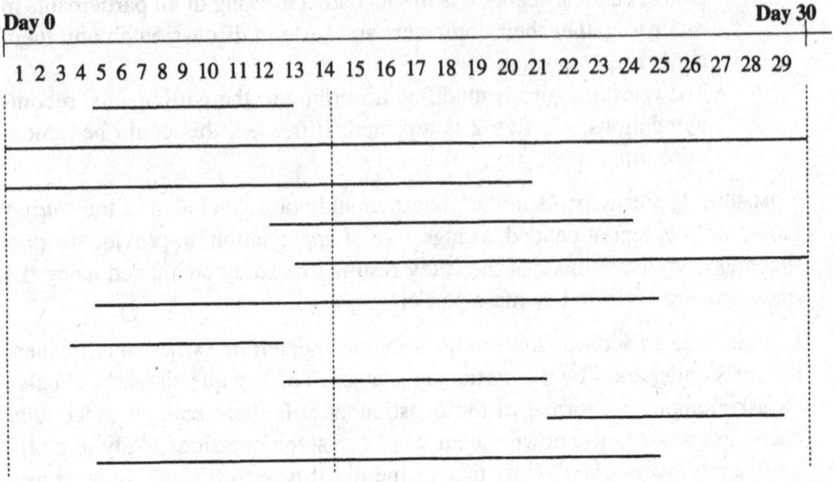

Monthly incidence (Day 0 to 30) = 8
Monthly prevalence (Day 0 to 30) = 10
Point prevalence (Day 14) = 7

FIGURE P9.   Schematic representation of prevalence and incidence. Each horizontal line corresponds to a case.

See also *apparent prevalence, prevalence rate.*

PREVALENCE IMMUNE: Syn: proportion immune

$$\frac{\text{Number of immune individuals}}{\text{Number of individuals in the population}}$$

COMMENT: Expression seldom used in North America. Often limited to an *estimate* * used when building an *infectious disease* * *model.* *

See also *herd immunity.*

PREVALENCE RATE:

$$\frac{\text{Total number of cases (or outbreaks)}}{\text{Number of epidemiologic units}} \text{ in the population during a period of time or at a given moment}$$

COMMENT 1: This *rate* * is usually based on a *sampling* * of the *population* * and is expressed per 100 or per 1000 or per any other number depending on the species and the nature of the problem. For example, abattoir condemnation results in chickens or turkeys in Canada is reported per 10,000 birds processed. This is because the number of condemned carcasses is normally very low and 10,000 represents a standardized flock size. The denominator is based on the relevant unit of interest. This *epidemiologic unit* * can be an individual, but it can also be part of a *herd** or flock (see *prevalence**).

COMMENT 2: The prevalence rate can be instantaneous (at a given moment; known as the point prevalence rate) or may be determined for a defined period of time (period prevalence rate).

EXAMPLES: The annual prevalence rate of cattle herds infected with brucellosis in France for 1983 was 3.1%; however, the point prevalence rate for these herds on December 31st, 1983 was 0.75%.

COMMENT 3: This rate can be calculated for diseases, infections, or any other conditions (see prevalence, comment 5).

COMMENT 4: Given the dynamic nature of most populations, when the prevalence rate is calculated for a long period of time (i.e., 1 year), it is preferable to use as denominator the average population for this time period.

See also *rate, prevalence, epidemiologic unit.*

PREVALENCE STUDY: See **Cross-Sectional Study**

PREVALENT CASE: Syn: existing case Diseased individual identified at a given time or during a certain period.

COMMENT: As compared to *incident case.** Prevalent cases include incident cases.

EXAMPLE: In 1994, 63 cases of housesoiling in cats (a chronic behavioral condition) were known in Guelph, Ontario, Canada.

See also *prevalence.*

PREVENTION: Set of measures that may be prophylactic (medical and sanitary), social, political, or economic, and designed to prevent the occurrence of a disease or any other detrimental health event, or to limit its progression and/or severity, with the intention of eventually eliminating it.

COMMENT 1: *Prophylaxis** is a form of prevention with medical and sanitary components. However, preventive measures are not limited to this. For example, speed limits are a very effective way of reducing severe and fatal injuries (nonmedical preventive measure).

COMMENT 2: The World Health Organization has defined three different levels of prevention: primary (reduction in *disease* incidence**), secondary (reduction in disease *prevalence**), and tertiary (reduction in disease severity). The transposition of these definitions to veterinary medicine is not universally accepted, especially for *tertiary prevention** (Figure P10).

COMMENT 3: Most veterinary practitioners are involved in some form of tertiary prevention (curative activities). This is particularly true in small animal and equine practices. However, changes in society's expectations of veterinary care, advances in science and technology, concerns over environmental deterioration and the globalization of world economic activities have supported a shift from tertiary to secondary and primary prevention. This is mainly occurring in commercial animal production. Prevention programs have put emphasis on *secondary prevention** (detection of disease processes before clinical disease occurs). Although *primary prevention** is often a core component of these programs, it is frequently neglected. This may be due to the fact that this form of prevention requires a continuous effort from different participants, and is often perceived as time consuming and disruptive.

COMMENT 4: Prevention is also referred to as disease control, which may, under certain circumstances, lead to disease *eradication.**

COMMENT 5: Prevention in veterinary medicine can be conceived according to human medicine concepts (person → individual animal; *public health** → *herd* health management**). However, because of particularities in the structure of animal *populations,** veterinarians have developed prevention programs that have unique features (especially for tertiary prevention).

See also *primary prevention, secondary prevention, tertiary prevention.*

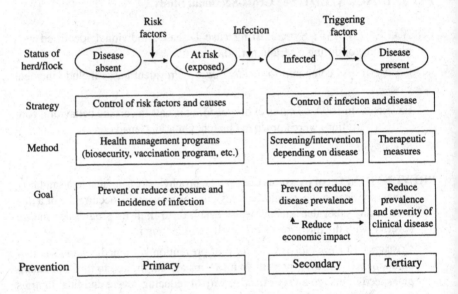

FIGURE P10.   The three different degrees of prevention of an infectious disease.

PREVENTIVE MEDICINE: Medical field dedicated to the prevention of disease occurrence.

COMMENT 1: Preventive or prophylactic measures include vaccination, strategic medication (antibiotics, probiotics, hormonal therapy, etc.), sanitation, nutrition supplements, etc.

COMMENT 2: Preventive medicine is an important component of *public health**, which also comprises social, political, and economic measures designed to prevent *disease** and improve the *health** of the community (preventive medicine may be targeted at individuals or communities).

See also *prophylaxis, public health, prevention.*

PREVENTIVE VETERINARY MEDICINE: Preventive medicine applied to animals.

COMMENT 1: As for *preventive medicine,** preventive veterinary medicine procedures can be applied to individuals or groups of individuals (for example, pens, barns, *herds**).

COMMENT 2: Preventive measures are similar to the ones listed for preventive medicine. However, some measures are more restricted to animal production, such as *biosecurity,** medicated early weaning, and multisite production.

COMMENT 3: When properly implemented, preventive measures lower *disease* incidence** and improve performances (feed conversion, average daily gain, herd or flock uniformity). Hence, preventive veterinary medicine is an important component of *health management.**

See also *preventive medicine.*

PRIMARY CASE: First case of a disease to have occurred in a region that was previously unaffected.

COMMENT: There can be more than one primary case in common source epidemics with subsequent secondary, tertiary, etc., cases involving *direct* or *indirect transmission.**

See also *index case.*

PRIMARY HOST: See **Definitive Host**

PRIMARY OUTBREAK: Initial outbreak of a transmissible disease occurring in an area previously free of this condition.

EXAMPLE: In 1981, in Côtes-d'Armor, France, the primary outbreak of foot-and-mouth disease was located on a farm in the commune of Henansal, and it led to 13 *secondary outbreaks.**

COMMENT 1: This expression would not apply for non*transmissible** diseases, such as nutritional deficiencies, chemical toxicity, and some genetic (e.g., no transmission between meat-line birds) or management-related conditions, as these diseases would not spread from a primary to a secondary location or group. However, the expression *point source epidemic** would apply.

COMMENT 2: The primary outbreak is not necessarily the first observed or recorded outbreak. It is also possible to have several primary outbreaks when the *agent** is introduced in different locations of a given region via one or several separate sources.

See also *outbreak, point source epidemic.*

PRIMARY PREVENTION: Set of measures designed to decrease disease incidence in a population, by preventing the introduction of disease agents and/or of related determinant factors in this population.

EXAMPLES: In the context of protecting a *herd** from known *infectious** agents: stringent *biosecurity** and sanitation; buying replacement animals from a reputable source; *screening** all animals introduced into the herd (including a *quarantine** period) for infectious agents for which tests are available.

In countries where *vaccination** against foot-and-mouth disease is allowed, vaccination of all cattle in an unaffected region, in order to prevent the emergence of a large number of *cases** if the virus were to be accidentally introduced. This primary prevention measure would facilitate disease containment and even *eradication** in this region.

Prophylactic chemotherapy against dirofilariasis (heartworms).

COMMENT 1: The basic aim of primary prevention is to avoid disease occurrence or, at least, to reduce disease *incidence**. The two preceding examples represent two different prevention schemes with different degrees of *efficiency.** However, they both have the same purpose.

COMMENT 2: Primary prevention is the most definitive form of *prevention** compared to the other two levels (secondary and tertiary). Many of its principles are many centuries old. For example, several concepts of biosecurity and sanitation can be found in the Bible. However, these principles are often neglected because the return on *investment** is rarely immediate or obvious (one could potentially have no serious problem even without implementing any prevention measures). Several primary prevention measures require consistency of application, are time consuming, and disrupt the flow of regular activities (e.g., cleaning and disinfection of vehicles after each farm visit, changing boots and coveralls between barns, pest management program, multisite production, etc.).

See also *prevention* (Figure P9), *secondary prevention, tertiary prevention.*

PRINCIPAL COMPONENTS ANALYSIS: Statistical procedure used to transform a large number of correlated variables into a smaller number of uncorrelated variables that are linear combinations of the original variables.

COMMENT 1: The purpose of principal components analysis is to search for linear equations, called principal components, that partition the total *variance.** The first principal component accounts for the maximum amount of variance; the second principal component (which is not correlated with the first component) accounts for the next largest amount of variance, etc.

COMMENT 2: The different components are a set of noncorrelated variables that should account for most of the variability in the original *measurements.** The components can then be interpreted by how strongly correlated certain individual measurements are within each component. This interpretation is based on graphical representations and numerical *parameters** designed to best assess the newly created variables.

COMMENT 3: Principal component analysis may be used as an exploratory *method** to describe the data before initiating other analyses. Like many statistical approaches, this method simplifies reality. Therefore, one must be careful when interpreting the results.

COMMENT 4: Simple or multiple *contingency table analysis** may be used for *qualitative variables.**

PRINCIPAL VECTOR: See **Main Vector**

PROBABILISTIC MODEL: Syn: random model, stochastic model Mathematical model for which the outcome is decided, at least in part, by hazard or which is driven, at least in part, by a random number generator.

COMMENT 1: The same conditions do not always give the same outcome.

COMMENT 2: These models can express the variation associated with the uncertainty surrounding the value of the parameters used.

EXAMPLES: The model of transmission of rabies in foxes. Each event in the life of the fox is randomly selected according to a law of probability which takes into account its distribution such as that known in reality.

PROBABILITY (OF AN EVENT): Value that weighs the chance associated with the occurrence of an event.

COMMENT 1: It is usually estimated by the ratio of the number of favorable incidents of this event over the total number of possible occurrences.

COMMENT 2: Probability is expressed as a numerical value included between 0 and 1. When an event is impossible, the probability is 0, whereas, when an event is certain, its probability is 1.

PROBABILITY SAMPLE: See **Random Sample**

PROBABILITY TREE: Tree that only includes chance nodes.

COMMENT: In a probability tree, the terminal branches result in a combined *probability** that is the product of probabilities from the same path.

See also *decision tree.*

PROBIT (TRANSFORMATION): A transformation of a proportion (p) into a number (y) by using the inverse cumulative distribution function of a standard normal random variable p representing the probability of obtaining a value equal to or less than y (Figure P11).

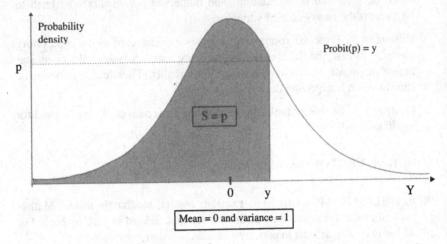

Probability
density

Probit(p) = y

p

S = p

0   y   Y

Mean = 0 and variance = 1

FIGURE P11.   Schematic representation of the concept of probit. The transformation of p to y consists of finding the value y for which the surface under the curve S is equal to the value p. This is essentially the probability of Y being less than y.

If F denotes the cumulative distribution function of a standard normal random variable, then probit $(p) = F^{-1}(p) = y$.

EXAMPLE: For a given drug dosage, X corresponds to a proportion of patients showing secondary effects (p). In probit modeling, probit (p) is modeled as a linear function of (X), i.e., probit$(p) = a + bX$.

COMMENT 1: Probit tables exist that will yield the value of y for a given value of p.

COMMENT 2: In older textbooks, the result of a probit transformation may be reported as $y + 5$ instead of y. This was done to avoid negative (< 0) results.

PROCEDURE: Set of successive rules and actions that should be implemented to reach an objective.

EXAMPLE: All the legal and technical aspects of pharmaceutical product registration represent a procedure that is outlined in a *protocol*.*

COMMENT: The evaluation of an action (*study,* * *health* * intervention) should focus on the procedure(s) before focusing on the results. Indeed, the *validity* * of these results is dependent on the procedure(s) executed to obtain them.

See also *protocol, method*.

PROFIT: Difference between income (revenue) and total (fixed + variable) costs.

COMMENT 1: Also referred to as earnings.

COMMENT 2: In the accounting sense of the term, net profit is the residual after deduction of all money *costs** (salaries, rent, raw materials, etc.), *interest** on loans, *depreciation** and taxes. Accounting profit and economic profit are only the same when all factors of production have been credited with their full *opportunity costs.**

See also *losses.*

PROJECT APPRAISAL: See **Ex-Ante Analysis**

PROJECT EVALUATION: See **Ex-Post Analysis**

PROPHYLAXIS: Set of measures (mostly hygienic or medical) employed to prevent the occurrence of disease.

COMMENT 1: Prophylaxis can be applied at *individual** or *population** levels and can comprise medical (e.g., biologics or pharmaceuticals) or sanitary (e.g., *quarantine,** disinfection) measures.

COMMENT 2: Prophylaxis is often most effective when adequate epidemiologic knowledge of the *disease** exists. However, in commercial animal production, for example, the implementation of stringent *biosecurity** measures is often sufficient to prevent the occurrence of most *infectious diseases,** including those for which little epidemiologic information exists.

COMMENT 3: When an objective of treatment is to reduce pathogen excretion and consequently reduce the *risk** of exposing naive animals to *infection,** therapy of affected individuals constitutes a prophylactic measure for the population.

COMMENT 4: Prophylaxis may also apply to noninfectious conditions, such as metabolic or nutritional diseases. For example, feeding management designed to reduce the *incidence** of ascites in broiler chickens.

See also *prevention.*

PROPORTION: A frequency ratio whose numerator is contained in the denominator (i.e., proportion $p = a/[a + b]$, where a and b are frequencies).

COMMENT 1: A proportion is used to estimate the *probability** of occurrence of an event.

COMMENT 2: Technically, a proportion is a dimensionless quantity (because the numerator and the denominator have the same dimension) ranging between 0 and 1. However, in practice, a proportion is often expressed as a percentage.

EXAMPLES: Number of cows in first gestation

Number of cows in gestation

The *prevalence rate** of mastitis in herd A in July was 0.18 (or 18%) because 45 of the 250 cows in this *herd** were affected with this *disease** during that month.

PROPORTION IMMUNE: See **Prevalence Immune**

PROPORTIONAL HAZARD MODEL: See Cox's Model

PROPORTIONAL QUOTA SAMPLE: See Proportional Sample

PROPORTIONAL RISK MODEL: See Cox's Model

PROPORTIONAL SAMPLE: Syn: **proportional quota sample** A sample in which the proportion of individuals in a stratum (e.g., age, breed, sex) is fixed by the frequency of individuals in the stratum of the source population.

EXAMPLE: In a region heavily populated by cattle, if 10% of the cattle are dairy, 50% are mixed, and 40% are beef, a proportional sample of cattle will be constrained to have the same *frequency* distribution** as that of the *population.**

COMMENT: Although the frequencies of the characteristics used to define strata may be constrained to be identical between the population and the *sample,** other nonconstrained characteristics need not have identical or even similar distributions between the two *groups.**

PROSPECTIVE STUDY: A study in which the population(s) of interest is followed over time to collect information on the risk factors and outcomes of interest.

EXAMPLE: In order to investigate respiratory disease *risk factors** of swine, 100 swine herds will be monitored for a period of 1 year.

COMMENT 1: Most *cohort studies** and *longitudinal studies** are prospective in nature.

COMMENT 2: A key feature of a prospective study is that the disease or outcome of interest has not occurred when the *study** starts.

COMMENT 3: The term prospective refers to the *method** by which the data are collected rather than to the specific design of the study.

COMMENT 4: Prospective studies may be *descriptive** (serve only to describe a population) or may be *analytical** (evaluate relationships between factors and outcomes of interest). Cohort and longitudinal studies are examples of analytical prospective studies.

COMMENT 5: The main advantage of conducting a study prospectively is that the investigator has much more control over the quality and completeness of the *data**.

COMMENT 6: In very select cases, provided that adequate historical records are available, it is possible to convert a *retrospective study,** (events that have already happened) into a "historical prospective study" in which the populations are followed through time using the historical records.

See also *longitudinal study, retrospective study*.

PROTECTIVE FACTOR: See Risk Factor

PROTOCOL: The policy and procedures employed in the implementation of a study.

COMMENT 1: It is not unusual in epidemiologic studies for the development of the protocol to take longer than the actual study.

COMMENT 2: A proper protocol should clearly specify the subjective and objective criteria used at all stages of conducting a study.

See also *experimentation, observational study, objective.*

PUBLIC HEALTH: The state of physical and mental well-being in a human population.

The set of activities designed to protect, promote and restore the public's health, with emphasis on the prevention of disease.

COMMENT: "In public health practice the *individual* * is not the patient, but the community is" (Schwabe, 1984).

See also *veterinary public health, preventive medicine.*

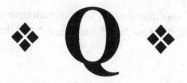

QUALITATIVE VARIABLE: Attribute or element that is either present or absent, or that may be divided into a limited number of nonmeasurable levels.

EXAMPLES: *Disease* * status: Present or absent.
Sex: Male or female.
Dog breed: Golden retriever, chow chow, etc.

COMMENT 1: For analytical purposes, each level of a qualitative variable may be coded using numerical values (e.g., disease present = 1, absent = 0; swine breed: Landrace = 1, Hampshire = 2, Large White = 3, Duroc = 4, others = 5).

COMMENT 2: Qualitative variables are said to be nominal when the levels are not ordered (male, female), and ordinal when they are (e.g., not present, rarely, sometimes, often, always present). The latter allows us to characterize the *variable* * according to a gradient of intensity.

See also *attribute.*

QUANTILE: Dispersion parameter allowing the division of the population of a quantitative variable into groups of equal size.

EXAMPLES: 3 quartiles define 4 groups of equal size (Figure Q1); 4 quintiles define 5 groups of equal size; 9 deciles define 10 groups of equal size; 99 centiles or percentiles define 100 groups of equal size.

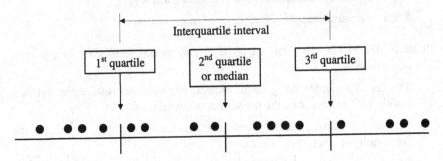

FIGURE Q1.   Representation of the notion of quantile.

QUANTITATIVE VARIABLE: Attribute or element whose variations can be measured using an appropriate scale.

EXAMPLES: Herd size measured in number of animals.
Height in meters.
Weight in kilograms.

COMMENT: The *sample distribution** of a quantitative variable is normally described by the *mean,** the *median,** the *range,** and the *standard deviation.**

See also *variable*.

QUARANTINE: The enforced isolation of people, animals, or animal products that are infected or may be infected, in order to prevent the infection from spreading to other animals or people.

EXAMPLE: Quarantine of animals imported from a country where the *disease** (e.g., rabies) is present into a country that is free of this disease.

COMMENT 1: (a) It may also refer to the isolation of noninfected animals that are at risk of infection, and (b) in food animal *populations**, a quarantine may also be in place for replacement animals in order to deliberately expose them to specific *agents** prior to their introduction into the *herd.**

COMMENT 2: The duration of quarantine is usually the maximum incubation period for the disease of concern.

COMMENT 3: *Monitoring** for the disease of concern is usually conducted during the quarantine period.

COMMENT 4: Quarantine may be applied to an individual animal, or at the farm, region or national level.

QUESTIONNAIRE: Series of questions designed to elicit information in the context of field investigations or observational studies.

COMMENT 1: Questionnaires may be produced and administered on paper or by electronic means.

COMMENT 2: In a questionaire, one may find three types of questions: *open-ended,* * *closed,* * and *semi-open-ended.* *

COMMENT 3: Questionnaires can be administered by mail, by an interviewer during a face-to-face interview, by telephone, or by computer (via internet). Questionnaires designed to be mailed and filled out directly by the respondent are the most prevalent form of questionnaire in veterinary medicine. The type of questionnaire used in a *study* * depends on several factors. The most significant factors are the *cost* * (determined in part by the number of people surveyed), the kind of questions (topics covered by the study), and the location of the study (for example, in some regions of the world, a large *proportion* * of people may not have access to a phone). The type of questionnaire used often has an impact on the magnitude of some *biases,* * as well as on the *response rate.* *

COMMENT 4: It is essential to pretest a questionnaire before its implementation.

COMMENT 5: Although often neglected in veterinary medicine, the *validation* * of the questionnaire is needed as part of the assessment of the *validity* * of the study.

See also *response rate, bias, pretesting.*

QUESTIONNAIRE FOLLOW-UP: Procedure designed to ensure the highest response rate possible for mailed questionnaires.

EXAMPLE: The Minnesota Center for Survey Research proposes a three-step approach:

1. An initial copy of the *questionnaire* * is sent with a cover letter and a stamped return envelope.
2. A reminder postcard or letter is sent to everybody on the mailing list 1 week after the initial mailing. This reminder serves two purposes: it includes a thank-you note (for responders) and a request for reply for people who have not yet responded.
3. A copy of the questionnaire sent in step 1 is mailed with another cover letter and a stamped return envelope to all who have not yet filled out and returned the initial questionnaire. This second copy is sent 2 weeks after the first reminder (step 2).

COMMENT: Other techniques have been shown to increase the *response rate.* * They include: hand stamped envelopes with commemorative stamps; hand signed cover letters; hand addressed envelopes; offering incentives to participate, such as a summary of the results, a small amount of money (e.g., $1.00);

precontacts (contacting study subjects in advance to request their participation. This is mainly successful when done by phone).

QUOTA SAMPLING: A sampling method designed to obtain proportional quota samples by making the frequency distribution of certain characteristics identical between the population and the sample.

See also *proportional sample.*

QUOTIENT: Syn: ratio The result of a division.

EXAMPLES: $10 \div 100 = 0.1$; 50 of 200 piglets were transferred from post-weaning to the grow–finish unit on Monday. Hence, a quarter (50/200) of all piglets were moved on that day.

COMMENT: In France, it is also used as the number of events observed by unit of time divided by a *standard population.** In this context, a quotient is similar to a *rate.** However, it differs from the usual rate in two ways: (1) the *population** represented in the denominator is the one at the beginning of the time period (and not the one at the middle of the period), and (2) quotients are mainly used to construct tables for fictitious populations. For example, when comparing two different control strategies using a standard population to facilitate the comparison.

See also *proportion, rate.*

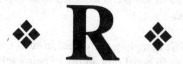

R

RANDOM: Expresses the lack of knowledge and capability of predicting or controlling a process or an event.

COMMENT 1: When referring to *sampling,** it indicates that each *subject** has an equal *probability** of being chosen and the choice is not controlled by the person in charge of sampling.

COMMENT 2: The existence of randomness as a part of nature is a question for philosophical debate. The application of the concept of randomness is key to the field of probability, which studies *random variables.** In medicine, the mathematics of probability are a very important aspect of the epistemology of modern *epidemiology,** which is also called predictive medicine. The need to predict is related to randomness because it arises when a decision has to be reached and no precise knowledge is available. Hence, probability is a means to deal with uncertainty.

COMMENT 3: Representative sampling has to be done randomly to be without *bias.** Bias is avoided because of the equal risk aspect of *random sampling.**

COMMENT 4: The only way to reproduce "chance" is to use a table of random numbers or an automatic random number generator. If not, insidious biases may occur.

COMMENT 5: It is not unusual to find in the scientific literature that samples selected without precise rules are considered to have been taken "at random." In fact, without using the procedures mentioned in comment 4, one can merely refer to a blind sample and not a *random sample.** Therefore, it would be more appropriate to reserve the use of the word random for cases where there is no ambiguity.

See also *random sample, random sampling, random selection, random variable, randomized trial.*

RANDOM MODEL: See **Probabilistic Model**

RANDOM SAMPLE: Syn: **probability sample** Sample characterized by random selection in which all individuals or units have a fixed and known probability of being chosen.

EXAMPLE: In a *population** of wild animals whose demographic structure is known, within each species, each *individual** has a given probability of being captured.

COMMENT 1: The assumption of random sampling is critical to *internal* and *external validity** in *observational studies.**

COMMENT 2: A random sample is assumed to be representative of the source population of *sample units.* *

RANDOM SAMPLING: Sampling performed in such a way that each individual in the population has an equal probability of being selected.

RANDOM SELECTION: Selection made such that each unit has a fixed probability of being selected according to the laws of probability.

EXAMPLE: Roulette at a casino.

RANDOM VARIABLE: Variable whose fluctuations follow a given probability law.

COMMENT 1: For each possible value of the *variable,* * there is a known probability of occurrence.

COMMENT 2: A random variable is characterized by its *probability* * *distribution* * (the relationship giving the probability according to the values of the variable), its *mathematical expectation* * and its *variance.* *

EXAMPLE 1: The protein level of milk is a random variable; its probability distribution is considered a *normal distribution.* *

EXAMPLE 2: Disease status (diseased/not diseased) may be looked at as a random variable if each level is coded (diseased = 1; not diseased = 0) and if a given probability is attached to each value.

RANDOMIZATION: Process of allocation in which the average probability of receiving a treatment or exposure is equal for each member of a group.

EXAMPLE: In a *randomized* clinical *trial* * to study the effect of itraconazole on feline nasal cryptoccocus, cats are randomly assigned to either the treatment group or the control group. The probability of assignment to either of the two groups is 50%.

COMMENT 1: Also, the process of assigning *individuals* * to exposure or treatment groups in which the *average* * probability of assignment to any *group* * is equivalent.

COMMENT 2: Any imbalances in a randomized experiment should be the result of chance, and not systematic *error.* *

COMMENT 3: Randomization is a carefully planned, replicable, and scientifically defensible allocation procedure. It is not equivalent to other convenience *methods* * of allocation (e.g., every other individual in a sequence receives a treatment).

RANDOMIZED: See **Random**

RANDOMIZED TRIAL: Trial in which individuals are distributed randomly into groups, one of these groups being a control group (absence of intervention, or placebo).

EXAMPLE: Vaccine trial in a calf farm: 50 calves are distributed into two groups (randomly), one that will receive the studied vaccine and the other a placebo.

COMMENT 1: The randomized trial mimics an *experimental study** in that the *study population** and the *distribution** of subjects into treatment and *control** groups are determined by the researcher.

COMMENT 2: The randomized trial is distinguished from the experimental study by the fact that environmental conditions of populations are not controlled by the observer.

COMMENT 3: The randomized trial is considered the most rigorous *method** of *hypothesis** testing in *epidemiology.**

RANGE: Dispersion characteristic of a theoretical or sample distribution, equal to the difference between the largest and the smallest values.

COMMENT: The range is usually expressed as the interval between the maximal and minimal values of the variable. It is of interest mainly for samples.

EXAMPLE: Weight of five carcasses: 29, 28, 25, 33, 24 kg. Range: 24 to 33 kg or 9 kg.

RANGE OF AN INTERVAL: Difference between the upper and the lower limit of an interval.

EXAMPLE: Class 1: 15 cm to less than 20 cm.
Class 2: 20 cm to less than 25 cm.
Range: 5 cm.

COMMENT: Classes may be of equal or unequal range.

See also *class, range.*

RANK: Sequential number associated with the sequential position of a value in a series that is classified in ascending order.

EXAMPLE: Classified *series** of values (in days) of the incubation period of rabies for a *group** of dogs. Series: 19, 21, 22, 25, 28, 28, 31, 37, 42; value 31 ranks 7th. Therefore, its rank is 7.

COMMENT: In computer science, rank refers to the number of linearly independent rows or columns of a matrix of numbers. It is also used for graphic purposes.

RATE: In epidemiology: A ratio that represents the magnitude of change in the occurrence of an event of interest (e.g., infection, disease, death, etc.) with respect to a population at risk over time.

In economics: The cost per unit of a service or commodity.

COMMENT 1: Rate was originally a fiscal term before becoming a legal, a banking and, finally, a demographic expression. Its usage is now common in most sciences, and has various connotations. In common language, it is used as a *ratio** whose numerator is part of the denominator. Such a broad denotation can be found in many scientific texts, including in the medical literature. Hence, expressions such as *attack rate,* * *mortality rate,* * and *culling rate* * are often simply *proportions* * and not true rates. To make matters worse, rate is often used differently by the same people depending on circumstances. This apparent flexibility can be, at times, very confusing.

COMMENT 2: When used as a proportion, it could represent, for example, the fraction of *individuals* * having a specific *disease* * in a *population at risk.* *

EXAMPLES: Rate of brucellosis infection in cattle $= \dfrac{\text{Number of infected cattle}}{\text{Total number of cattle at risk}}$

Rate of brucellosis infected herds $= \dfrac{\text{Number of infected herds}}{\text{Total number of herds at risk}}$

COMMENT 3: Rates and proportions are known as ratios. However, some authors prefer to limit the definition of ratio to the relationship between two independent and different entities (numerator not part of the denominator).

COMMENT 4: Rates are often expressed in percent, per thousand, per ten thousand, etc.

COMMENT 5: Based on the *epidemiology* * definition stated above, a rate corresponds to a speed of occurrence of an event over time. The numerator corresponds to the totality of observed events (death, birth, disease, etc.) and the denominator corresponds to the individual-time at risk for a given period. Hence, time appears in the denominator:

$$\dfrac{\text{Number of cases that occur during a given time}}{\text{Animal-time at risk}}$$

This rate describes the average speed with which the event under *study* * appears. In the equation above, the denominator represents the sum of the time at risk for all the animals susceptible to contract the disease in the observed *population.* * Animals that are already sick (and that can no longer contract the disease) are not considered in the calculation of the denominator. When a disease can reoccur in the same individual (e.g., mastitis), the observation period is often fragmented in intervals allowing one occurrence per animal. For example, one could calculate several rates of mastitis, one for each 30-day interval postpartum.

COMMENT 6: An estimate of the denominator may be obtained by adding the number of animals at risk at the beginning of the study period to the number at risk at the end, dividing the sum by 2.

COMMENT 7: Rates with an animal-time denominator are used when the population is very dynamic (many additions and/or withdrawals). Such rates can only be interpreted at the population level (i.e., a rate of 0.67 per animal-month should not be interpreted at the individual level).

See also *ratio, animal-time.*

RATE DIFFERENCE: See Attributable Risk

RATE OF CHANGE OF THE INCIDENCE RATE: Degree of variation in the incidence rate over time.

COMMENT: See Figure R1. The slope of the curve, at each point, represents the velocity of the incidence rate, and is thus equivalent to the acceleration of incidence. In the *epidemic** process described in Figure R1, the velocity of incidence increases for the first 3 months (V1, the slope is increasing); is stable during the 4th month (V2, the slope is zero); and then decreases (V3, the slope is decreasing).

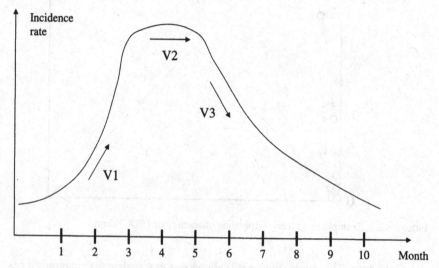

FIGURE R1. Evolution of disease incidence during an epidemic.

RATIO: The relative size of two quantities expressed by dividing one (numerator) by the other (denominator).

COMMENT 1: *Proportions,** percentages, and *rates** are ratios. However, the numerator of a proportion is always included in the denominator, whereas this is not necessarily the case for all ratios.

EXAMPLES: *Stillbirth** *rate:** 123 stillbirths/2300 piglets born over a 1-week period in a farrowing unit. Hence, the stillbirth rate was 5.3% for this period.

A 3:2 female-to-male ratio on a farm, also known as *sex-ratio.**

COMMENT 2: See comment 3 under the definition of *rate.**

$$\frac{\text{Number of dairy cows in a region}}{\text{Number of dairy farms in that region}} = \text{mean number of cows per farm.}$$

RECEIVER OPERATING CHARACTERISTIC CURVE: Syn: ROC curve
Graphical representation of the curve constituted by points corresponding to the sensitivity and the specificity of a test according to a chosen cutoff value.

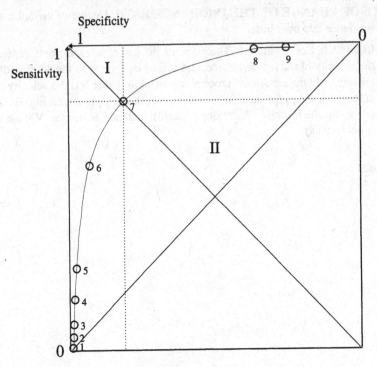

FIGURE R2.   Example of a receiver operating characteristic (ROC) curve.

COMMENT: This curve (Figure R2) allows one to visualize the antagonism between *sensitivity** and *specificity** for the same test. According to the specified cut-off value, decisions favor the use of either specificity (inferior part by the curve, 1 to 6) or sensitivity (superior part of the curve, 8 and 9). At point 7, sensitivity and specificity are equal. This point, the intersection of the ROC curve and the diagonal, is usually where the curve is the closest to the superior left corner and the sum of the two *errors, alpha** and *beta,** is lowest. Two quadrants can be defined from this point. All points situated in quadrant 1 (superior left) correspond to a test having a larger diagnostic efficiency than the one represented by the ROC curve. All points situated in quadrant II (inferior right) correspond to a test having a lower diagnostic efficiency.

RECEPTIVITY: In France: The potential for an individual to harbor a pathogen, allowing its development or multiplication.

In English: This word is not used in this context (see comment 1).

EXAMPLES: Adult pig infected by Aujeszky's virus; pig infected by the African swine fever virus.

COMMENT 1: The term receptivity is not found in English epidemiologic texts. However, it is a very useful concept despite potential confusion with the term indicating a female's willingness to breed during estrus (common usage in veterinary medicine). This is why, if used in English, it is recommended to be specific by adding *infection** (infection receptivity) or *infestation** (infestation receptivity) for clarity.

COMMENT 2: The species is a major determinant of receptivity.

COMMENT 3: Receptivity does not necessarily imply the ability to transmit the pathogen.

COMMENT 4: Receptive individuals may or may not be susceptible to the pathogen. For example, domestic pigs are receptive (virus multiplication) and susceptible (clinically affected) to African swine fever. However, wart hogs and bush pigs are receptive but are not susceptible to this virus. Cattle, horses, and sheep are not receptive and, therefore, are not susceptible to this agent.

COMMENT 5: Receptive individuals may become *vectors** or *carriers.** The species to which these individuals belong is an important determinant of their infection or infestation receptivity. Other *intrinsic** and *extrinsic factors** may also be involved.

COMMENT 6: Prevention measures (vaccination, strategic medication) act by increasing the threshold of infection/infestation receptivity of a *population.**

COMMENT 7: Receptivity can be quantitatively assessed (e.g., number of microbes needed [e.g., $>10^4$ *E. coli*] to establish infection). The outcome of *contamination** of an individual depends on the degree of *infectivity** of the *agent** and on the degree of infection/infestation receptivity of this individual.

See also *susceptibility*.

RECORD: A collection of data that relates to a particular client, animal, or group of animals.

EXAMPLE: Sow farrowing card with sow identification number, farrowing date, number of piglets born alive, number of mummies, number of stillborns, and treatments (including vaccines) administered to the sow and the piglets, etc.

COMMENT: The aggregation of records from all animals or groups of animals in a farm represents the data component of a *recording** system. Data manipulation and the production of pertinent reports are the other two main components of computerized recording systems.

RECORDING: Systematic collection of data regarding one or several events of interest in a population.

COMMENT 1: This word is normally part of expressions, such as recording scheme and recording system. Many computerized recording or record-keeping systems are available today in veterinary medicine:

In swine: PigCHAMP, PigTale, Swine Graphics, etc.
In dairy cattle: DAISY, DairyCHAMP, etc.
In companion animals: VetStar, PSI, THIS, etc.
In poultry: Agri-Stats.

COMMENT 2: Recording normally implies the permanent preservation of data or information.

COMMENT 3: Recording of data is now an essential component of veterinary practice, in particular in commercial animal production. Several factors have influenced the development of recording systems: larger farm operations; the integration of animal production; the growing involvement of veterinarians in *health management,* * mainly regarding production problems that do not have an infectious origin; and society's expectation of services going beyond traditional veterinary medicine.

RECURRENCE: Reoccurrence of clinical signs of a disease in an individual that had recovered from this disease, following or not following a new infection or infestation (Figure R3).

> EXAMPLES: Following a new *infection** or *infestation:** Recurrence can be observed with *diseases** caused by pathogens having antigenically and immunogenically different serotypes: human or avian influenza, foot-and-mouth disease, etc.
>
> No new infection or infestation: Infectious anemia in horses, malaria in humans, etc.

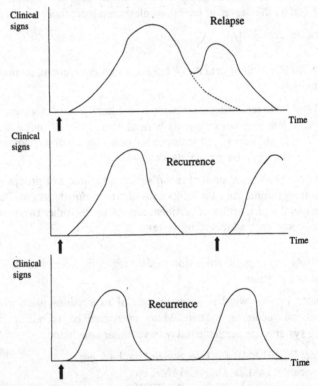

FIGURE R3.   Illustration of the difference between relapse and recurrence.   Arrow indicates contact with the pathogen.

COMMENT: Recurrence differs from *relapse** (no new infection or infestation). In general, a relapse occurs only once and during the convalescent period, whereas recurrence characterizes a *phenomenon** that may occur repeatedly after the initial recovery. For some authors, however, recurrence and relapse are considered synonomous.

RECURRENT DISEASE: Disease characterized by a series of recurrences separated by periods of remission.

EXAMPLE: Recurrent fever due to various *Borrelia* species.

COMMENT: *Recurrence** may occur once or several times. In general, however, the word recurrent is associated with numerous reoccurrences separated by periods of remission that may last days to months depending on the *disease.**

See also *recurrence, relapse.*

REFERENCE POPULATION: See **General Population**

REFERENCE PRICE: See **Shadow Price**

REGRESSION ANALYSIS: A statistical analysis based on a linear or nonlinear model used to describe or explain a variable as dependent on or predicted by one or many other variables called independent or explanatory.

COMMENT 1: Regression analysis allows one to test the existence of a relationship between *dependent* and *independent variables.**

COMMENT 2: The following is a multiple linear regression model:

$$y = \beta_0 + \beta_1 x_1 + \beta_2 x_2 + \beta_3 x_3 + ... + \beta_k x_k + \varepsilon$$

This model supposes that for all values of x_1, x_2, ..., x_k, the above equation gives an approximation of the true relationship between y (a continuous variable) and these x's. Linear refers to linearity in the unknown *parameters** β_0, β_1, β_2, ... ,β_k. The symbol ε represents the deviation between the calculated value obtained from the model and the observed value, and it is assumed that $E(\varepsilon) = 0$ with var $(\varepsilon) = \sigma^2$.

COMMENT 3: To *estimate* the parameters β_0 ... β_k, the most commonly used *methods** are the *least squares method** and the *maximum likelihood method.** Other than the assumption of independence, no assumptions on the distribution of the response variable y are needed to estimate the parameters by the method of least squares. However, this is not the case with the method of maximum likelihood.

COMMENT 4: The relationship can be nonlinear. For example, $y = e^x$.

COMMENT 5: When the *dependent variable** y is dichotomous (case–control, death/survival), one should consider *logistic regression.**

See also *least squares method, maximum likelihood method.*

REINFECTION: A second infection by the same pathogen occurring in the same animal.

COMMENT 1: To be differentiated from *secondary infection** (different pathogen).

COMMENT 2: May refer to an infection in a different organ within the same animal after the initial infection has ended. For example, an *E. coli* infection producing airsacculitis in chickens and reinfection with the same *agent** resulting in joint *disease.**

See also *recurrence*.

RELAPSE: Reoccurrence of clinical signs of a disease in a convalescent individual or group.

COMMENT: It concerns the reactivation of the pathogen responsible for the initial clinical expression (to be differentiated from *recurrence**).

See also *recurrence* (Figure R3).

RELATIVE ERROR: Ratio of the absolute error over the true value.

EXAMPLE: True value: 200 g
Value measured: 206 g
Absolute error: 6 g
Relative error = (206 − 200)/200 = 6/200 = 3%

See also *absolute error*.

RELATIVE FREQUENCY: Ratio of the number of events recorded to the number of individuals in a population or sample.

EXAMPLE: Table C3 (*cumulative relative frequency**).

COMMENT 1: The relative frequency may be expressed as a *proportion** between 0 and 1 or, more frequently, as a percentage.

COMMENT 2: To be differentiated from frequency (Table C3).

RELATIVE PRECISION: Ratio of the precision of an estimate to the estimated value.

COMMENT 1: Given the same precision, the relative precision on an estimated rate improves as the *frequency** of the event of interest increases.

COMMENT 2: The relative precision is expressed as a percentage. The lower its value, the better the precision.

RELATIVE RATE: Syn: incidence rate ratio, incidence density ratio Ratio of the rate in an exposed population to the rate in an unexposed population.

EXAMPLE: If the rate of illness in one cohort is 1.56 per 100 calf-years, and the rate of illness in another cohort is 0.76 per 100 calf-years, then the relative rate is 2.05.

COMMENT: The relative rate should not be considered as necessarily equivalent to the *relative risk,** which is a ratio of two *risks,** rather than *rates.** The two closely approximate each other when the *disease** is rare.

RELATIVE RISK: Ratio of the incidence of an outcome of interest in individuals exposed to a hypothesized risk or causal factor, to the incidence in individuals not so exposed.

RR = incidence rate (exposed)/incidence rate (nonexposed) (Table R1)

COMMENT 1: The relative risk is a measure of the strength of the *association** between an exposure and an outcome, which is an important criteria in the establishment of a causal relationship.

The RR can *range** from 0 to infinity. Given a factor A and a *disease** B:

• if RR < 1; this is an indication that A may be a protective factor;
• if RR = 1; this would indicate that there is no association between A and B (based on this information alone).
• if RR > 1; factor A could be a *risk* or *causal factor.**

COMMENT 2: The incidence information used for the calculation of the relative risk may be in the form of a true *rate** or a *cumulative incidence rate.**

COMMENT 3: Example of calculation (see data presented under the term *attributable risk**).

$$\text{Relative risk} = \frac{\text{Cumulative incidence rate}}{\text{(no measure of hygiene)}} = 13.33\%/5\% = 2.7$$
$$\qquad\qquad\qquad\frac{}{\substack{\text{Cumulative incidence rate}\\ \text{(hygiene measures present)}}}$$

When the incidence of the disease is rare, the value of the *odds ratio** is close to the one of the relative risk. Indeed, using the following two-by-two table:

	Diseased	Nondiseased
Exposed	a	b
Nonexposed	c	d

Relative risk = [a/(a+b)]/[c/(c+d)]; when the incidence of the disease is low, the number of diseased individuals is negligible compared to the number of nondiseased. Hence, if the number of diseased individuals is omitted from the denominator of each cumulative incidence rate, the relative risk = $\dfrac{a/b}{c/d} = \dfrac{a \times d}{c \times b}$, which is the formula for the odds ratio.

COMMENT 4: The relative risk is calculated from data obtained in *prospective studies** (*cohort studies**). With *retrospective studies** (*case–control**), the odds ratio is calculated as an estimate of RR.

TABLE R1. Relationship between relative risk, attributable risk, and attributable fraction

I_e = incidence rate in a group exposed to a given risk factor
$I_{\bar{e}}$ = incidence rate in a nonexposed group
I_{pop} = incidence in the total population

Relative risk (RR) = $\dfrac{I_e}{I_{\bar{e}}}$

Attributable risk = $I_e - I_{\bar{e}}$

Attributable fraction = $\dfrac{I_e - I_{\bar{e}}}{I_e}$ or (RR − 1) / RR

Population attributable fraction = $\dfrac{I_{pop} - I_{\bar{e}}}{I_{pop}}$ or $(RR_{pop} - 1) / RR_{pop}$

Where RR_{pop} = [(a + c) / n] / [c / (c + d)] or $\dfrac{I_{pop}}{I_{\bar{e}}}$

See also *case–control study, cohort study.*

RELIABILITY (OF A TEST): Quality of a test reflecting its tendency to give the same results on repeated measurements of a sample.

COMMENT 1: A reliable test gives repeatable results, usually over time, locations or populations, but does not ensure *accuracy** (Table A1, accuracy).

COMMENT 2: Reliability has been used as a synonym for (1)(preferred) *precision,* *reproducibility,* *repeatability,* and *consistency,* and (2) accuracy in some references (Table A1).

REMOVAL: Withdrawal of animals from a herd or flock for various reasons.

COMMENT 1: Removal is expressed as a number of animals removed over a given period of time, which is dependent on the species and type of production. For example, in dairy and pig operations, it is normally 1 year.

COMMENT 2: Removal includes all culled and dead animals. In some types of production (e.g., dairy), it may also include animals sold.

REMOVAL RATE:

$\dfrac{\text{Number of sold, culled and dead animals}}{\text{Average herd inventory}}$ during a given period of time

COMMENT 1: This term is normally applied to reproductive animals (gilts in swine production; heifers in dairy production, etc.). It is usually presented as an annual *rate,** although it is also calculated based on a production cycle such as over one lactation period in dairy cattle. In grow–finish facilities, it is calculated over one production cycle, and only culled and dead animals are part of the numerator.

COMMENT 2: This rate assumes a relatively stable denominator. Under such condition, it should be equivalent to the *replacement rate.* *

REPEATABILITY (OF A TEST): Measure of the closeness of agreement between values obtained from repeated measurements performed on samples or individuals under specific conditions, usually by the same operator or laboratory.

COMMENT 1: A repeatable test gives consistent results but does not ensure *accuracy* * (Table A1, accuracy).

COMMENT 2: Repeatability corresponds to intralaboratory variation (σ_r^2).

COMMENT 3: In France, for example, a standard exists (AFNOR NF X 06041) regarding the limit of variability of repeatability:

$$r = 1.96\sqrt{2\sigma_r^2}$$

REPLACEMENT RATE:

$$\frac{\text{Number of animals introduced into herd}}{\text{Average herd inventory}} \text{ during given period of time}$$

COMMENT 1: This terminology applies to reproductive animals (gilts in swine production; heifers in dairy production, etc.). It is usually presented as an annual *rate,* * although it is also calculated based on a production cycle, such as over one lactation period in dairy cattle.

COMMENT 2: This rate assumes a relatively stable denominator. Under such condition, it should be equivalent to the *removal rate.* *

See also *removal rate.*

REPORTABLE DISEASE: See **Notifiable Disease**

REPRESENTATIVE SAMPLE: A sample whose distribution of one or more criteria is similar to the distribution of these criteria in the source population.

COMMENT 1: The concept of a representative *sample* * is meaningless without specification of the criteria on which *representativeness* * is based.

COMMENT 2: *Random sampling* * is not a guarantee of representativeness with respect to *individual* * criteria; this is analogous to the principle that randomization to *groups* * does not guarantee equal distribution of all factors between the groups.

COMMENT 3: This is an unbiased *sample.* *

REPRESENTATIVENESS: Quality of a sample to faithfully represent, based on one or more chosen criteria, the population from which it has been extracted.

COMMENT 1: Representativeness of a *sample* * is essential if one wants to extrapolate results to the *population.* *

COMMENT 2: *Random sampling** is considered the best unbiased approach to obtain a representative sample from a population. Without *randomization,** the *risk** of a *selection bias** increases, which may reduce the representativeness of the sample.

COMMENT 3: Unfortunately, efforts to increase representativeness may lead to a reduction in data *validity.** For example, a random selection of *herds** to obtain production or *disease**-related data from producers may lead to incomplete information due to a variation in the degree of participation depending on the producer and/or because of the poor quality of existing farm records available for some of the selected herds. In contrast, data obtained from a convenience sample may have a superior internal validity but may not be representative of the entire population. In this case, a comparison between the convenience sample and the general population for *parameters** where data are available for both may allow the assessment of the degree of representativeness of the sample. For example, data on *mortality rates,** abattoir condemnations, herd size, etc. may be available for large areas (county, state, country), which would allow the investigator to determine the representativeness of a convenience sample for these particular *variables.** Because of the nature of the data being collected, one may have to compromise on the representativeness of the sample to optimize data validity.

REPRODUCIBILITY (OF A TEST): Measure of the closeness of agreement between values obtained from repeated measurements performed on samples or individuals under specific conditions, usually by different operators or laboratories.

COMMENT 1: This notion includes the concept of reproducibility (e.g., repeated measurements by different operators or laboratories) and *repeatability** (e.g., repeated measurements taken by the same operator).

COMMENT 2: A reproducible test gives repeatable results but does not ensure *accuracy** (see Table A1, Accuracy).

COMMENT 3: When applied to the same operator or laboratory, repeatability is preferred to reproducibility.

COMMENT 4: Reproducibility corresponds to the "variability among laboratories."

COMMENT 5: The variance associated with reproducibility is equal to the sum of the variance among and within laboratories.

Reproducibility index = $(\sigma^2_R/(\sigma^2_r + \sigma^2_R)$
Where: r = repeatability, and R = reproducibility

COMMENT 6: In France, a standard exists (AFNOR NF X 06041) regarding the limit of variability of reproducibility:

$$R = 1.96\sqrt{2\sigma_R^2}$$

RESERVOIR: Syn: reservoir host, reservoir of infection Any animate (humans, animals, insects, etc.) or inanimate object (plant, soil, feces, etc.) or any combination of these serving as a habitat of a pathogen that reproduces itself in such a way as to be transmitted to a susceptible host.

EXAMPLES: Animal reservoir:

The rat as a reservoir of *Leptospira*, the *agent** responsible for leptospirosis in cattle, pigs, etc.

Chickens carrying *Histomonas meleagridis*, the agent responsible for histomoniasis in turkeys.

Waterfowl carrying the influenza virus (AIV), responsible for devastating *epidemics,** such as the one in Pennsylvania in 1983–1984, which resulted in losses of over 200 million US dollars in addition to about 62 million dollars in eradication *costs.** A similar epidemic was reported in Mexico in early 1995.

Inanimate reservoir:
The soil harboring spores of *Clostridium chauvoei*, the agent responsible for blackleg, a *disease** principally of cattle.

Reservoir with more than one component:
Warthogs and ticks (African swine fever). The African swine fever (ASF) virus is maintained in a region by a cycle of *infection** between warthogs and soft ticks. Both are needed for the survival of the ASF virus. Bushpigs can also serve as reservoir of this agent.

A rodent and its burrow (plague caused by *Yersinia pestis*). When a rodent carrying *Yersinia pestis* dies in its burrow, the stable soil conditions, enriched by nutritive elements coming from the decomposition of the dead rodent, are favorable to the multiplication of the bacteria.

COMMENT: A species is likely to be an effective reservoir, in the context of *disease transmission,** under the following circumstances:

• The infectious agent does not affect the reservoir host.
• The reservoir host is highly infected. In the case of a viral infection, viremia is prolonged (> 1 week).
• The *population** density of this reservoir host is high.

However, a pathogen may also be maintained in nature via the continuous and necessary occurrence of the disease in a susceptible population. For example, considering rabies in foxes; although all affected foxes die from rabies, the virus is maintained within the fox population due to the continuous fox-to-fox transmission.

RESERVOIR HOST: See Reservoir

RESERVOIR OF INFECTION: See Reservoir

RESISTANCE (OF AN INDIVIDUAL): The ability of an individual to defend itself against a pathogen.

EXAMPLES: An adequate immune response following rabies vaccination confers resistance against the rabies virus. The protected individual is said to be resistant. Pigs lacking the specific receptors in the intestinal epithelial cells that are required for binding K88 pili are resistant to infection by K88+ enterotoxigenic *Escherichia coli*.

Leukosis-resistant strains of poultry.

COMMENT 1: Resistance may be individual or species dependent.

COMMENT 2: Resistance is also commonly used in the context of drug resistance, which is the ability of a microorganism to withstand the effects of a drug.

RESPONSE RATE:

$$\frac{\text{Number of individuals participating in a survey}}{\substack{\text{Total number of individuals who would have been surveyed,} \\ \text{had they all participated}}}$$

COMMENT: Many authors exclude from the denominator all individuals who could not be located (i.e., individuals included in the initial *sample,** but who did not have the opportunity to participate). It is highly recommended to specify how many people could not be reached, if any, when reporting the response rate.

EXAMPLE: A *questionnaire** was mailed to 334 cat owners as part of a *study** on inappropriate elimination behavior. Twenty-one people could not be located. Of the 313 individuals who received the questionnaire, 242 replied.

Response rate = 242/334 or about 72.5% of the study sample.

or

Response rate = 242/313 or about 77.3% of individuals in the study sample who could be reached.

RESPONSE VARIABLE: See **Dependent Variable**

RETROSPECTIVE STUDY: A study in which historical records about the population(s) of interest are used as the basis for studies of risk factors and outcomes of interest.

EXAMPLE: A *case–control study** in which hospital records of cows presented for surgical corrections of an abomasal displacement and cows presented for other surgical conditions were used to determine if there was a breed predilection for abomasal displacement.

COMMENT 1: A key feature of a retrospective study is that the *disease** or outcome of interest has occurred when the *study** starts.

COMMENT 2: The term retrospective refers to methods in which the *data** are collected rather than to the specific design of the study.

COMMENT 3: Retrospective studies may be descriptive (serve only to describe a *population**) or may be analytical (evaluate relationships between factors and outcomes of interest). Case–control studies are an example of an analytical retrospective study.

COMMENT 4: The main advantages of conducting a study retrospectively are that they are inexpensive and the results are available very quickly.

REVENUE: All cash inflows, taxable and nontaxable.

RISK: Probability that an event (disease, pathological phenomenon) will occur at a given time or during a given time period.

In risk analysis: The integration of the likelihood of occurrence of an event and of the magnitude of its impact on animal and/or human health.

COMMENT 1: Risk can be modified by exposure to *extrinsic factors** or by modification of *intrinsic factors.**

COMMENT 2: Risk is a *probability** that is an estimated value. Risk should not be confused with *incidence rate.**

COMMENT 3: Risk assessment is becoming a popular *method** for decision making in the health sciences.

See also *risk analysis.*

RISK ANALYSIS: The formal process for evaluating, managing, determining, and communicating the impact of a risk in a population.

COMMENT 1: Risk analysis includes (1) risk assessment, (2) risk management, and (3) risk communication (Figure R4).

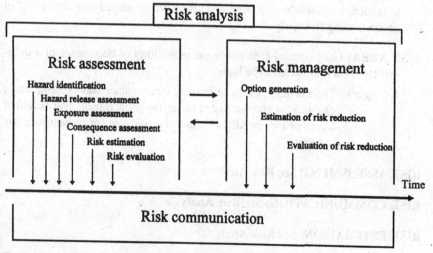

FIGURE R4. Schematic representation of the principal stages of risk analysis.

Risk assessment answers the following questions: what can go wrong? how likely is the event to occur? and what are the consequences if it occurs? Risk assessment can be both quantitative and qualitative. Quantitative risk assessment uses all available data to develop the *probability** of events occurring and associated measures of uncertainty. Risk assessment should be based on all available scientifically valid data and the estimation process should be transparent.

Risk management is a pragmatic decision-making process aimed at the adoption of actions or policies to mitigate *risks.** It answers two questions: should any actions be taken? and if so, what action should be taken? Risk management uses information from a risk assessment to develop a strategy to reduce risk and increase safety, taking into account other social considerations such as politics, public opinion, and international relations.

Risk communication is the unambiguous exchange of information among individuals or affected groups concerning any phase of the risk analysis process. It is an open, two-way exchange of information and opinion about risk, leading to a better understanding and better risk management decisions.

COMMENT 2: Risk analysis is a well-established, usually highly quantitative procedure that has been applied broadly across many disciplines such as finance, engineering, and international diplomacy. In the health sciences, it has been most widely used in the *environmental health** sciences. Recently, in veterinary medicine, risk assessment has become increasingly utilized to evaluate risks posed by microbial pathogens in a *food safety** context and for decision making concerning international trade and imports. Risk assessment is useful not only in the development of quantitative measures of risk but also in identifying the most important gaps in our knowledge concerning a particular risk. The risk analysis process is best thought of as an iterative process whereby the risk assessment is updated as we develop better data concerning the risk in question and this new information is used to refine risk management strategies. *Hazard** identification, risk mitigation strategies, risk characterization, *cost–benefit analysis,** and safety are all related concepts useful in understanding risk analysis.

RISK AREA: Geographical area where the probability of occurrence of a detrimental event is expected to be high.

EXAMPLES: The Lorraine region of France, where rabies was present, was a risk area for nonvaccinated cattle; the geographical distribution of *Glossina spp.* in Africa defines the risk area for trypanosomiasis in cattle.

RISK ASSESSMENT: See **Risk Analysis**

RISK COMMUNICATION: See **Risk Analysis**

RISK ESTIMATION: See **Risk Analysis**

RISK EVALUATION: See **Risk Analysis**

RISK FACTOR: Factor associated with an increase in the probability of occurrence of an outcome of interest (e.g., disease, reduced performance, or productivity, etc.).

EXAMPLES: Poor ventilation leading to a high *incidence** of respiratory problems.

Introduction of cattle infected with bovine leukosis into a herd resulting in its *contamination.**

Excessive temperature variation over a short period of time (< 1 day) associated with an increase in the incidence of diarrhea in piglets.

COMMENT 1: This expression is used in the literature in at least two different ways. Some authors consider a risk factor as any factor that is statistically associated with the outcome of interest, whether or not *causality** has been demonstrated or is even probable. Such a factor could actually be a *risk marker.**

Other authors consider that a risk factor is a determinant of a given outcome, i.e., a certain degree of causality exists between the risk factor and the outcome, or is at least very probable. The implication is that, to be a risk factor, a factor must contribute to the events leading to the outcome.

COMMENT 2: Many authors will consider as risk factor one that is associated with a decrease in the probability of occurrence of an outcome. Such a factor is also referred to as protective factor.

COMMENT 3: For some authors, a risk factor is a factor that is modifiable (i.e., can be prevented, removed, reduced, or altered).

COMMENT 4: The *relative risk** is an epidemiologic measure of the strength of the relationship between a risk factor and an outcome (can be estimated by the *odds ratio**). The magnitude of the effect can be assessed by determining the *attributable risk,** the *attributable fraction,** and the *population attributable fraction.**

COMMENT 5: An *interaction** between several risk factors is often needed to produce the observed outcome.

See also *risk marker, determinant cause.*

RISK INDICATOR: See **Risk Marker**

RISK MANAGEMENT: See **Risk Analysis**

RISK MARKER: Syn: **risk indicator** A factor, usually a surrogate for a causal factor, associated with an increased probability or rate of occurrence of a health outcome.

EXAMPLE 1: Age is a risk marker for the clinical expression of maedi-visna in sheep.

EXAMPLE 2: Living in a habitat with old and flaking paint is a risk marker for lead toxicosis.

COMMENT: This term is restricted by some authors to refer exclusively to *intrinsic* (i.e., nonmodifiable) *host factors.* *

ROBUST: Quality of a statistical procedure whose results remain valid even when there is some departure from the underlying assumptions for this test.

EXAMPLE: The *t* test is robust with respect to the kurtosis of the *distribution.* *

ROC CURVE: See **Receiver Operating Characteristic Curve**

ROLLING AVERAGE: See **Moving Average**

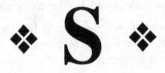

SAMPLE: A subset of a population selected for inclusion in a study.

COMMENT 1: Also, a collection of *sample units* * derived from a *sampling frame.* *

COMMENT 2: See specific types of *sampling strategy* * for further detail.

SAMPLE MEAN: If $x_1, x_2, ..., x_n$ constitute a sample, the mean is the sum of all n x's divided by the sample size *n*.

COMMENT 1: The sample mean is a measure of central tendency for *normal distribution.* *

COMMENT 2: In practice, the sample mean is often calculated even when *sampling* * is not *random.* *

COMMENT 3: Often inappropriately used. It is highly sensitive to extreme values. For example, in Ontario in 1991 the mean percent carcass condemnation in turkeys due to airsacculitis was 3.5% while the *median* * was only about 0.55%. This was due to a few severe *outbreaks* * recorded on a limited number of farms. Hence, given a negatively or positively skewed (asymmetrical) *distribution,* * the sample mean does not indicate the point of most frequent occurrence.

SAMPLE MEETING ELIGIBILITY CRITERIA: A sample whose units have all met prespecified conditions regarding eligibility for inclusion in a study.

COMMENT: The restrictiveness of the eligibility criteria will have an influence on the generalizability or *representativeness** of the results.

SAMPLE SIZE: Number of statistical units or individuals in a sample.

COMMENT: The sample size is usually determined based on the desired degree of *precision** of the *study** (descriptive) or on its required power (inferential). Sample sizes depending on study criteria are available in the form of tables. The size of a *sample** is calculated according to the *probability** of occurrence of an event of interest in the *population** or in function of the expected differences between *groups.**

See also *precision, power.*

SAMPLE UNIT: The basic element that is sampled.

COMMENT 1: The sample unit can be an animal, a group of animals (i.e., a pen, a herd), etc.

COMMENT 2: In a *cluster sample,** the sample unit is the *cluster,** whereas the *statistical unit** is the element of the cluster.

COMMENT 3: In *multistage sampling,** the sample unit of the first stage is called the primary unit, the sample unit of the second stage is called the secondary unit, etc.

See also *sampling, cluster sampling, statistical unit* (Figure S6).

SAMPLE VARIANCE: See Variance of a Sample

SAMPLED POPULATION: Fraction of the eligible population effectively retained in the sample after application of a sampling procedure.

EXAMPLE: 2000 farms (of the *eligible population**) chosen randomly.

COMMENT 1: This is a subset of the *target population.**

COMMENT 2: For practical reasons, the sampled population may differ from the *study population** selected at the beginning of the project or from the *final study population,** because part of the original *sample** may not be accessible (i.e., refusal to participate, lost to follow-up) or may not be retained in the *study** (i.e., incomplete *records**).

See also *population* (Figure P3).

SAMPLER EFFECT: Measurement error caused by the individual collecting information.

EXAMPLE: Interviewer bias: when an interviewer knows the outcome under study, he/she may be more likely to probe for exposure histories.

COMMENT: This is a measurement *bias.**

See also *bias.*

SAMPLING: The process of selecting elements from a population in order to construct a subset (sample) to be used for making inferences about the population.

See also *sample*.

SAMPLING APPROACH: See **Sampling Strategy**

SAMPLING BASE: See **Sampling Frame**

SAMPLING BIAS: See **Bias**

SAMPLING DESIGN: See **Sampling Strategy**

SAMPLING ERROR: See **Sampling Variation**

SAMPLING FRACTION: Syn: **sampling risk** Ratio of the sample size to the population size.

> EXAMPLE: The sampling fraction for a *survey** on pseudorabies (Aujeszky's disease) was 4% (60 of the 1500 pig farms located in a region were included in the *study**).

COMMENT 1: The sampling fraction is not indicative of the *representativeness** of the *sample.**

COMMENT 2: It is often wrongly referred to as the sampling rate.

SAMPLING FRAME: Syn: **sampling base** The assemblage of individuals (or groups) on which sampling is performed.

> EXAMPLE: All registered dairy farms in a region (see Figure P3, *population**).

See also *population, source population*.

SAMPLING RISK: See **Sampling Fraction**

SAMPLING SCHEME: See **Sampling Design**

SAMPLING STRATEGY: Syn: **sampling approach, sampling design** Detailed description of the selection process used to obtain a sample from a population.

> EXAMPLE: In a finite *population,** assuming that a list of all *individuals** is available, one could use a *random** number table to select a subset of individuals. This is a simple random sampling scheme.

COMMENT 1: One should always strive to develop a random sampling design. However, this is not often achieved under field conditions.

COMMENT 2: It is an intrinsic component of study design since it determines the nature and *precision** of *extrapolations** from the *sample** to the *population.** The type or method of *sampling** (nonprobability sampling, simple random sampling, systematic random sampling, stratified random sampling, *cluster sampling,** *multistage sampling,** etc.) is the core of the sampling strategy.

COMMENT 3: The sampling strategy should always be part of the *protocol** of an epidemiologic *study.**

SAMPLING VARIATION: Random variation of the estimate of the distribution parameters of a random variable under study; defined as the difference between the sample estimate and the actual values in the population of origin.

COMMENT: This variation is due to the sampling error.

EXAMPLES: In the case of a normally distributed *random variable** (weight in the male population of a given species), the difference between $E(x)$ and μ.

Given a *population** from which two *samples** (1 and 2) were drawn; Sample 1 yielded an average weight of 10 kg. Sample 2 yielded an average weight of 15 kg. Because the same *statistical units** were not in both samples, the average weight varied from Sample 1 to Sample 2.

SANITARY MEASURES: See **Sanitary Prophylaxis**

SANITARY PROPHYLAXIS: In France: Prophylaxis using only sanitary measures. This expression is not used in English. The term sanitary measures would be preferred.

EXAMPLES: *Quarantine** and restriction of animal (or people) movement, disinfection, and *population** screening with elimination of affected *individuals** (e.g., *eradication** programs for bovine tuberculosis).

COMMENT 1: Sanitary and medical measures of prophylaxis are usually complementary (e.g., combination of quarantine and vaccination when introducing animals into a population) but can be antagonistic. For example vaccination may interfere with screening tests in eradication campaigns (e.g., BCG vaccination of cattle against tuberculosis and tuberculin testing; *Brucella* vaccines and serological testing).

COMMENT 2: *Biosecurity** measures are part of sanitary prophylaxis.

COMMENT 3: Sanitary prophylaxis may be implemented as part of a strategy to *control** or *eradicate** a particular *disease** present on a farm or in a region, or to prevent the introduction of such disease.

SAPROPHYTE: A microorganism or organism that feeds on inert organic material.

EXAMPLES: Various fungi, protozoa, and bacteria living in the external environment.

COMMENT 1: Some saprophytes can have *pathogenic** (for example, some clostridial spp.) or sensitizing (some mycobacterial spp.) actions when introduced into an organism.

COMMENT 2: To be differentiated from a *commensal** that lives in a *host** and not in the external environment.

SCREENING: Systematic examination of individuals or groups of individuals of a population in order to ascertain the prevalence of certain characteristics or a given health problem that may not be apparent in any member of the population.

EXAMPLES: Screening for: bovine tuberculosis using an intradermal test, bovine brucellosis based on a serological test, mercury levels in wildlife and in domesticated animals in Northern Canada.

COMMENT 1: Screening may be limited to areas where *cases** of a *disease** of interest have already been identified. This is a form of strategic screening where, for example, only animals from *herds** located within a 5-km radius of a herd found to be positive for a given disease would be tested. However, in general, screening is applied to all individuals in a *population** (*mass screening**) or at least to a large sample of the population. It may also be limited to individuals from a certain segment of the population. For example, all replacement animals in swine herds.

COMMENT 2: Screening may be performed at the individual or group level (e.g., pen, herd). In the latter case, the detection of a single affected individual may be sufficient to consider that the corresponding group is affected, even if the other members of the group are not necessarily affected. This approach is useful when the screening *method** is known to have a relatively low *sensitivity.** Tests performed on pooled *samples** (e.g., mixing of several sera, milk from bulk tank) are also commonly used for screening at the group level.

COMMENT 3: The quality of the screening procedure depends on the *predictive values** (positive and negative) of the test, which are dependent on the sensitivity and *specificity** of the test as well as the within-herd *prevalence** of the disease or *health** characteristic** of interest.

COMMENT 4: Screening differs from establishing a *diagnosis,** even if the same tests may be used in both cases. The fundamental difference is that the presence of *clinical signs** normally prompts diagnostic procedures on the affected individuals, whereas screening, although often implemented after a disease has been identified in a population, includes all individuals or groups of a population independently of their clinical status. This impacts on the performance of the test, whose predictive values depend on whether it is used as a diagnostic tool or as a screening test. Indeed, the positive predictive value of a test decreases as the prevalence of the disease decreases (see also *positive predictive value,** Figure P7). Because the prevalence of disease among individuals showing clinical signs is much more likely to be higher than in the population at large, one can assume that the predictive value of a positive test will be higher when it is used for diagnostic purposes than when it is employed for screening the population.

COMMENT 5: Some authors may refer to preventive screening in reference to the screening of a population with a preventive medical program in prospect.

COMMENT 6: The screening procedure may be limited to one condition or may include several at the same time.

See also *diagnosis, positive and negative predictive values, sensitivity, specificity.*

SEASONAL VARIATION: Syn: annual periodic variation Significant fluctuation of the incidence of an event occurring within a 1-year period, and which reoccurs every year.

EXAMPLES: The incidence of pseudorabies (Aujeszky's disease) and transmissible gastroenteritis in swine increases during winter, while the incidence of myxomatosis is highest during summer and fall.

A reduction in conception rate in swine, known as seasonal infertility, is associated with irregular returns to estrus. Indeed, the gradual increase in day-length toward summer solstice is related to reduced fertility of females mated during the summer months.

COMMENT 1: Some diseases undergo regular seasonal fluctuations in *incidence** (Aujeszky's disease, myxomatosis), whereas others hardly show any fluctuation throughout the year (clinical cases of bovine viral leukosis).

COMMENT 2: The factors responsible for these fluctuations may be known (transmission of myxomatosis by mosquitoes) or unknown (Aujeszky's disease).

COMMENT 3: In the above definition, the word significant underlines statistically and biologically meaningful variations. In the context of animal production, the threshold of significance varies depending on the relative importance of the variable in terms of productivity.

SECOND QUARTILE: See Median

SECONDARY CASE: Case of disease linked directly or indirectly to a primary case.

See also *primary case.*

SECONDARY INFECTION: Infection by a pathogen following an infection by a different infectious agent.

EXAMPLE: A pig infected with *Bordetella bronchiseptica* that also becomes infected with *Pasteurella multocida*, resulting in atrophic rhinitis.

COMMENT 1: To be differentiated from *reinfection,** which is a second infection with the same *agent.**

COMMENT 2: The agent involved in the secondary infection will differ from the first agent in varying degrees. For example, they may be two totally different types (*Pasteurella* versus pseudorabies (Aujeszky's disease), genuses (*Bordetella* versus *Pasteurella*), species (*Mycoplasma gallisepticum* versus *Mycoplasma synoviae*), or serotypes (*Actinobacillus pleuropneumoniae* serotype 1 versus serotype 5).

COMMENT 3: It is often difficult, under field conditions, to determine which agent came first and which one came second. Also note that the secondary infection is not necessarily required to trigger disease. In the example above, both *Bordetella* and *Pasteurella* can produce disease on their own.

See also *intercurrent.*

SECONDARY OUTBREAK: Outbreak linked, directly or indirectly, to the first observed outbreak, without the introduction of the causal agent from a source other than the primary outbreak.

EXAMPLE: In 1981, in Côtes-d'Armor, France, 14 outbreaks of foot-and-mouth disease were observed, the *primary outbreak** and 13 secondary outbreaks.

See also *point source epidemic, primary outbreak.*

SECONDARY PREVENTION: Set of measures designed to detect disease processes before clinical disease occurs and to stop these processes, hence reducing the prevalence of such disease in the population.

EXAMPLES: *Screening** of *herds** to detect diseased or *infected* individuals, followed by therapy or any other relevant interventions.

Determination of somatic cell counts in dairy cows to detect *subclinical** mastitis, followed by treatment of cows with high cell counts.

Systematic examination of postpartum cows followed by antibiotherapy if required.

Determination of metabolic profiles on dairy farms to prevent or minimize hypocalcemia, acetonemia, etc.

COMMENT 1: The goal of secondary prevention is only reached if the screening stage leads to an action plan designed to prevent, or at least reduce, the clinical expression of the disease. Without such follow-up, the screening procedure would be equivalent to a simple *cross-sectional study.**

COMMENT 2: In contrast with *primary prevention,** the disease is normally present at the subclinical stage, and performance indicators, such as average daily gain and milk production, may be altered. Therefore, the analysis of farm *records,** part of *herd* health management,** can be viewed as a secondary prevention procedure if it is followed by corrective actions.

See also *prevention, primary prevention, tertiary prevention, screening.*

SECONDARY VECTOR: A vector that, under natural conditions, is of secondary importance compared to the usual primary vector in transmitting a pathogen.

EXAMPLES: Broad sense: Contaminated dust (from the road, sheepfold) and human brucellosis due to *B. melitensis.*

Strict sense: *Aedes atroparvus* and yellow fever.

COMMENT: An important ecological modification (spontaneous or provoked) may lead to the usual vector disappearing, resulting in a corresponding decline in the associated disease, unless a secondary vector is available to replace the primary one (*competing cause**).

SELECTION BIAS: See **Bias**

SELECTIVE SCREENING: Screening applied to a specific segment of a population.

EXAMPLE: Screening all cattle purchased at auctions for tuberculosis or brucellosis, because they are considered a high *risk** group.

COMMENT: To be differentiated from *mass screening.**

SELECTIVE SLAUGHTER: Disease control method based on the elimination of animals believed to be infected from an affected population.

EXAMPLES: *Method** used to control bovine brucellosis and tuberculosis in France, Canada, and the United States.

Method occasionally used by swine producers in Canada to *eradicate* porcine pleuropneumonia at the *herd** level. The procedure involves antibiotic coverage of the entire herd designed to "freeze" the *infection** (reduce, if not block, the *transmission** of the pathogen) during the serological *screening** of the herd and the *removal** of seropositive individuals (see also *test and removal**).

COMMENT 1: The *effectiveness** of this approach is greatly enhanced if a very *sensitive* screening test is available, and if the incubation period or latent period is long. These criteria allow for the screening and isolation of positive animals followed by their slaughter before they get to transmit the pathogen to a large proportion of the *population.**

COMMENT 2: When the number of infected animals in a population is high, or when the latent period is short, selective slaughter may be more expensive to perform than complete *depopulation,** because of the *costs** associated with repeated screening and removal of positive animals. To these *expenses,** one should also add *losses** resulting from various restrictions often imposed on farms during this process, which may last several months (e.g., restriction on sale of offspring).

SEMI-QUANTITATIVE VARIABLE: In France: Quantitative variable whose values have been regrouped in a limited number of ordinal classes.

This expression is not used in English.

EXAMPLE: Weights (*quantitative variable**) of pigs in a grow–finish unit that have been regrouped in six ordinal categories: 60 to < 65 kg; 65 to < 70 kg; 70 to < 75 kg; 75 to < 80 kg; 80 to < 85 kg; ≥ 85 kg.

COMMENT: Do not confuse with an *ordinal variable,** which is *qualitative.**

See also *discrete variable.*

SENSITIVITY OF A MEASUREMENT SCALE: In France: Ratio of the variation of the magnitude of a measurement over a given variation of the quantity to measure.

This expression is not used in English.

EXAMPLE: In a serological test, a set of twofold dilutions (1:2, 1:4, 1:8, 1:16, 1:32, etc.) has a better sensitivity than a set of 10-fold dilutions (1:10, 1:100, 1:1000, etc.).

SENSITIVITY (OF A TEST): Ability of a test to correctly detect individuals with the disease or infection of interest.

EXAMPLE:

Diagnostic test	Disease present	Disease absent (healthy)	
Positive	180 a	b	160
Negative	20 c	d	640

Sensitivity: $a/(a + c) = 180/(180 + 20) = 0.9$ or 90% *Proportion** of diseased animals that are correctly identified by the test.

Specificity: $d/(b + d) = 640/(160 + 640) = 0.8$ or 80% Proportion of disease-free animals that are correctly identified by the test.

COMMENT 1: For most tests, an inverse relationship exists between sensitivity and *specificity.** This occurs when the *distribution** of the *parameter** being tested in diseased animals overlaps with its distribution in healthy (disease-free) animals. Therefore, with a highly sensitive test, the *risk** of having *false negatives** is low (c) but the risk of having *false positives** may be high (b) (Figure S1).

EXAMPLE: The enzyme-linked immunosorbent assay (ELISA) is generally more sensitive but less specific than seroneutralization.

COMMENT 2: Sensitivity and specificity can only be determined if a healthy and a diseased group of animals are available and identified as such, based on one or more *gold standards.** Those are the two intrinsic *characteristics** of a test. They should not be confused with *predictive values.**

COMMENT 3: If more than one test is used on the same animal or *herd,** the results can be interpreted either in series or in parallel. A parallel interpretation means that animals that are positive to any of the tests will be considered positive, which maximizes the sensitivity of the diagnostic procedure but lowers its specificity. In contrast, a series interpretation means that only animals positive to all the tests will be labeled positive, which, of course, increases specificity at the expense of sensitivity.

COMMENT 4: The sensitivity of a test applied to *individuals** differs from the sensitivity interpreted at the herd level. Herd sensitivity is defined as the proportion of diseased herds that are found to be positive by the test, i.e., the number of positive animals meets or exceeds a predetermined cutoff point number of positives. Hence, at the herd level, sensitivity increases with the number of individuals being tested and with the actual *prevalence** of the disease in the herd. However, it decreases as the cutoff point number of positive animals needed for declaring the herd diseased increases. For example, given a test with an individual sensitivity of 95% and a specificity of 99%, the herd sensitivity would be 66% if 10 animals were tested compared to 96% if 30 were tested (assuming that one positive individual among those tested is sufficient to declare the herd positive and that the prevalence of positive animals in each herd is 10%). With an actual within-herd prevalence of 30% and with all other parameters being the same, the herd sensitivity would be 96% for 10 tests per herd and 100% for 30.

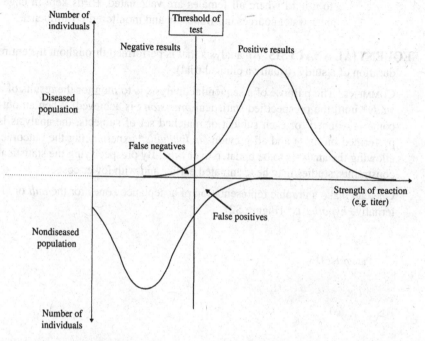

FIGURE S1. Relationship between sensitivity and specificity of a test depending on the threshold of the test. A lower threshold leads to a higher sensitivity (fewer false negatives) but a lower specificity (more false positive). In this particular example, the test favors sensitivity to the determinant of specificity.

SENTINEL: Animal that is free of, and susceptible to, a specific condition, and that is monitored during and/or after being exposed to other animals or an environment suspected of harboring this condition.

COMMENT 1: In veterinary medicine, sentinel is a word almost exclusively associated with animals. However, some authors also refer to veterinary clinics or farms as sentinels, being viewed as a recording mechanism selected or posted explicitly to record relevant occurrences in an active surveillance program.

The condition of interest is often an infectious disease. However, the presence of noninfectious problems, such as toxic gases and radiation, may also be monitored in a similar fashion.

COMMENT 2: The monitoring could be over a period of several weeks, months, or even years. However, the period of exposure may be as short as a few minutes or hours. For example, in the case of the poult enteritis mortality syndrome (PEMS), a transmissible enteric disease of turkeys, young sentinel turkeys are exposed to a PEMS-suspect flock for often less than 24 hours; they are then removed from the flock and monitored in a disease-free environment for a period of 2 weeks.

EXAMPLES: Domesticated rabbits exposed in cages to detect myxomatosis. Rams that are not vaccinated for brucellosis and that are exposed to a herd where all females are vaccinated. Birds kept in cages near water sources in Minnesota and monitored for influenza.

SEQUENTIAL ANALYSIS: An analysis that is performed throughout the entire duration of a study (usually a clinical trial).

COMMENT: The purpose of a sequential analysis is to monitor the results of a *study** until the prespecified statistical *precision** is achieved. When an outcome is reached for each subject or matched set of subjects, the analysis is performed on these and all previous *individuals** experiencing the outcome, allowing the analysis to be updated over time. By prespecifying the statistical constraints, studies may be terminated earlier and with lower costs.

One can make a graphic representation of acceptance zones for the *null* or alternative *hypothesis** (Figure S2).

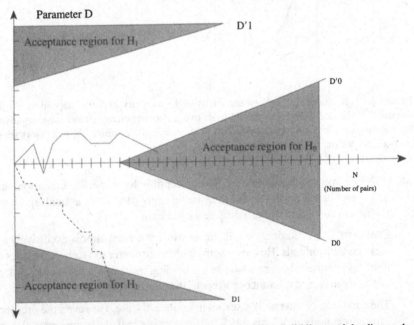

FIGURE S2.   Schematic representation of sequential analysis. Solid line, path leading to the acceptance of the null hypothesis (H_0); dashed line, path leading to the acceptance of the alternative hypothesis (H_1). D1 and D'1 = limits to reject H_0; D0 and D'0 = limits to reject H_1.

SERIES: Set of consecutive numerical data resulting from the observation of a specific characteristic for each unit of a sample or a population.

EXAMPLE: All carcass weights recorded in a slaughter plant on a given day.

COMMENT: An ordered series is a series for which values are in a defined order (increasing or decreasing). A chronological series or *time series** is a series ordered according to dates, hours, etc.

SERO-EPIDEMIOLOGY: Term used sometimes to designate an epidemiologic study based on the analysis of serum collected on a sample from a population.

EXAMPLE: Many descriptive studies dealing with *infectious diseases** are done by searching for antibodies in the serum (bovine viral leukosis, bovine viral diarrhea, etc.).

COMMENT: Sera collected for purposes other than the current study can introduce major *biases** into the study results.

SEX-RATIO: Proportion based on the number of males and females observed at birth.

COMMENT: This expression is seldom used in veterinary *epidemiology.** Of greater interest (particularly in animal production) is the ratio females:males used for reproduction. For example, sow:boar ratios of 20:1 to 25:1 are often recommended in commercial swine operations.

SHADOW PRICE: Syn: reference price An artificial price calculated to measure the value of a good or service as a function of its opportunity cost.

EXAMPLES: A *cost–benefit analysis** of a national *disease**-control program that would result in an increase of the current surplus supply of beef, would use a shadow price, as the value of the extra beef would likely be less than the current *market price.** A price fixed a priori by a government as part of its agricultural policies.

COMMENT: This price is determined when there is a discrepancy between the market price and the real value of the good or service of interest. It is often derived using linear programming techniques.

See also *benefit–cost ratio, opportunity cost.*

SHEDDING (OF AN INFECTIOUS AGENT): Discharge of an infectious agent into the environment by an infected individual.

COMMENT 1: Shedding may occur via excretion, secretion, open wounds (skin or mucous membrane) and exhalation.

EXAMPLES: Foot-and-mouth disease virus is shed by exhalation, mouth lesions, and secretion (saliva, semen, and milk). Coronavirus is shed in the feces of infected animals.

COMMENT 2: The rate of discharge of an infectious agent may vary considerably depending on the agent, the host, and the environment.

COMMENT 3: Shedding is an attribute of *contagious diseases.**

SICKNESS: See **Disease**

SILENT CARRIER: Carrier that does not shed the infectious agent.

EXAMPLE: Person harboring a hydatid cyst.

See also *carrier.*

SILENT INFECTION: See **Inapparent Infection**

SIMILARITY: A geometrical measure of closeness between two individuals.

COMMENT: It is measured as 1 minus the *distance.**

See also *distance.*

SIMPLE CORRELATION: See **Coefficient of Correlation**

SIMPLE GROWTH: Increase of a number at a given annual rate applied only to the initial number.

EXAMPLE: Given an initial number of 1000 at an annual growth rate of 10%. Simple annual growth: 100. At the end of the 1st year: 1100. At the end of the 2nd year: 1200. At the end of the 3rd year: 1300, etc.

COMMENT 1: This can apply to an amount of money, a price, an animal *population,** etc.

COMMENT 2: As opposed to *compound growth.**

SIMPLE INTEREST: Interest calculated by applying the percentage rate only to the initial amount, such that the numerical value of periodic growth is always the same.

See also *compound interest, interest rate.*

SIMPLE RANDOM SAMPLE: A sample drawn in such a way that every unit has the same probability of being selected.

EXAMPLE: One can obtain a simple random sample of 123 *individuals** from a *population** of 4567 individuals by using a table of random numbers or by a computer generating 123 random numbers, which are used to select the *sample.**

See also *random sample.*

SIMPLE SAMPLE: Sample resulting from one-stage sampling.

COMMENT: Simple samples are to be distinguished from stratified or multistage samples.

See also *multistage sampling, stratified random sample.*

SIMULATION: Implementation of a model, typically mathematical, for the purposes of predicting real occurrences.

EXAMPLE: Simulation of the progression of foot-and-mouth disease from the first *case** that occurred in the Isle of Wight in the spring of 1981, in order to estimate the risk of *contamination** for the remainder of England.

COMMENT: Simulation is often performed using mathematical and/or informatic tools. For example, during the design of a *health** implementation plan, it is possible to simulate the various stages in order to evaluate the probability of success or failure.

SIZE: The total number of units of interest in an assemblage.

EXAMPLE: The size of a dairy herd is the sum of all the cows in the herd.

COMMENT: When used in the context of a *sample size,** it corresponds to the number of units [part of individuals (e.g., legs), individuals, pens, herds, etc.] selected or available. Herd size, as in the example above, is often referred to in terms of the number of reproductive females (e.g., 300-sow herd; 100-cow herd).

SKIP PATTERN: Direction(s) provided in a questionnaire to guide respondents when one or several questions do not apply to them.

EXAMPLE: Excerpt from a questionnaire requesting information about the farrowing section of farrow-to-finish swine farms:

Q-4. How many crates and pens do you have per farrowing room? *(Please fill in the blanks)*

ROOM 1:_____CRATES AND PENS
ROOM 2:_____CRATES AND PENS
ROOM 3:_____CRATES AND PENS
ROOM 4:_____CRATES AND PENS
ROOM 5:_____CRATES AND PENS
ROOM 6:_____CRATES AND PENS
MORE THAN 6 ROOMS (PLEASE SPECIFY):

The following two questions relate to crates. If you have PENS ONLY, please go to question 7

Q-5. Do you normally adjust the crate width for the sow according to her size?

1. YES
2. NO
3. NO, BUT I USUALLY PUT THE LARGEST SOWS IN THE WIDEST CRATES

Q-6. ...
Q-7. ...

COMMENT: Arrows can also be used as part of the skip pattern to direct the respondent to the next relevant question. When present in a *questionnaire,** skip patterns should be carefully reviewed during *pretesting.**

See also *pretesting.*

SLAUGHTER: Deliberate killing of infected or potentially infected animals (in contact with infected individuals) in an attempt to prevent the spreading of the infection to a noninfected population.

COMMENT: It is usually followed by a thorough washing and disinfection of the premises (including equipment) followed by a downtime period before restocking.

See also *selective slaughter, depopulation.*

SLOW VIRUS: Virus responsible for diseases with a very long incubation period (in general, over a year) and a very slow progression.

EXAMPLE: Maedi-visna virus of sheep.

SOFTWARE: Collection of instructions, written in a computing language, that is used to direct the computer to accomplish specific tasks.

COMMENT 1: These instructions are called computer programs.

COMMENT 2: There are three major types of software:

1. Application: This is the general term for programs that have been written to perform specific user-oriented tasks, such as programs allowing the establishment or evaluation of the dietary need of cattle or programs that perform the payroll in an office.
2. End user: It is composed of prebuilt programs, called packages, which are available to help the users design their own computer-based application (for example, spreadsheet, word processor, database manager).
3. Operating systems software: These are sets of programs that ease the task of working with the computer system itself. The operating system acts as an interface between application or end-user software and the computer (for example, DOS, UNIX).

SOURCE OF INFECTION: Broad sense: Host, object, or environment that is at the origin of the transmission of a disease.

Restricted sense: Host or environment sustaining the infectious agent (e.g., reservoir) which is at the origin of the transmission of a disease.

COMMENT: Sources of infection are generally divided into four categories: living *hosts,** dead animals, animal by-products, *environment.** Sources that make up living hosts include diseased, incubatory, convalescent, and *healthy carriers.** Sources that comprise animal by-products include animal protein (blood, plasma, viscera), meat and bone meal, eggs, milk, etc. Environmental sources include soil, equipment, and buildings.

See also *reservoir.*

SOURCE POPULATION: Syn: underlying population Fraction of the general population from which comes the sampling frame.

EXAMPLE: All dairy farms located in the North part of a country (*study**** at the *herd**** level) (see also Figure P3, *population****).

See also *sampling frame*.

SPEARMAN CORRELATION: A measure of general tendency in a chronological series.

COMMENT: To each value of a chronological series (*time series****) corresponds a chronological *rank**** and, after *classification**** of the values by increasing order, an ordering rank. These two ranks are then compared and the Spearman correlation is calculated by:

$$r = 1 - \frac{6\Sigma d_i^2}{n(n^2 - 1)}$$

where *dj* is the rank difference and *n* the number of values in the series.

SPEARMAN RANK CORRELATION: Measure used with ordinal paired variables to estimate correlation.

COMMENT 1: It is calculated in a similar fashion to *Spearman correlation,**** although in this case it considers the difference between the ranks of the two variables in the pair.

EXAMPLE: When comparing variables obtained from a *questionnaire**** inquiring about degree of satisfaction.

COMMENT 2: There are other rank correlation estimation methods (i.e., gamma, Kendall's, Stuart's, Somer's, etc.). These methods vary mainly in their treatment of pairs in agreement.

SPECIFIC RATE: Rate limited to a particular category (such as age, race, sex, disease) of the population under study.

EXAMPLES: Specific mortality rate of calves from birth to 8 days; specific rate of mammary tumors in the dog.

SPECIFICATION BIAS: See Bias

SPECIFICITY: Ability of a test to correctly detect individuals free of the disease or infection of interest.

COMMENT 1: See *sensibility**** for details regarding the calculation and interpretation of specificity for tests applied at the *individual**** level.

COMMENT 2: The specificity of a test applied to individuals differs when it is interpreted at the *herd**** level. Herd specificity (for a given test) is defined as the proportion of disease-free herds (i.e., negative) in which the number of positive animals is below a predetermined cutoff point number of positives. Hence, at the herd level, specificity decreases with the number of individuals being tested. However, it increases as the cutoff point number of positive animals needed for declaring the herd diseased increases. For example, given a test with an individual sensitivity of 95% and a specificity of 99%, the herd specificity would be 90% if 10 animals were tested, compared to 74% if 30 were tested (assuming that one positive individual among those tested is sufficient to declare the herd positive). If two positive animals were needed before a herd could be declared positive, and assuming that all other parameters remain the same, the herd specificity would be 100% for 10 tests per herd and 96% for 30.

SPORADIC CONDITION: See **Sporadic Disease**

SPORADIC DISEASE: Syn: sporadic condition Disease that occurs irregularly and haphazardly in time and space and, in general, not frequently.

EXAMPLE: In France, equine infectious anemia over the last 20 years.

COMMENT: A few isolated *cases** (sporadic cases) or *cluster** of cases may be observed.

See also *endemic* (Figure E1).

SPOT PREVALENCE: See **Point Prevalence**

SPREAD OF DISEASE: Spatial dissemination of a disease over time in a population.

EXAMPLE: Dissemination of African swine fever from a farrowing unit to several grow–finish facilities following a stockyard auction.

COMMENT: The dissemination or movement of a disease in a *population** is largely determined by its mode of *transmission** (*horizontal,** vertical,** vector,** direct,** indirect**) (Figure S3).

See also *horizontal transmission, point source epidemic.*

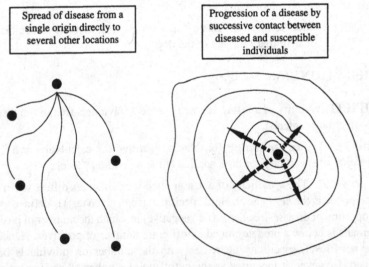

> Spread of disease from a single origin directly to several other locations

> Progression of a disease by successive contact between diseased and susceptible individuals

FIGURE S3. Schematic representation of two different patterns of spread of disease.

STAGES OF DISEASE: See **Disease Cycle**

STAMPING OUT: See **Depopulation**

STANDARD DEVIATION: A measure of the dispersion of a random variable defined as the square root of the variance.

EXAMPLES: A study comparing two methods of dosage performed on a set of sera gives the following results:

	1st method	2nd method
Mean	20	20
Standard deviation	5	10

The two *methods** give the same results for the mean, but the *dispersion,** measured by the standard deviation, is two times smaller for method 1 than for method 2. We conclude that method 1 is more precise than method 2.

COMMENT 1: The standard deviation is expressed in the same unit as the *random variable.**

COMMENT 2: The standard deviation divided by the square root of the sample size is called standard error.

See also *variance, precision of an estimate*

STANDARD ERROR: See **Standard Deviation**

STANDARD NORMAL VARIABLE: Random variable that follows a normal (Gaussian) distribution with mean equal to zero and standard deviation equal to 1.

COMMENT: It is tabulated in many textbooks. To find the *probability** of observing values smaller than a given value x_0 for a normal *variable** with *mean** μ and *standard deviation** σ, we need to transform x_0 into

$z = (x_0 - \mu) / \sigma$

and read the corresponding probability from the standard normal distribution table.

See also *normal distribution, standard deviation.*

STANDARD POPULATION: Population, real or fictitious, whose characteristics (age, sex, etc.) are known and that is used to make two or more populations comparable by adjusting them for some of these characteristics.

EXAMPLES: *Population** made by averaging data from all cattle herds in a region. In a *study** comparing two populations, a standard population may be created by pooling all observations from both populations.

In a study on hip dysplasia, a standard population was used to adjust for breed, sex, and age in a comparison between an urban and a rural dog population.

See also *standardization*.

STANDARDIZATION (OF RATES): Method enabling a comparison between different populations or groups of individuals by preventing potential distortion from factors such as host attributes (e.g., age, sex, breed).

EXAMPLE: Standardization can be direct or indirect (Figure S4).

COMMENT 1: Reasons for standardization:

1. A confounding factor is present.
2. A single summary *statistic** for a *population** is more easily compared with other summary statistics than are entire schedules of specific *rates.**
3. If some strata (*stratum,** sing.) are comprised of small numbers of individuals, the associated specific rates may be too imprecise and unreliable for use in detailed comparisons.
4. For small populations or groups, specific rates may not exist.

COMMENT 2: Warnings about standardization:

1. Specific rates (for each stratum of *host** *attribute** or of the parameter of interest) are essential for an accurate and detailed study of the variation of the phenomenon under study (e.g., mortality rates, etc.) among population strata.
2. If the specific rates vary in different ways across the various strata, then no single method of standardization will indicate that these differences exist. Standardization will, in fact, tend to mask these differences.

COMMENT 3: The selection of the *standard population** for direct standardization is not critical since the stratum-specific rates are known. However, in the case of the indirect approach, the selection of the standard population (to provide stratum-specific rates) is important because this approach removes most but not all of the effects of different *distributions** of the factor of interest in each group.

Given OBS P_i = observed distribution of factor of interest; OBS R_i = observed stratum-specific rates; STD R_i = Stratum-specific rates of standard population; STD P_i = Standard population distribution:

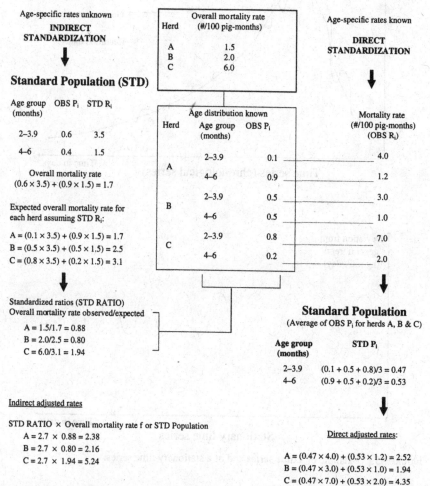

FIGURE S4. Comparison of mortality rates between three continuous growing–finishing facilities (pigs of two different age groups present at the same time on the premises) depending on whether age-specific rates are known or not. OBS P_i: observed distribution of factor of interest; OBS R_{-i}: observed stratum-specific rates; STD R_i: stratum-specific rates of standard population; STD P_{-i}: standard population distribution.

STATIONARY TIME SERIES: Chronological series without any general trend (Figure S5).

COMMENT 1: A chronological series with a general trend becomes stationary once the trend component is removed.

COMMENT 2: Before one can assess *autocorrelation** in a chronological series, it has to be made stationary.

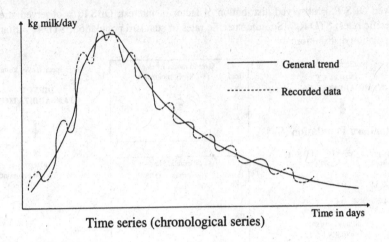

Time series (chronological series)

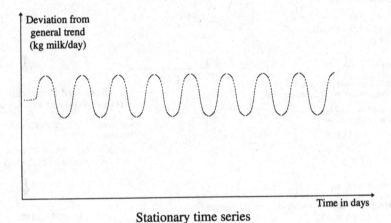

Stationary time series

FIGURE S5. Example of a time series and of a stationary time series.

STATISTIC: A quantity computed from the data obtained from a sample and used to represent the sample or the underlying population from which the sample was obtained.

COMMENT: A statistic may be descriptive (*descriptive statistics**): description of the values taken by one or many *variables** within a predefined *group;** or inferential, aimed at extrapolating the values taken by the variables or at establishing the relationships between the variables based on *studies** performed on a representative *sample** of the *population.**

STATISTICAL ASSOCIATION: Syn: **statistically significant association** An association between two factors that has a quantifiable probability of occurring under a null hypothesis.

COMMENT 1: Typically the *null hypothesis** is one of independence between the two factors, and the *probability** specifically pertains to the probability that an *association** of the given magnitude or more extreme would occur under the null hypothesis and an implied statistical *model.**

COMMENT 2: An association between two factors may in reality result from a true dependence between the factors, from *bias,** or from *random* error** (chance). Associations that are unlikely to be ascribed to chance (i.e., have a low probability of occurrence) when the null hypothesis of no association is assumed are frequently called significant associations.

COMMENT 3: A statistical association does not necessarily imply a causal relationship. Conversely, a causal relationship does not necessarily mean that a statistical association will be observed.

See also *causality.*

STATISTICAL INFERENCE: Process of drawing conclusions about the characteristics (or nature) of a population based on the characteristics of a random sample from that population.

EXAMPLE 1: If 20% of a group of randomly chosen cattle in a region tested positive to bovine parvovirus, one could infer that approximately 20% of all cattle from that region are *infected** with this virus.

COMMENT: Statistical inference requires that certain assumptions be satisfied in order for the conclusions to be valid.

STATISTICAL TEST: A rule that tells one how to choose between two competing hypotheses based on observations obtained from a random sample of individuals from a population of interest.

COMMENT 1: The two *hypotheses** are the *null hypothesis** (H_0) and the alternative hypothesis (H_1). According to the observed values obtained from the *sample,** the decision will be made in favor of one or the other of the two hypotheses. This *procedure** includes *errors** due to sampling variability. Possible situations are presented in Table S1.

COMMENT 2: A very important aspect of this method of *inference** is the *sample size** relative to the *population** size. Inferences are made following theorems proved in mathematical probability theory.

TABLE S1. **Different situations relative to reality and the conclusions of a statistical test**

		Reality	
		H_0	H_1
Decision	Accept H_0	$1 - \alpha$	β
	Reject H_0	α	$1 - \beta$

Note: The *alpha (type 1) error** corresponds to the rejection of H_0 when it is true. The *beta (type 2) error** corresponds to accepting H_0 when it is false. The quantity 1-beta is the *power** of the test.

COMMENT 3: In practice, many statistical tests are being used even when the samples have not been randomly drawn.

See also *alpha (type 1) error, beta (type 2) error, power.*

STATISTICAL UNIT: A basic countable element of a larger population on which measurements are taken.

COMMENT 1: A *population,** in a statistical sense, is a set of independent statistical units.

COMMENT 2: A statistical unit does not always correspond to an animal; it can be a pen, a cage, a house or barn, a *herd** or flock, a farm, a company, a region, etc.

COMMENT 3: To be differentiated from *sample unit** in *cluster sampling** (Figure S6).

See also *population, cluster sampling, sample unit.*

A   B

Stratified   Cluster
sampling   sampling

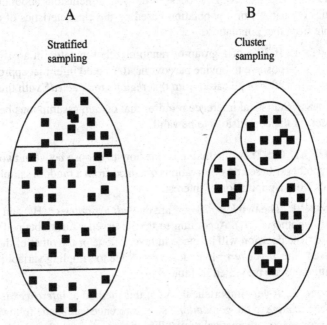

FIGURE S6. Schematic representation of the difference between sample unit and statistical unit. In A, the sample unit within each stratum is the individual; the individual is also the statistical unit. In B, the *cluster** is the sample unit, while the individual is the statistical unit.

STATISTICALLY SIGNIFICANT ASSOCIATION: See Statistical Association

STATISTICS: A branch of mathematics and probability theory that is used to sample, analyze, and infer from data.

A set of numerical data.

STILLBIRTH: Mortality occurring shortly before (prepartum) or during the birth process (intrapartum).

COMMENT: Unless a necropsy is performed, it is often difficult to differentiate pre- or intrapartum deaths from early postpartum deaths.

See also *neonatal mortality*.

STOCHASTIC MODEL: See **Probabilistic Model**

STOCK:

1. Accumulation of a commodity.
2. Genetic lines available to a breeding company.
3. A share in the ownership of a business.
4. The raw material used to produce an output or product.

COMMENT: A multitude of definitions are attached to the word stock. For example, Webster's II New Riverside University Dictionary lists 22 different meanings. The four definitions listed above are frequently used in veterinary medicine, in particular in food animal practice (e.g., livestock production).

STRATA: See **Stratum**

STRATIFICATION: The process of subdividing a study population into strata.

COMMENT: The rationale for stratification is that within strata *individuals** are either exactly alike on the stratification factors (e.g., sex) or are more homogeneous within strata relative to between strata (*stratum,** sing.) (e.g., individuals less than 1 year old versus individuals greater than 1 year old). If the *distribution** of the stratification factor(s) is identical within strata, such as sex, then no further confounding by the stratification factor exists. Hence, in the absence of confounding by any other factor and any other *biases,** an unbiased stratum-specific *effect measure** can be obtained. If any remaining distribution of the stratification variable remains within strata (such as when strata are defined by ranges of age), then obtaining an unbiased stratum-specific measure requires the assumption of no remaining (residual) confounding within the stratum by the stratification variable(s).

See also *stratum, cluster* (Figure C4).

STRATIFIED RANDOM SAMPLE: Syn: **stratified sample** Sample obtained by random selection of units within prespecified and distinct strata.

EXAMPLE: A stratified sample of dairy cattle in Canada could be obtained by taking separate random samples of dairy cattle within each of the Canadian provinces.

COMMENT: Sampling within each stratum does not have to be proportional to the size of the stratum (Table S2).

Age (years)	Population	Proportional sampling	Nonproportional sampling
0 to <1	100	10 (10%)	5 (5%)
1 to <2	50	5 (10%)	5 (10%)
2 to <3	30	3 (10%)	5 (17%)
≥3	20	2 (10%)	5 (25%)
Total	200	20 (10%)	20 (10%)

STRATIFIED SAMPLE: See **Stratified Random Sample**

STRATIFIED SAMPLING: Sampling in which the random selection of statistical units is performed within different strata.

COMMENT 1: Strata (*stratum,* * sing.) are based on important *characteristics** associated with the *variable** under study.

EXAMPLE: *Random selection** of animals to be studied from each age category (stratum).

COMMENT 2: Should be distinguished from *cluster sampling.** In a stratified sample, strata are first defined according to the variables under study, and then random selection of the *statistical units** is performed within each stratum. In cluster sampling, clusters of units are available and some of them, randomly selected, will have all of their statistical units studied.

STRATUM (Plural: strata): Two or more subsets of a study population defined by mutually exclusive characteristics.

COMMENT: Strata are reserved for partitioning *study populations** by *variables** that are *confounders** or effect modifiers, and should be distinguished from two or more levels of an exposure factor whose effect is to be estimated, rather than controlled.

EXAMPLE: In a study of the effect of an environmental carcinogen on risk of mammary cancer, animals may be placed in appropriate discrete age and sex strata.

See also *cluster* (Figure C4).

STRUCTURED INTERVIEW: Mode of information gathering where the investigator asks orally, and in a systematic and consistent manner, a series of preworded questions.

COMMENT 1: Structured interviews can be conducted in person or over the phone.

COMMENT 2: To be differentiated from an *unstructured interview.** The investigator or interviewer must ask the *questions** according to instructions. He or she is also expected to record the answers according to specified instructions. These tasks require adequate training, which may last several weeks, including observing experienced interviewers, interviewing people related to the project followed by critiques of the interview, and a trial period before the actual *study** begins.

See also *unstructured interview*.

STUDENT'S *t* TEST: A statistical test that compares two means calculated from two independent samples assuming that the underlying populations are normally distributed.

Given two *series** of observations $(x_1, x_2, ..., x_{n1})$ and $(y_1, y_2, ..., y_{n2})$

$$t = \frac{m_1 - m_2}{\sqrt{\dfrac{s^2}{n_1} + \dfrac{s^2}{n_2}}}$$

with $(n_1 + n_2 - 2)$ *degrees of freedom,** and where

$$m_1 = \Sigma \frac{x_i}{n_1}$$

$$m_2 = \Sigma \frac{y_i}{n_2}$$

$$s^2 = \frac{(n_1 - 1)s^2_1 + (n_2 - 1)s^2_2}{n_1 + n_2 - 2}$$

COMMENT: The above formulas are used under the assumption of homogeneity of *variance.**

EXAMPLE: If one wants to compare the production of dairy cows affected with clinical mastitis (M+) to cows without clinical mastitis (M–) (Table S3).

TABLE S3. Comparison of milk production in liters

Group 1 M+	Group 2 M–
128	143
133	145
123	138
141	148
129	137
	154
	140

$m_1 = 130.8$	$m_2 = 143.6$	$n_1 = 5$
$s^2_1 = 45.2$	$s^2_2 = 36.3$	$n_2 = 7$

$s^2 = (4*45.2 + 6*36.3)/10 = 39.86$
$t = -12.8 / 3.70 = -3.46$

The *level of significance** of *t* changes with the *sample size.** With an *alpha error** of 0.05 and 10 degrees of freedom $(n_1 + n_2 - 2)$, under the *null hypothesis,* t* should be smaller or equal to 2.23. For a two-sided test, if the observed absolute value of t is larger than 2.23, the *probability** that the observed difference between the two means is due to *sampling fluctuations** is less than 5%. In this example, one can conclude that an *association** exists between clinical mastitis and the level of milk production.

STUDY: Methodical search for information aiming to learn and/or understand.

COMMENT 1: Study is a more general term encompassing *surveys.**

COMMENT 2: Two design criteria can be used to create a basic classification of epidemiologic studies:

1. Artificial manipulation of the study factor(s)
2. Random allocation of the categories of study factor(s) when the study factor(s) are artificially manipulated.

Three mutually exclusive types of epidemiologic studies are described using these two criteria (Figure S7).

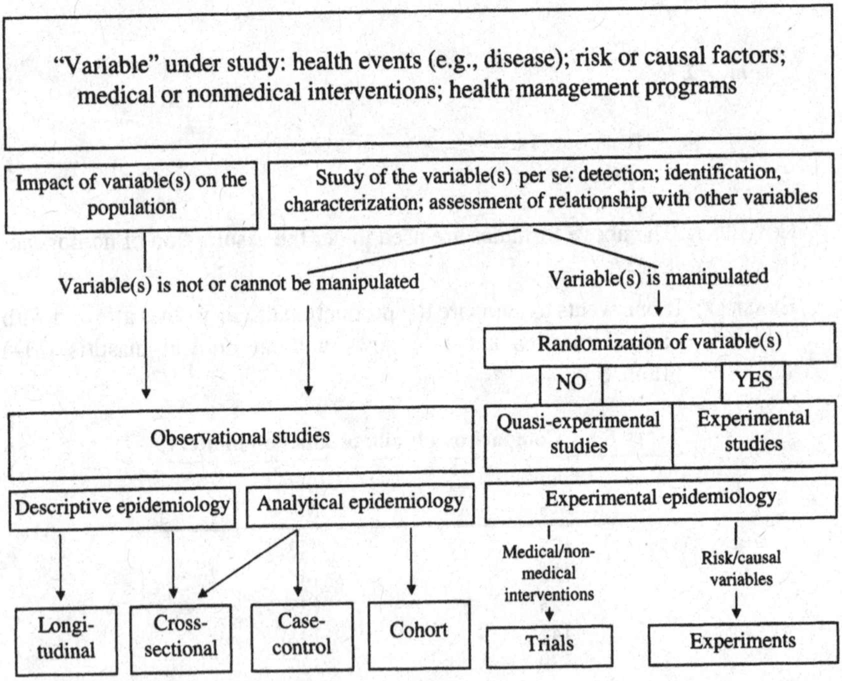

FIGURE S7. Different types of epidemiologic studies.

STUDY POPULATION: Part of the sample that will effectively undergo observation, after applying exclusion criteria (e.g., refusal to cooperate, dangerous animals, herd size, availability of farm records, etc.).

EXAMPLE: 1892 farms from the original 2000 included in the sampling (108 refused to participate in the study).

See also *population* (Figure P3), *target population* (Figure T1).

SUBCLINICAL: Without clinical manifestations.

> EXAMPLES: Subclinical mastitis can only be detected via an indirect test such as the California mastitis test. Hypomagnesemia in cows without neuromuscular signs.

SUBCLINICAL DISEASE: Condition that cannot be clinically detected, often throughout its duration.

> EXAMPLE: Subclinical mastitis. This condition may reduce productivity but good record keeping and diagnostic tests, such as microbiological cultures and somatic cell count, are needed to determine the presence of the problem.

> See also *inapparent disease, infection, subclinical infection.*

SUBCLINICAL INFECTION: Infection that does not produce clinical signs but generates detectable biological reactions.

> EXAMPLES: Subclinical mastitis is not associated with clinical signs but results in an increase in the number of leukocytes in the milk.
>
> Detection of antibodies to *Actinobacillus pleuropneumoniae* type 5 in 12-week-old pigs using ELISA.

> COMMENT: Some confusion exists in the literature between subclinical infection and *inapparent infection.** Some authors use these terms synonymously. Others ascribe a loss of productivity to subclinical infection but not to inapparent infection.

> See also *infection, inapparent infection.*

SURVEILLANCE: See **Epidemiologic Surveillance**

SURVEY: A comprehensive investigation designed to describe one or more characteristics of a population.

> EXAMPLE: Serological survey of Aujeszky's disease (pseudorabies) based on a *one-stage* cluster *sampling** in a given county.

> COMMENT 1: A survey is essentially a *descriptive study** based on *measurements** obtained from blood sampling, swabbing, *questionnaires,** etc. It never uses experimental *methods.** It may be referred to as an epidemiologic survey.

> COMMENT 2: Some authors use the word survey as synonymous to questionnaire. However, as can be seen in the example mentioned above, a survey does not necessarily include a questionnaire.

SURVEY NETWORK: Set of survey units included in an epidemiologic study and chosen according to certain criteria.

> EXAMPLE: A diagnostic laboratory reporting system is a survey network for reporting the occurrence (generally *prevalence**) of animal *diseases.**

> COMMENT 1: In veterinary *epidemiology,** a *survey** unit is often a *herd.**

COMMENT 2: There are different levels of survey networks depending on the *objective** of the survey: The objective of a primary survey network is generally descriptive and identifies *trends** and generates *hypotheses.** A secondary survey network identifies *risk factors** for the disease under investigation; a tertiary survey network develops, evaluates, and tests the *associations** of risk factors identified by the secondary network.

SURVIVAL FUNCTION: Syn: survivorship function; cumulative survival rate Function representing the probability of surviving for a specific period of time.

COMMENT 1: It may also be used to refer to the curve illustrating the function (syn: survival curve) (Figure S8).

COMMENT 2: *Mortality** of a *population** or a *cohort** is described with respect to the complementary event of death, which is survival.

COMMENT 3: To determine the survival function, one calculates the *probability** that an *individual** is still alive for successive time periods, from a chosen starting time (time $t = 0$) and during a period of observation T. The probability of surviving at least at the time 0 is 1, and that of surviving for an infinite time is zero.

COMMENT 4: The mean is normally used to describe the *central tendency* of a *distribution.** However, with survival distributions the *median** is often better because a few individuals with exceptionally long or short lifetimes may disproportionately influence mean survival time.

COMMENT 5: In most cases, it is assumed that the *risk** of death is independent from time period to time period.

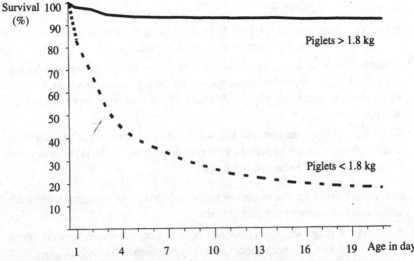

FIGURE S8.   Survival curves of two cohorts of piglets depending on birth weight.

COMMENT 6: Survival functions can be estimated by parametric and nonparametric *methods.** The two nonparametric methods of *estimation** of the *survival rate** (or probability of remaining alive) are the *Kaplan–Meier** and *actuarial methods.**

SURVIVAL MODEL: Model that expresses time before the occurrence of a dichotomous event in longitudinal or cohort studies following the onset of an event which is used to define time 0.

EXAMPLE: Prognosis *study** for cancer *patients** following various treatments.

COMMENT 1: These models include the *survival function,** which describes duration without the event of interest, and the hazard function, which describes the event occurring at a given time.

COMMENT 2: The outcome under study is often death, which explains where the name survival model comes from.

COMMENT 3: Parametric and semiparametric survival models can be found.

COMMENT 4: These *models** are of interest because they offer the possibility to study factors explaining the increase or decrease in the *risk** of occurrence of the event of interest as it relates to time.

COMMENT 5: Survival models should be differentiated from nonparametric methods of *estimation** of survival functions *(actuarial method,** Kaplan–Meier method*)*.

See also *survival function, Cox's model, actuarial method, Kaplan–Meier method.*

SURVIVAL RATE:

$$\frac{\text{Number of survivors to a disease at the end of a given time period}}{\text{Number of individuals affected with the disease of interest during this period}}$$

EXAMPLE: In a herd of 100 calves, 20 of 40 calves with colibacillosis died. Therefore, the survival rate is 50%.

COMMENT: Survival rate = 100% – *case fatality rate.**

See also *rate.*

SURVIVAL RATE IN A POPULATION: See **Cumulative Survival Rate**

SURVIVORSHIP FUNCTION: See **Survival Function**

SUSCEPTIBILITY: The state of being readily affected by a pathogen.

COMMENT 1: This lack of *resistance** to a pathogen may be acquired, individual, inherited, species related, age specific, etc.

EXAMPLE: Piglets are more susceptible to Aujeszky's disease (pseudorabies) than boars and sows.

COMMENT 2: Given the same exposure to a pathogen, the degree of susceptibility may vary greatly within a species or a group (e.g., litter).

SYMBIONT: Syn: symbiote Organism that lives in a durable and reciprocally profitable relationship with another living being.

See also *commensal* (Table C2).

SYMBIOTE: See **Symbiont**

SYMPTOM: Broad sense: Spontaneous manifestation of disease, as subjectively assessed by the patient or as determined by an observer (e.g., clinician).

Restricted sense: Spontaneous manifestation of disease, as subjectively assessed by the patient.

EXAMPLES: Vertigo, nausea, pain.

COMMENT: In the general literature, and in everyday conversation, symptom may be used as synonymous with clinical sign. However, in the English medical literature, subjective symptoms felt by the *patient** are differentiated from clinical signs, that can be studied or provoked by an observer. Hence, in English medical terminology, symptoms cannot be evaluated in veterinary medicine because veterinary patients are unable to communicate their subjective impressions other than through a change in behavior, which is a clinical sign.

SYNDROME: Recognized set of clinical signs and/or functional, biochemical or morphologic modifications of an individual, constituting a diseased state and that could be induced by various causes or is of uncertain origin.

EXAMPLE: The vagal indigestion syndrome in cattle, with abnormalities of forestomach motility and electrolyte disturbances, can be associated with localized inflammatory peritoneal disease, but also with various mechanical and primary neurologic and/or digestive factors.

COMMENT: Identification or definition of a syndrome does not constitute arrival at a definitive *diagnosis,** but only recognition of the common *association** of the observed set of signs/modifications. The commonality of association may reflect common *characteristics** or modes of action among possible causes and/or the spectrum of options for response on the part of the diseased *individual.**

SYSTEM: Set or group of interacting, interrelated, or interdependent elements relating to one another in such a way that they act like a unique entity, with an input and output, and have a common purpose.

EXAMPLE: An integrated swine company can be considered a system with breeding stock, feed mills, farrowing units, nurseries, grow–finish units, technical services, and processing plants.

COMMENT 1: A system is defined by its boundaries (one farm, several farms, etc.).

COMMENT 2: Systems analysis is a mathematical modeling process designed to examine or simulate a system. Hence, it addresses the complex relationships inherent to systems. Models may be designed to determine optimal solutions or to simulate the system given predefined sets of *variables.** According to Dent et al. (1978), systems analysis involves six interconnected steps: (1) definition of the system and *objectives** for modeling, (2) analysis of data, (3) construction and (4) *validation** of the model, (5) sensitivity analysis (values of relevant *parameters** are systematically modified within a given range of interest to determine their impact on the outcome), and (6) use of the *model** in decision support.

SYSTEMATIC SAMPLE: A sample in which ordered individuals are selected at fixed points in an interval.

> EXAMPLE: Selecting every fourth cow in a dairy herd that passes through the door of a milking parlor.

COMMENT: The *statistical units** are either ordered in the source *population** or become eligible for sampling in a sequential manner. The total population size is first divided by the *sample size** to obtain a fixed constant k, which represents the inverse of the population sampling proportion. The first of k *individuals** is randomly sampled, and then every kth individual is systematically sampled.

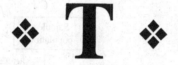

T

TARGET POPULATION:
1. Population to which results of the study will be applicable or extrapolated.
2. Population that an epidemiologic intervention or a health program wishes to reach.

COMMENT 1: Ideally, the target population should be the *population at risk.** For practical reasons (i.e., ability to select or assemble individuals), one may have to consider different types of *populations** (see Figure P3, population):

- a *general population,** that comprises all individuals, including the nonaccessible;
- a more restricted population, including only accessible subjects (underlying or *source population**);
- an *eligible population,** whose members are the only ones likely to be selected as part of the *sampling** process (considering inclusion and exclusion criteria) (Figure T1).

According to the selection criteria, the target population can be more or less restricted: the epidemiologist's challenge is then to evaluate the possible difference(s) between the effective target (target population) that constitutes the *sample,* * and the target she/he would have wished to reach.

COMMENT 2: The expressions reference population and target population are used interchangeably by some authors. However, the word reference is more commonly used to indicate a *control group** in comparative studies (e.g., in a *case–control study** there will be cases and controls or reference group).

COMMENT 3: For *extrapolation** purposes, the target population should be the one that provides the necessary *sampling base** for the *study.* *

See also *population at risk, study population, general population, eligible population, source population.*

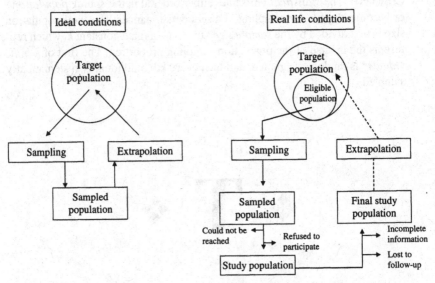

FIGURE T1.   The different categories of population under ideal and real life conditions. Under ideal conditions, each member of the target population would be available for sampling, which would facilitate any extrapolation from the results of the study (based on a limited sample) to this population. Under real life conditions, the eligible population (for sampling purposes) is often a fraction of the target population, which may limit the interpretation of the data.

TERTIARY PREVENTION: Set of measures designed to reduce the impact of clinical disease.

Human medicine: set of measures designed to reduce impairments, disabilities and pain from disease, to prevent intercurrent diseases, and to reduce disease related deaths.

EXAMPLES: Set of therapeutic measures such as antibiotic therapy and fluid therapy; changes in management such as increased ventilation in the face of a pleuropneumonia outbreak in swine; electrolytes added to the drinking water.

COMMENT 1: It may seem contradictory to equate therapy with *prevention.* * In fact therapeutic interventions are meant to prevent the full expression of *disease,** such as death, for example. It is still today a very important component of veterinary practice, in particular in small animal and equine medicine. However, veterinarians working in commercial animal production are increasingly focusing on *primary** and *secondary prevention** activities.

COMMENT 2: The World Health Organization's definition of tertiary prevention in humans puts emphasis on reducing the impact of disease and also on enhancing the patient's rehabilitation. It is mainly individual centered. In veterinary medicine, this definition applies well to pets. However, in animal production, tertiary prevention activities are more *population** based and the economic component of the decision-making process is more determinant.

See also *prevention.*

TEST AND REMOVAL: Screening designed to detect affected individuals with the objective of eliminating them as part of an eradication program.

EXAMPLE: In an effort to eliminate cattle infected with tuberculosis or brucellosis from a *herd**, one could proceed with two *screenings** separated by 2 to 3 months. Hence, the test and removal of infected cattle is followed by the same procedure at a later date in order to detect any infected cattle that may have been missed the first time around because they were incubating the *disease** but were not detectable yet.

COMMENT 1: In the case of bacterial *infections,** it may be possible to "freeze" the infection by treating all animals in the herd while testing and removing positive individuals. For example, this strategy has been successful in eradicating porcine pleuropneumonia from herds with a low to moderate *prevalence** based on the first screening. For high prevalence (> 30% positive), depopulation–repopulation is often the only viable option.

COMMENT 2: The duration of the time interval between the two screenings is critical. If it is too long, it may allow the infection to spread further in the herd, which would result in failure of the test and removal procedure.

TEST OF HOMOGENEITY: A generic term for a test that attempts to evaluate whether or not two or more items, such as distributions, parameters of distributions, proportions or rates, are similar.

COMMENT 1: There are many tests of homogeneity. Homogeneity of *variance** is an assumption of the *analysis of variance,** of covariance and of the two-sample *t* test for the means.

COMMENT 2: Another application of a test of homogeneity is in the evaluation of the consistency of the relationship between a *risk factor** and a *disease** of interest across different levels of another factor, when one wants to make sure that there is no effect modifier.

EXAMPLE: Study of the relationship between the preventive treatment of dairy cows during the dry period and mastitis depending on lactation number. The test of homogeneity allows one to see if this relationship remains the same from one lactation to another.

COMMENT 3: When the test is not significant, the *hypothesis** of similarity of the relationship is accepted. For the example above, one would conclude that there is no *interaction** between the preventive treatment and the number of lactations.

COMMENT 4: Tests of homogeneity are sometimes used as tests of goodness of fit.

COMMENT 5: When comparing or estimating *risks,** if homogeneity is present, *Mantel–Haenszel's test** and formulas can be used.

THEORETICAL EPIDEMIOLOGY: Division of epidemiology that studies and uses mathematical models in order to establish prediction on occurrence of disease or health states, to better understand epidemiologic mechanisms, and to test hypotheses concerning these mechanisms.

EXAMPLES: Use of the Reed–Frost model to study *transmission** of rabies in a fox *population.**

*Model** of mastitis in dairy herds to investigate biologic and economic results from different control strategies.

COMMENT 1: Theoretical studies use *mathematical models** to mimic the reality or simulate field conditions.

COMMENT 2: Theoretical epidemiologic models are highly dependent on the quality of the information used in their elaboration.

THIRD QUARTILE: In a given series, the value of the variable that is higher than 75% of all values but that is lower than 25% of them.

COMMENT: See the example and the comments attached to the definition of *first quartile.**

See also *quantile* (Figure Q1).

THRESHOLD: Level that must be reached for an effect or a change to occur.

EXAMPLES: *Epidemic threshold;** cutoff point for a diagnostic test; *level of significance** in statistics.

COMMENT: Threshold level may refer to the spatial density of *susceptible** individuals required to trigger an *epidemic,** to the minimum number of units of an *infectious** agent needed to effectively allow transmission, or to the level arbitrarily selected (cutoff point established for a continuous variable) above which a change is deemed to have occurred. Several other applications of this word exist in the medical field, such as renal threshold, auditory threshold, neuron threshold, etc.

THRESHOLD OF DETECTION: The smallest quantity of a substance for which a test gives a positive result.

COMMENT 1: The detection ability of a serological test is sometimes defined in relation to a standard, such as a standard serum. For example, one may say that test X has a threshold of detection equivalent to a 1/200 dilution of the standard serum. This concept can also be expressed in different ways. For example, one could say that an enzyme-linked immunosorbent assay (ELISA) applied to bulk milk can detect one infected cow among 40 healthy ones.

COMMENT 2: Laboratory workers often use the word *sensitivity** in reference to threshold of detection. Hence, a test with a low threshold of detection would be said to be sensitive. This application of the word sensitivity is, of course, very different from its epidemiologic meaning, which can lead to confusion.

See also *sensitivity*.

THRESHOLD OF SIGNIFICANCE: Probability threshold used for deciding to reject or not reject the null hypothesis.

COMMENT 1: The threshold of significance should ideally be selected after weighing the relative costs of *alpha* (type I) and *beta* (type II) *errors,** although the most commonly used thresholds are 5% and 1%.

COMMENT 2: If a test is significant at the 5% level, then sampling variability alone would have less than a 5% chance of producing the observed values (or values more extreme) when the *null hypothesis** is true. Therefore, the probability of incorrectly rejecting the null hypothesis (i.e., committing a type I error) is approximately 5%.

TIME SERIES: Syn: chronological series Consecutive numerical values taken by a variable over time.

COMMENT: For a given *disease,** the analysis of the time series can lead to the concept of *trend** (slow modification of the *frequency** during a relatively long time period), cyclical fluctuation, or seasonal fluctuation of the *incidence.**

See also *stationary time series* (Figure S5).

TOTAL INCOME: Revenues, including all sales of products and sales of capital and miscellaneous items.

COMMENT: Total income appears on the *income statement.**

See also *income statement*.

TOTAL PRODUCTION COST: Total of fixed (indirect) and variable (direct) costs attributable to producing a specified amount of a specific product.

COMMENT 1: All components of total production cost can be found in the *profit** and *loss** statements.

COMMENT 2: The *average cost** is obtained by dividing total production cost by the number of units produced.

COMMENT 3: The relationships between total *variable cost,** total *fixed cost,** and total production cost are illustrated using total cost functions.

See also *variable cost, fixed cost.*

TOXIGENIC POTENTIAL: Syn: toxogenic potential A measure of the ability of an organism to produce toxins capable of inducing pathologic change in a susceptible host.

EXAMPLE: *Bacillus anthracis* and *Clostridium botulinum* both possess high toxigenic potentials.

TOXOGENIC POTENTIAL: See Toxigenic Potential

TRACEBACK: Epidemiologic strategy of locating the origin of a case or an outbreak (Figure T2).

COMMENT: This is an important strategy used as part of *disease** investigations. Determining when and where an animal or a *group** of animals has stayed often requires that an identification system be in place (such as eartags with codes identifying the vendors, tattooing and registration of the animals, etc.). Tracing the movement of animals, people, and equipment is an essential component of traceback and *follow-up investigations.**

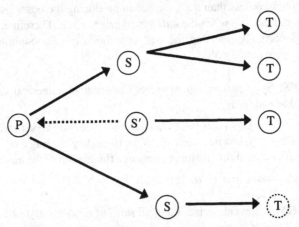

FIGURE T2. Schematic representation of traceback and follow-up investigations. A traceback investigation from S' leads to the primary outbreak (P). A follow-up investigation results in the identification of secondary (S) and tertiary outbreaks (T), as well as in the prevention of a tertiary outbreak Ⓣ.

See also *traceback investigation, follow-up investigation.*

TRACEBACK INVESTIGATION: Syn: traceback survey Probe of a disease outbreak to determine its origin.

COMMENT: A traceback investigation is designed to identify the source of an *outbreak** and, consequently, other outbreaks having the same origin.

TRACEBACK SURVEY: See **Traceback Investigation**

TRANSMISSIBLE DISEASE: See **Communicable Disease**

TRANSMISSION OF A DISEASE: Action/event/process whereby a pathogen is passed from one individual to another.

EXAMPLES: Rabies transmission; transmission of strangles.

COMMENT 1: Classically we differentiate *horizontal transmission** from *vertical transmission,** and *direct transmission** from *indirect transmission.**

COMMENT 2: The chain of transmission is described by reference to sequential steps and concepts (*source of infection,** excretion, mode of transmission, mechanism of penetration, *susceptibility** of the potential *host**).

COMMENT 3: Biological transmission (by a biological *vector**) is differentiated from mechanical transmission (by a *mechanical* or *passive vector*).*

COMMENT 4: For each disease, among the different modes of transmission (e.g., *direct contact,* indirect contact,** vector), there is generally (but not exclusively) a single mode that is the primary or "usual" mode of transmission. The usual mode is the one responsible for transmission of most *cases** of a disease; under otherwise stable circumstances, suppression of the usual mode promotes *elimination of the disease** (for example, bite of a carnivore with rabies, flea bite for *Yersinia pestis* transmission, coitus for dourine).

TRANSPORT HOST: Syn: paratenic host Host that ensures the survival and/or the transportation of a parasite without the parasite undergoing any maturation.

EXAMPLE: Earthworms and *Dictyocaulus* sp. larvae.

COMMENT: This is an optional host (i.e., it is not indispensable to the development of the pathogen).

See also *definitive host.*

TREND: Persistent variation in a specific direction across ordinal levels.

COMMENT 1: In a *time series** analysis, trend is considered to be a long-term systematic variation, as opposed to short-term fluctuations.

COMMENT 2: Do not confuse with *seasonal variation** or pluri-annual variation.

COMMENT 3: A trend can be linear or nonlinear.

EXAMPLE 1: Progression of Aujeszky's disease in France from 1979 to 1983.

Year	Number of outbreaks
1979	95
1980	137
1981	166
1982	213
1983	344

EXAMPLE 2: Risk of pulmonary cancer showed an increasing trend across increasing levels of radon exposure.

TRIAL: Study aiming at the evaluation of an intervention, in comparison to a reference situation, conducted on a population in its natural environment, and in which the progress of the process is under the control of the scientist.

COMMENT 1: A trial normally differs from an *experimental study** in two aspects:

1. The objective of a trial is to evaluate a *health** intervention (drug, vaccine, *prevention** measure, health system), whereas an experimental study aims at studying a *health factor** (*pathogenic** factor, or natural protective factor).

2. The degree of control the observer has over the environment of the subjects under observation (less control in a trial compared to an experiment). If, as in an experiment, the observer controls the intervention, the *comparability** between groups (*cases** and controls), which is necessary to interpret the results, may be acceptable. For example, in a *randomized trial,** the comparability is ensured via the *random** *distribution** of individuals in each group. However, practical or ethical constraints may prevent the researcher from achieving true randomness (first criterion of comparability). The second criterion of comparability (identical environmental conditions for groups for the duration of the *study** period) is never respected at the same level as in an experimental study, because *populations** are studied in their natural environment, and therefore cannot be controlled as well by the observer.

COMMENT 2: Trials can be undertaken on human, animal, or vegetable populations, and trials can be divided into types based on study design (Figure T3).

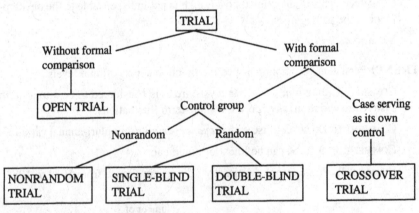

FIGURE T3. Different types of trial.

TRIGGERING FACTOR: Factor inducing an event.

EXAMPLES: Transportation triggering estrus in sows or revealing *latent infections** resulting in *diseases** such as porcine pleuropneumonia and erysipelas; ambient temperature variation inducing diarrhea in young animals.

TWO-SIDED TEST: Syn: bilateral test Statistical test in which the null hypothesis is rejected when values of the test statistic are larger than an upper critical value or smaller than a lower critical value.

COMMENT: The choice between a one-sided and a two-sided test depends on the alternative *hypothesis.** If we want to know whether two *parameters** are statistically different, then a two-sided test would be appropriate. If we want to know whether one parameter is smaller than another, larger than some constant, or smaller than some constant, then a one-sided test is appropriate.

EXAMPLE: When comparing the *prevalence** of *disease** in two regions it is possible for either region to have a higher prevalence, therefore the appropriate test is a two-sided test.

See also *statistical test, one-sided test.*

TYPE 1 ERROR: See **Alpha Error**

TYPE 2 ERROR: See **Beta Error**

TYPE 3 ERROR: See **Gamma Error**

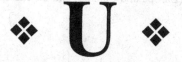

UNDERESTIMATION: An estimate that is lower than the true value.

EXAMPLE: When *matching** in a *case–control study** and failing to control for the confounding introduced by matching, *bias** toward the null effect measure occurs, resulting in an underestimate of the true effect measure.

COMMENT: Underestimation is also used when only a fraction of all cases of a particular condition are reported. For example, if 1000 cases of diarrhea have occurred, but only 500 have been reported, the reported information would be an underestimation of reality. This often occurs with *notifiable diseases.**

UNDERLYING POPULATION: See **Source Population**

UNIFACTORIAL DISEASE: See **Monofactorial Etiology**

UNIFACTORIAL ETIOLOGY: See **Monofactorial Etiology**

UNILATERAL TEST: See **One-Sided Test**

UNIMODAL DISTRIBUTION: See **Modal Distribution**

UNIVARIATE: See **Monovariate**

UNSTRUCTURED INTERVIEW: Mode of information gathering in which the investigator provides the respondent with the opportunity to freely elaborate on one or several topics of interest.

COMMENT 1: This approach is often used when limited knowledge exists about a problem or an issue, and when the investigator wants to obtain information prior to developing one or several *hypotheses.* * A face-to-face meeting is normally conducted. However, the same approach could be used over the phone.

COMMENT 2: To be differentiated from a *structured interview.* *

USUAL RESERVOIR: Predominant reservoir ensuring the maintenance of a pathogen under natural conditions.

EXAMPLES: Mice and *Leptospira bataviae*.
Squirrels (USA); gerbils, also known as sand rats (Sahara); and black rats (India) are all considered usual reservoirs in their respective *environment** for *Yersinia pestis*, the *agent** responsible for bubonic plague.
Foxes (Europe and Canada) and the rabies virus.

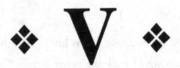

VACCINATION COVERAGE: Proportion of vaccinated individuals in a population.

This expression is seldom used in veterinary medicine in North America.

COMMENT 1: When the population is large, the vaccination coverage may not reach 100% of the exposed *population.** This is mainly true in wildlife. In commercial animal production, 100% coverage is often achieved at the *herd** level.

For example, in a 1500-sow operation, a vaccination program could be designed to ensure that all sows entering the gestation unit have been vaccinated against specific *agents*,* according to the regional distribution of *diseases*.*

COMMENT 2: The main factor determining vaccination coverage is the *method** of vaccination [injection (intramuscular, subcutaneous); eyedrop/intranasal; ingestion (drinking water, bait); coarse spray; wing web in poultry].

COMMENT 3: Vaccination coverage is usually determined by *sampling** the population and establishing the percentage of *individuals** who have seroconverted. For example, serology performed on chickens from a 100,000-bird flock revealed that 97% were seropositive to Marek's disease 3 weeks post-vaccination.

COMMENT 4: 100% vaccination coverage does not necessarily imply 100% protection, which is termed vaccinal *efficacy*.* A measure of vaccinal efficacy is the *attributable fraction.**

See also *herd immunity, population exposed.*

VALIDATION: The process of verifying legitimacy or relevance of some entity with regard to its purpose or intended use.

EXAMPLES: A randomly selected group of farms may be compared against regional farm *characteristics** to determine the *sample's** validity with regard to its *representativeness.** A statistical *model** is developed using a randomly selected portion of a large data set. The model's validation is accomplished by rerunning it using the remainder of the data set and determining if its results remain stable.

COMMENT: The validation process may require comparisons between different tests, data sets, etc., sometimes performed under different conditions (operators, laboratories).

VALIDATION STUDY: A study performed to test the validity of a prediction, inference, or observation based on observational research.

EXAMPLE 1: *Validation** of a *model** using certain *risk factors** to predict the presence or absence of sepsis in calves. One hundred calves were used to construct the model, and 200 different calves were used in the validation study.

EXAMPLE 2: Validation of *causes** of mortality recorded in a computerized recording system prior to using the information in the context of an *observational study.**

COMMENT 1: Validity refers to the ability of a diagnostic test, *survey** or *analytical study** to produce, on average and over time, an accurate result.

COMMENT 2: The construction of a predictive model of *disease** must be followed by a validation study (example 1). In this case, the validation study normally involves a greater number of *observations** than the study that led to the predictive model. In example 2, the validation study precedes the observational study and generally requires fewer observations.

See also *validation*.

VALIDITY (OF A TEST, AN EPIDEMIOLOGIC STUDY): Ability of a test, an examination or an epidemiologic study to measure what it is supposed to measure, without being influenced by other sources of systematic or random errors.

COMMENT 1: A valid test always gives nonbiased results but does not ensure *accuracy** (see Table A1, accuracy).

COMMENT 2: Good validity presumes high *sensitivity** and *specificity.**

COMMENT 3: The validity of a test constitutes only a particular case of *validation** which can also be applied to an object (instrument of measure), a medical intervention, or a concept (explanatory model).

COMMENT 4: In an epidemiologic *study,** internal and external validity are considered (Figure V1):

1. Internal validity: Characterizes the quality of the conclusions relative to the *population** under study. It pertains first to the quality of the statistical *inference** from the sample under study to the *eligible population** (problems of precision, selection bias, measurement bias, bias due to a *confounder**), and second, the quality of the interpretation toward the target population. Care must be taken that these *biases** do not lead to totally erroneous conclusions.

2. External validity: Relates to the possibility of extrapolating the conclusions (assuming that the internal validity has been confirmed) to other populations (others times or places). Consideration must be given to the risk that the conclusions may only be valid for the population under study.

See also *population, sampling*.

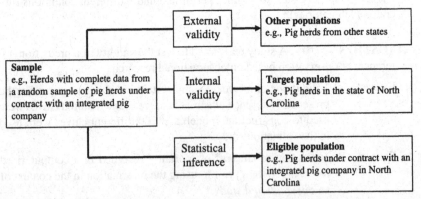

FIGURE V1. Schematic representation of the relationship between different populations and validity of study results obtained from a sample.

VARIABLE: Attribute or observable event that can vary.

COMMENT 1: Variables can be classified depending on their attributes:

Quantitative variables*:
quantitative variable with discrete values: number of gestations.
continuous quantitative variable: weight, size.
ordinal quantitative variable: weight classified in mutually exclusive groups.

Qualitative variables*:
nominal qualitative variable: sex, species.
ordinal qualitative variable: never, sometimes, often, constantly.

Status in the *statistical* analysis:
independent variable.*
dependent variable.*
control variable/uncontrolled variable.

These classes are not all mutually exclusive, and other adjectives may be used to better define the word "variable" (derived, intervening, predictor, confounding, moderator, dummy, *random,** etc.)

COMMENT 2: Technically, the word "variable" should only apply to quantitative attributes or events. In practice, however, qualitative ones are also considered as variables. The elements of such variables are often coded for analytical purposes (*disease** = 1, nondisease = 0; severity of clinical signs: 0 = absent, 1 = minimal, 2 = moderate, 3 = severe, 4 = fatal).

VARIABLE COSTS: Costs which vary according to the level of production or the activity level of an enterprise.

EXAMPLES: Annual *expenditure** on fuel, seed, fertilizer, harvesting, casual labor, feed, insurance on livestock, veterinary, medical, and marketing are considered to be variable costs within a farm business.

COMMENT 1: Variable costs are a function of the amount produced, and are not incurred if the operator does not attempt to produce a product.

COMMENT 2: As the length of the planning period increases, costs considered fixed in the short term become variable. In the long run, all costs are considered variable.

See also *fixed costs.*

VARIANCE (OF A SAMPLE): The amount of dispersion of a set of measurements of a variable calculated as the mean of the squared deviations from the mean of this variable.

COMMENT: When the variance is estimated, the sum of squares of the deviations is divided by the degrees of freedom $(n - 1)$. In this case, the sample variance is symbolized by s^2 while the symbol for the population variance is σ^2 (variance considering all observations).

For observations $x_1, \ldots x_n$, the sample variance is

$$s^2 = \frac{\Sigma(x_i - \bar{x})^2}{n - 1}$$

where n is the number of observations, $\bar{x}$ is the mean and x_i the value taken by the variable for the ith observation.

See also *dispersion*.

VARIATE: See **Random Variable**

VECTOR: The true meaning of vector is "one who carries" (Latin: *vector*, from *vehere*: to carry). Broad and restricted definitions are possible.

Broad definition: Anything that allows the transport and/or transmission of a pathogen.

EXAMPLES: The following are vectors (broad definition) of foot-and-mouth disease: an infected cow introduced into an unaffected herd, a dog that travels from farm to farm, a producer visiting his neighbor, reused wrappings (e.g., food bags), a delivery truck, etc.

Within this definition, one can also distinguish between animate vectors (the first three examples above) and inanimate vectors (the last two examples above). These latter could also be called *vehicles** or *fomites:** we would then differentiate between vectors (animate) and vehicles or fomites (inanimate).

COMMENT: What appears essential in this idea is the notion of support (Latin: *supportare*), irrespective of what is "on" or "in" the vector. The consequences of this depend on the vector's behavior.

Strict definition (ecological sense): A living creature which, because of its ecological relationship to others, acquires a pathogen from one living host, and transmits it to another.

EXAMPLES: *Aedes aegypti*: yellow fever; *Ixodes ricinus*: tickborne encephalitis; *Anopheles*: malaria; lice: typhus.

COMMENT: The ecological relationship is usually associated with food supply. In the great majority of cases, these vectors are invertebrates, particularly arthropods.

VECTOR COMPETENCE: See **Vector Efficiency**

VECTOR EFFICIENCY: Suitability of a vector for the transmission of a pathogen.

COMMENT 1: This concept is usually applied to blood-feeding arthropods. The vector efficiency of an arthropod varies for a given pathogen as a function of time and place. It is dependent on several factors: vector competence (the intrinsic biological ability of a *vector** to support the development or replication of the pathogen), trophic preferences, the frequency of meals, the longevity of the vector, the duration of the extrinsic incubation, the density of the vectorial *population,** the dispersion of the vector, its possible *resistance** to control measures, etc. All these factors will affect the likelihood that the *agent** will be transmitted from one *host** to the next. Hence, vector efficiency is determined by vector competence and by ecological or *extrinsic factors.**

COMMENT 2: To be efficient, a vector of an *arbovirus** has to be both competent and subjected to ecological conditions favorable for *transmission.** An a priori competent vector living under ecological conditions that are not favorable for transmission of the virus is a *potential vector.** Conversely, an a priori slightly competent vector can nevertheless play an important role if the ecological conditions are very favorable for transmission (e.g., if the vector is very abundant or closely associated with the vertebrate host).

VEHICLE (OF A DISEASE): An object, substance, or nonreceptive living being serving as an intermediary in transmitting a pathogen from the organism hosting it to a receptive host.

COMMENT 1: The *indirect transmission** of a *disease** can be ensured by vehicles or *vectors.**

COMMENT 2: Some authors oppose this use of the terms vehicles and vectors, preferring to restrict the use of the terms vehicle and *fomite** to inanimate *carriers,** and the term vector for living transmitters.

VENN DIAGRAM: A figure illustrating the various possibilities of union and intersection of two or more sets (Figure V2).

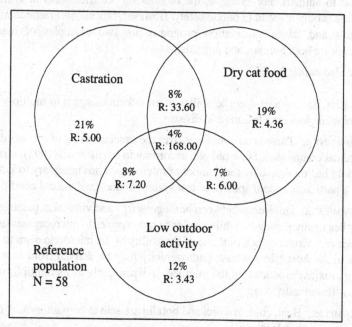

FIGURE V2.   Venn diagram representing three *risk factors** related to the feline urological syndrome in male cats, and the *distribution** (in %) of these factors in the male cat *population of reference** (Willeberg, 1977). This Venn diagram is presented as an example only. Recent findings suggest that dry food may not be an important risk factor. *Confounders** (not considered here) may partly explain the results shown here.

R = estimated *relative risk** for each factor or combination of risk factors.

VERTICAL TRANSMISSION: Transmission of a pathogen from a parent to a descendant, based on reproduction.

EXAMPLES: Transmission of the virus of lymphocytic choriomeningitis of the mouse; occasional transmission of enzootic bovine leukosis virus from a diseased cow to its calf.

COMMENT 1: This transmission can take place through the gametes (*hereditary diseases**), transplacentally (*congenital disease**), during parturition or, for arthropods, from one phase of arthropod development to another (egg, larva, adult for ticks: transtadial transmission).

COMMENT 2: Diseases of genetic origin (hemophilia, daltonism, etc.) are included in this definition.

VETERINARY PUBLIC HEALTH: Those aspects of veterinary medicine that concern the physical and mental well-being of humans.

EXAMPLES: Zoonotic disease control, safety of foods from animals, comparative medicine, human–animal bond, environmental medicine.

COMMENT: In the context of veterinary public health, some activities may be designed to protect or improve only human health, but they may also be beneficial to animals. For example, the *monitoring** of trichinosis in swine carcasses is only relevant to public safety. However, brucellosis *eradication** programs and rabies vaccination programs are two examples of measures benefiting both humans and animals.

See also *public health*.

VIRULENCE: The host-specific ability of an infectious agent to multiply in the host while inducing lesions and disease.

COMMENT 1: There is no consensus over the exact meaning of this word in the medical community. For example, according to Joklik et al. (1992), virulence should be "measured by the number of microorganisms necessary to kill or alter a particular animal species or test system under standardized conditions."

COMMENT 2: Difference between *pathogenicity** and virulence: pathogenicity applies to any pathogen, while virulence only applies to microorganisms. Furthermore, virulence is a function of the ability of the microorganism to multiply in the *host.** In contrast, pathogenicity may be derived from substances (e.g., toxins) produced by the microbe, independently of its multiplication in the affected individual.

EXAMPLES: Heat, cold, arsenic, and botulin are said to be *pathogenic** but not virulent.

COMMENT 3: A microorganism may multiply intensively in an individual without producing clinical signs or detectable lesions. In this case, the *agent** is said to be invasive but avirulent (e.g., some *arboviruses**) (see also *invasiveness**).

COMMENT 4: Agents can exhibit differing degrees of virulence depending on a particular genus or species.

COMMENT 5: An individual must possess some degree of *susceptibility** to the *infectious** agent in order for it to be virulent in that individual.

EXAMPLE: *Vibrio vulnificus* is not a shellfish pathogen, but it is a human pathogen. However, most infections in humans are avirulent; they remain subclinical or mildly clinical and are often ignored. Nevertheless, this organism can be highly virulent in the immunocompromised host, those with impaired hepatic function, and those suffering from elevated serum iron levels. Under such circumstances, the *case fatality rate** is high.

See also *pathogenicity.*

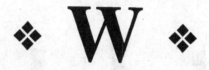

WEIGHTED KAPPA: See **Kappa Statistic**

WELFARE: The degree of harmony between an individual and its environment, in association with its physical and mental health.

COMMENT 1: Proper welfare assumes that the animal is able to adapt to its *environment** without suffering. A working definition of suffering is "a wide range of unpleasant emotional states."

COMMENT 2: Over the past several years, the idea has emerged that welfare is, or should be, mainly or solely dependent on what the animal "feels." This has led to a surge in field and controlled environmental research designed to determine animals' likes and dislikes.

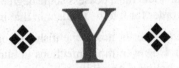

YEAR EFFECT: Concept of change in the frequency of an outcome or event of interest depending on the year.

COMMENT 1: This effect is well known in oenology (study of wines).

COMMENT 2: Often used to refer to changes in the *frequency** of *health** status over time regardless of the age of the animal (Figure Y1). In particular, this effect is observed in relation to meteorological conditions.

See also *confounder, effect modification.*

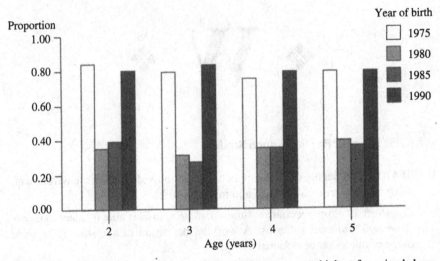

FIGURE Y1.   Hypothetical example where disease frequency was highest for animals born in 1975 and 1990 compared with 1980 and 1985 regardless of their age.

❖ Z ❖

ZOONOSIS: Disease or infection that can be naturally transmitted between other vertebrate animals and people.

EXAMPLES: Rabies, Lyme borreliosis, echinococcosis.

COMMENT 1: The word is derived from the Greek roots zoo, or animal, and nosos, or illness, thus, literally, *diseases** from animals (i.e., not exclusively infectious diseases).

COMMENT 2: Zoonoses may be classified in various ways, including the direction of *infection** (people to other animals, or vice versa), types of *agent** (parasitic, viral, bacterial), or according to the role of *vectors** or the external *environment** in their *transmission** cycles (e.g., direct, cyclo-, meta-, and sapro-zoonoses).

COMMENT 3: Variations on the definition above, which is that espoused by the World Health Organization, include (1) "diseases of animals that may be transmitted to [people]" (Dorland's dictionary); (2) "those diseases of [people] shared in nature by other vertebrate animals" (Schwabe, in *Veterinary Medicine and Human Health*); and (3) "those aspects of human medicine that depend on the (human–animal) relationship" (Fiennes, in *Zoonoses and the Origins and Ecology of Human Disease*).

Z TEST: Syn: comparison of means with known variances A statistical test that compares two observed arithmetic means, when the variance of the distribution of each of the two groups is known.

COMMENT: This test is applicable only if n_1 and n_2 (sample size of the groups) are greater than 30. This statistic is obtained with the following formula:

$$\varepsilon = \frac{(m_1 - m_2)}{\sqrt{\dfrac{\sigma_1^2}{n_1} + \dfrac{\sigma_2^2}{n_2}}}$$

Where m_1 = mean of the first sample
m_2 = mean of the second sample
σ_1^2 = variance of the first distribution
σ_2^2 = variance of the second distribution
n_1 = sample size of the first sample
n_2 = sample size of the second sample

After having calculated this statistic, the probability of the null hypothesis being true is looked up in a table.

References

Adeprina. 1983. Session Analyse des Données et Informatique. Paris: INA. Cours polycopié.

Armitage, P. 1971. Statistical Methods in Medical Research. Oxford: Blackwell Scientific Publications.

Bannock, G., R.E. Baxter, and E. Davis. 1992. Dictionary of Economics, 5th ed. Harmondsworth: Penguin Books.

Blood, D.C., and V.P. Studdert, (eds). 1988. Baillière's Comprehensive Veterinary Dictionary. London: Baillière Tindall.

Boehlje, M.D., and V.R. Eidman. 1984. Farm Management, New York: John Wiley and Sons.

Brealey, R.A., and S.C. Myers. 1981. Principles of Corporate Finance. New York: McGraw Hill.

Bridier, M., and S. Michaïlof. 1980. Guide Pratique d'Analyse de Projets. Paris: Economica.

Brigham, E.F. 1979. Financial Management: Theory and Practice. Hinsdale: The Dryden Press.

Butler, B., and A. Isaacs. 1993. A Dictionary of Finance. Oxford: Oxford University Press.

Daget, P., and M. Godron. 1979. Vocabulaire d'Ecologie. Paris: Agence de Coopération culturelle et technique, Centre international de la langue française. Distributed by Hachette.

Dagnélie, P. 1973. Théorie et Méthodes Statistiques. Vol. 1: La Statistique Descriptive et les Fondements de l'Inférence Statistique. Gembloux: Les Presses agronomiques de Gembloux: A.S.B.L.

Dagnélie, P. 1975. Théorie et Méthodes Statistiques. Vol. 2: Les Méthodes de l'Inférence Statistique. Gembloux: Les Presses agronomiques de Gembloux: A.S.B.L.

Dagnélie, P. 1975. Analyse Statistique à Plusieurs Variables. Gembloux: Les Presses agronomiques de Gembloux: A.S.B.L.

Dajoz, R. 1974. Dynamique des Populations. Paris: Masson.

Daniel, W.W. 1983. Biostatistics: a Foundation for Analysis in the Health Sciences, 3rd ed. New York: John Wiley and Sons.

Dent, J.B., M.J. Blackie, P.S. Teng, B.A. Stynes, R.C. Close, I.C. Harvey, F.R. Sanderson, R.E. Gaunt, and A.J. McCully (eds.). 1978. Epidemiology and crop loss assessment. Proceedings of a workshop held at Lincoln College, Canterbury, New Zealand, August 29–31, 1977.

Dictionnaire Usuel de l'Environnement et de l'Écologie. 1981. 2 vol. (A–E) (F–Z). Paris: Guy le Prat.

Dorland's Illustrated Medical Dictionary, 28th ed. 1994. Philadelphia: W.B. Saunders.

Eidman, V.R., and M.D. Boehlje. 1976. Farm Management, 2nd ed. New York: John Wiley and Sons.

Fabia, J., J.F. Boivin, P.M. Bernard, S. Ducic, and M. Thuriaux. 1988. Dictionnaire anglais-français et français-anglais des termes utilisés en épidémiologie. International Journal of Epidemiology 17(Suppl. 1): 1–49.

Fénelon, J.P. 1981. Qu'est-ce que l'Analyse de Données. Paris: Lefonen.

Feinstein, A.R. 1987. Clinimetrics. Philadelphia: W.B. Saunders.

Fienberg, S.E. 1987. The Analysis of Cross-Classified Categorical Data., 2nd ed. Cambridge: MIT Press.

Fleiss, J.L. 1981. Statistical Methods for Rates and Proportions, 2nd ed. New York: John Wiley and Sons.

Fletcher, R.H., S.W. Fletcher, and E.H. Wagner. 1988. Clinical Epidemiology: The Essentials, 2nd ed. Baltimore: Williams and Wilkins.

Garnier, M., and V. Delamare. 1967. Dictionnaire de Termes Techniques de Médecine. Paris: Maloine.

Goldberg, M., Y. Charpak, A. Chevalier, C. Godard, S. Gottot, P. Guenel, C. Lepetit, and D. Luce. 1990. L'Épidémiologie sans Peine. Paris: Frison-Roche.

Greenland, S. (Ed.). 1987. Evolution of Epidemiologic Ideas: Annotated Readings on Concepts and Methods. Chestnut Hill: Epidemiology Resources Inc.

Grenier, B. 1990. Décision Médicale. Paris: Masson.

Gyles, C.L., and C.O. Thoen. 1986. Pathogenesis of Bacterial Infections in Animals. Ames: Iowa State University Press.

Hawkins, R.O., R. Craven, K. Klair, R. Loppnow, D. Nordquist, and W. Richardson. 1997. FINPACK Users' Manual. St. Paul: Center For Farm Financial Management, University of Minnesota.

Hoey, L., and R. Lambert. 1981. Eléments d'Épidémiologie pour le Clinicien. Lyon: C.N.R.S.

Illingworth, V., E.L. Glaser, and I.C. Pyle. 1990. Dictionary of Computing. 3rd ed. Oxford: Oxford University Press.

Jammal, A., R. Allard, and G. Loslier. 1988. Dictionnaire d'Épidémiologie. Paris: Maloine.

Jenicek, M., and R. Cléroux. 1983. Épidémiologie: Principes, Techniques, Applications. Paris: Maloine.

Joklik, W.K., Willett, D.B., Amos, D.B., and Wilfert, C.M. (eds). Zinsser Microbiology, 20th ed. Norwalk, CT: Appleton and Lange.

Kelsey, J.L., W.D. Thompson, and A.S. Evans. 1986. Methods in Observational Epidemiology. New York: Oxford University Press.

Kleinbaum, D.G., L.L. Kupper, and H. Morgenstern. 1982. Epidemiologic Research: Principals and Quantitative Methods. New York: Van Nostrand Reinhold Company.

Kraemer, H.C. 1992. Evaluating Medical Tests: Objective and Quantitative Guidelines. Newbury Park: Sage.

Kramer, M.S. 1988. Clinical Epidemiology and Biostatistics: A Primer for Clinical Investigators and Decision-Makers. Berlin: Springer-Verlag.

Last, J.M. 1983. A Dictionary of Epidemiology. New York: Oxford University Press.

Last, J.M. 1988. A Dictionary of Epidemiology, 2nd ed. New York: Oxford University Press.

Last, J.M. 1995. A Dictionary of Epidemiology, 3rd ed. New York: Oxford University Press.

Leclerc, A., L. Papox, G. Bréart, and J. Lellouch. 1990. Dictionnaire d'Épidémiologie. Paris: Frison-Roche.

Lee, E.T. 1980. Statistical Methods for Survival Data Analysis. Belmont: Lifetime Learning Publications.

Lellouch, J., and P. Lazar. 1974. Méthodes Statistiques en Expérimentation Biologique. Paris: Flammarion Médecine Sciences.

Lessard, P.R., and B.D. Perry. 1988. Investigation of Disease Outbreaks and Impaired Productivity. The Veterinary Clinics of North America. Food Animal Practice. Philadelphia: W.B. Saunders.

MacMahon, B., and T.F. Pugh. 1970. Epidemiology, Principles and Methods. Boston: Little, Brown and Co.

Manuila, A., L. Manuila, M. Nicole, and H. Lambert. 1970. Dictionnaire Français de Médecine et de biologie. Paris: Masson.

Martin, S.W., A.H. Meek, and P. Willeberg. 1987. Veterinary Epidemiology. Principles and Methods. Ames: Iowa State University Press.

Massé, L., and G. Massé. 1973. Statistique Sanitaire et Sociale. Paris: Foucher.

Mims, C.A. 1987. The Pathogenesis of Infectious Disease, 3rd ed. London: Academic Press.

Ott, L. 1984. An Introduction to Statistical Methods and Data Analysis, 2nd ed. Boston: Duxbury.

Putt, S.N.H., A.P.M. Shaw, A.J. Woods, L. Tyler, and A.D. James. 1987. Veterinary Epidemiology and Economics in Africa. Addis Ababa: ILCA Manual No. 3.

Robert, P. 1976. Dictionnaire Alphabétique et Analogique de la Langue Française: Le Petit Robert S.N.L. Dictionnaire. Paris: Le Robert.

Rothman, K.J. 1986. Modern Epidemiology. Boston: Little, Brown and Company.

Rothman, K.J. (Ed). Causal Inference. 1988. Chestnut Hill: Epidemiology Resources Inc.

Rumeau-Rouquette, C., G. Bréart, and R. Padieu. 1985. Méthodes en Épidémiologie. Paris: Flammarion.

Sackett, D.L., R.B. Haynes, G.H. Guyatt, and P. Tugwell. 1991. Clinical Epidemiology: A Basic Science for Clinical Medicine, 2nd ed. Boston: Little, Brown and Company.

Schlesselman, J.J. 1982. Case–Control Studies. New York: Oxford University Press.

Schmid, C.F. 1983. Statistical Graphics. Design Principles and Practices. New York: Wiley-Interscience.

Schwabe, C.W. 1984. Veterinary Medicine and Human Health, 3rd ed. Baltimore: Williams and Wilkins.

Schwabe, C.W., H.P. Riemann, and C.E. Franti. 1977. Epidemiology in Veterinary Practice. Philadelphia: Lea and Febiger.

Schwartz, D. 1969. Méthodes Statistiques à l'Usage des Médecins et des Biologistes. Paris: Flammarion.

Schwartz, D., R. Flamant, and J. Lellouch. 1970. L'Essai Thérapeutique chez l'Homme. Paris: Flammarion Médecine Sciences.

Shoukri, M.M., and V.L. Edge. 1996. Statistical Methods for Health Sciences. New York: CRC Press Inc.

Silem, A., and J-M. Albertini. 1989. Lexique d'Économie. Paris: Dalloz.

Slettbakk, T., A. Jørstad, T.B. Farver, and D.W. Hird. 1990. Impact of milking characteristics and teat morphology on somatic cell counts in first-lactation Norwegian cattle. Prevent. Vet. Med. 8:253–267.

Smith, R.D. 1991. Veterinary Clinical Epidemiology: A Problem-Oriented Approach. Stoneham: Butterworth-Heinemann.

Soukhanov, A.H., and Ellis, K. (eds). 1984. Webster's II New Riverside University Dictionary. Boston: The Riverside Publishing Company.

Teutsch, S.M., and Churchill, R.E. (eds). 1994. Principles and Practice of Public Health Surveillance. New York: Oxford University Press.

Thrusfield, M. 1986. Veterinary Epidemiology. London: Butterworths.

Thrusfield, M. 1995. Veterinary Epidemiology, 2nd ed. London: Butterworths.

Villemin, M. 1975. Dictionnaire des Termes Vétérinaires et Zootechniques, 2nd ed. Paris: Vigot.

Weisberg, S. 1985. Applied Linear Regression, 2nd ed. New York: John Wiley and Sons.

Weiss, N.S. 1986. Clinical Epidemiology: The Study of the Outcome of Illness. New York: Oxford University Press.

Willeberg, P. 1977. Animal disease information processing: Epidemiologic analyses of the feline urological syndrome. Acta Vet. Scand. Suppl. 64:1–48.